CELLULAR PATHOLOGY

As Based upon Physiological and
Pathological Histology

CELLULAR PATHOLOGY,

As Based upon Physiological and Pathological Histology

BY

R U D O L F LUDWIG KARL

V I R C H O W

TRANSLATED FROM THE SECOND GERMAN EDITION BY

FRANK CHANCE

WITH

A NEW INTRODUCTORY ESSAY BY

L. J. RATHER, M.D.

PROFESSOR OF PATHOLOGY

STANFORD UNIVERSITY MEDICAL CENTER

DOVER PUBLICATIONS, INC.
NEW YORK

This Dover edition, first published in 1971, is an
unabridged and unaltered republication of the
English translation (of the second German edition)
originally published by J. B. Lippincott and Com-
pany, Philadelphia, in 1863.
This edition also contains a new Introduction
by L. J. Rather.

International Standard Book Number: 0-486-22698-0
Library of Congress Catalog Card Number: 76-143679

Manufactured in the United States of America
Dover Publications, Inc.
180 Varick Street
New York, N. Y. 10014

The Place of Virchow's
"Cellular Pathology" in Medical thought.

BY L. J. RATHER

I

RUDOLF VIRCHOW—pathologist, sanitarian, medical reformer, anthropologist, ethnologist and statesman—was born in Pomerania, a part of Prussia, on 13 October 1821. Virchow's father, a farmer and minor town official, supervised the boy's early education, which was acquired in a private school and from a tutor until he entered the Köslin Gymnasium in 1835. After receiving a certificate of maturity (*Abitur*) in 1839 Virchow immediately began the study of medicine at the Friedrich Wilhelms Institut in Berlin, where he received his medical degree in 1843. He was then appointed assistant to Robert Froriep, prosector at the Charité Hospital in Berlin, and in 1846 became his successor. In 1847 he was qualified as a teacher at the University of Berlin. In the same year, together with Benno Reinhardt, he founded the *Archiv für pathologische Anatomie und Physiologie und für klinische Medizin* (now known as *Virchows Archiv*). He was the sole editor of some one hundred and seventy volumes of the *Archiv* which appeared after the death of Reinhardt in 1852 up to the time of his own death fifty years later. Virchow's social and political interests became apparent in 1848 when at the request of the Prussian Minister of Culture he investigated an epidemic of typhus fever in Silesia. His report to the government, emphasizing as it did the need for democratic reforms in Silesia, together with other liberal and anti-monarchistic activities on his part (he played a modest role on the barricades in the

v

Berlin demonstrations of 1848) brought him into disfavor with the regime. After an attempt in 1849 by conservative governmental forces to remove him from his prosectorship at the Charité, Virchow accepted a call to Würzburg (in then independent Bavaria) as professor of pathology. He was only twenty-eight years old, yet already had behind him a course of lectures in pathology at the Charité Hospital which had brought him a measure of renown, the co-editorship with Rudolf Leubuscher of the short-lived reform journal *Medizinische Reform* (1848–49) and the routing of the humoralistic speculations of the leading pathological anatomist of the time, Karl von Rokitansky. After seven productive years at Würzburg he accepted a call to Berlin as professor of pathological anatomy, general pathology and therapy, and director of the newly founded Institute of Pathology. His political and social interests now reasserted themselves. In 1862 he was elected to the Prussian House of Delegates. He became one of the founders and leaders of the liberal Progressive Party, and held a seat in the Reichstag from 1880 to 1893. His public-health activities included an important and influential report in 1873 on the sanitation of Berlin. During this same period he became one of the founders of the German Anthropological Society. He was prominent in the Berlin Anthropological Society as well, and an editor of the ethnological journal, *Zeitschrift für Ethnologie*. His writings reveal him to be an opponent of the growing anti-Semitic and racist trend in Germany. In 1879 he visited the site of Troy, the result of his investigations appearing in two monographs, one on the geography of Troy, and the other on Trojan graves. Virchow's fame was now world-wide. In 1893 he gave the Croonian lectures in London, in 1896 he was made a commander in the Legion of Honor in France, in 1897 he gave the opening lecture marking the founding of the German Society of Pathology at Düsseldorf, and in 1898 the Huxley lectures in London. In 1899 his fiftieth year as professor was the occasion of widespread celebration throughout the academic world. When he died in Berlin on 5 September, 1902 from a heart ailment (complicating a fracture of the neck of the femur sustained in a fall from a streetcar), it was said that Germany had lost her leading pathologist, anthropologist, sanitarian and liberal in one stroke.[1]

II

Rudolf Virchow was one of the chief architects of the structure of modern medicine, and his book on cellular pathology, first published in 1858 and here presented in Frank Chance's English translation (published in London in 1860) of the second German edition of 1859, is still a cornerstone of the edifice. But Virchow's *Cellular Pathology, as Based upon Physiological and Pathological Histology* is neither a systematic treatise on pathology nor even a systematic exposition of the author's views on the new direction to be taken in the field of pathology. It is simply the record of twenty lecture-demonstrations given by Virchow in February, March and April of 1858 to an audience of physicians at the newly founded Institute of Pathology in Berlin, an audience familiar with the current state of medical science, if not with the historical developments leading up to that state. The work was then published, with little revision according to Virchow, in August 1858. To a modern audience, unfamiliar with both the current state and the historical background of mid-nineteenth-century medicine, some features of the book will seem obscure and others perhaps deceptively obvious. It might be supposed, for example, that the novelty of the work consists in Virchow's preoccupation with cells rather than organs or tissues. But this could have been no novelty to Virchow's audience, for an equal amount of attention to cells had been given in Lebert's three-volume *Physiologie pathologique* (1845),[2] the third volume of which is a superbly illustrated atlas of pathological cytology; in Vogel's *Pathologische Anatomie* (1845);[3] and in Wedl's *Grundzüge der pathologischen Anatomie* (1854).[4] There was a difference, of course, in Virchow's treatment of the subject, and it will be mentioned later. Again, Virchow's references throughout the book to the views of "neuro-pathologists" and "humoro-pathologists," competing with his own, were perfectly clear to his medical audience but are likely to mislead a modern one. The following paragraphs will therefore sketch the main lines of development of medical thought down to Virchow's time and set forth in the briefest possible fashion the state of that thought in the mid-nineteenth century, with special reference to the central theses of Virchow's "cellular" pathology.

III

In the sixteenth century two of the subdisciplines that had (since the Arabic systematization of Greek medical thought and its transmission to Europe) constituted the whole of medicine received two new names: physiology and pathology.[5] Formerly known as the study of the "naturals" and the "contra-naturals," respectively, their subject matter was largely derived from the second-century Greek physician Galen. The change of name merely represented a terminological shift from Latin back to Greek and carried with it no change in subject matter. In the case of pathology this continued, as before, to deal with the signs, symptoms, nature, causes and effects of disease in general. The prevailing medical theory was that of Galenic humoralism. In the sixteenth and (to a far greater extent) in the seventeenth centuries inroads into Galenic humoralism were made from the side of the new chemistry and physics, and so arose the schools of medical thought known as the iatrochemical and iatrophysical. The effects of these schools of thought were less revolutionary than evolutionary. So also were the effects of the new discoveries in anatomy and physiology, beginning with those of Vesalius in the sixteenth century and extending through those of the great sevententh-century cultivators of anatomy and physiology, of whom Harvey is the most outstanding. The gradualism with which changes were introduced into the structure of medical thought is sometimes overlooked, partly due to historical foreshortening, partly to a failure to grasp the fact that there was and is such a structure.

Galenic humoral medicine with respect to both theory and practice nevertheless lost ground throughout the seventeenth and eighteenth centuries, and in the latter century the chemical humoralism of the iatrochemists itself began to appear outmoded as chemistry progressed. Toward the end of the eighteenth century, in the work of John Hunter, a third form of humoralism began to appear on the medical scene. Its full development was reserved for the first half of the nineteenth century. This new form of humoralism intended to derive all formative, regenerative, nutritive, in a word, structural changes in the organs and tissues of the body in health and disease, including those now known as hypertrophy, atrophy, inflammation and neoplasia, from changes in the intrinsic character of, or in local influences acting on, an amorphous, fluid living substance distributed throughout the body by the blood vessels. This fundamental living substance came to be known by many names—coagulating or plastic lymph, blastema, cytoblastema, plasma, etc.—and had had its forerunners in the "radical moisture" and "balsam of nature" of much earlier medical writers. The circulating plastic or formative substance in the blood stream, ultimately derived by transformation of food, was supposed to pass out into the tissues as needed through the intact walls of small blood vessels. The vascular system was generally conceded in Virchow's time to constitute a closed circuit throughout, the "exhalant" and "secretory" open endings of the microvasculature still accepted by Bichat in the closing years of the eighteenth century having been generally rejected. Pathological formative processes were regarded as quantitative or qualitative perversions of physiological processes, e.g. atrophy and hypertrophy meant literally, as their names imply, "nutritive" deficiency or excess, respectively. This school of thought is sometimes referred to as that of the hematopathologists or, to distinguish it from modern hematopathology (a branch of cellular pathology), of the "hemal" pathologists. Virchow refers to its proponents as humoro-pathologists (*Humoral-pathologen*) in the present work.

Virchow also frequently refers to—and usually attacks—"neuropathological" views. Here too the reader must be on his guard not to take this as a reference to neuropathology in the modern sense of a subdiscipline of cellular pathology. These "neuro-pathologists," or "neural" pathologists as they have been called, were the last representatives of "solidism," the attempt to ground the essence and control of healthy and diseased life processes in the solid, rather than in the fluid constituents of the body. The outstanding eighteenth-century "neural" pathologist was the Scot William Cullen. By his own admission, he had derived his medical doctrine from a leading idea in the work of Friedrich Hoffmann (1660–1742), professor of medicine at Halle. Simultaneously with Cullen, the idea that the nervous system exercised final control over bodily processes, including normal and abnormal formative and nutritive processes, was being cultivated by many others, of whom Unzer and Prochaska are two of the most outstanding.[6]

Within the school of the neural pathologists there were many shades of opinion and sometimes little more was insisted on than the existence of a large measure of control over physiological and pathological processes exerted by the cerebro-spinal and sympathetic nervous systems via control of the vascular pathways. Other neural pathologists attempted to show that nerve endings acted in some way directly on the tissues (Virchow's argument in Lecture XII should be read with this in mind). The hemal and neural viewpoints were by no means mutually exclusive. A study of the work of such representatives of neural pathological thought as Henle[7] and Spiess,[8] two of Virchow's contemporaries, will show that they shared many of the assumptions of the hemal pathologists regarding the course of normal and abnormal bodily processes.

Furthermore, whether they followed one line of thought or the other, medical investigators of the first half of the nineteenth century were greatly concerned with the structural alterations of the body in disease, i.e. with pathological anatomy. This field had been intensely cultivated in recent times, especially within the French school of clinician pathological anatomists by such men as Laënnec and Corvisart, after the appearance in 1766 of Morgagni's justly esteemed book on the correlation of clinical and post-mortem findings had called attention to the harvest that might be forthcoming.[9] The effect of this wave of interest in pathological anatomy had been to convince most physicians of the importance and ubiquity of "organic," as opposed to merely functional or "dynamic" changes in the body brought about by disease. Hemal and neural pathologists alike felt under an obligation to furnish rational explanations of organic or structural changes. The result was that neural pathologists usually drew to a greater or lesser extent from the hypotheses of the hemal pathologists in order to explain nutritive and formative disturbances in the body, while hemal pathologists of course accepted the well-established role of the nervous system in many of the functional disturbances of disease, those not associated with lasting structural changes.

IV

We now raise the question of the ultimate structural units of the "tissues," as the so-called similar parts of Galen came to be called in the seventeenth century and thereafter. It was assumed that in animal organisms these units and the tissues as a whole were somehow formed from a plastic substance transuding from the small vessels under normal circumstances, and exuding under abnormal. Prior to the nineteenth century we find that the basic structural unit is called a "fiber." The doctrine has a firm base in some elementary facts of observation at both the gross and microscopic levels, and its history reaches into antiquity at least as far back as Erasistratus.[10] Reil's well-known essay of 1795, in the first issue of the *Archiv für die Physiologie,* sets forth a theory of fiber formation that neatly fitted into the newly emerging early-nineteenth-century version of humoral physiology and pathology.[11] Fibers arose from an amorphous, fluid mother substance through a process that was an organic equivalent of inorganic crystallization. The crystallized fiber was an array of particles of animal matter and constituted the "simplest organ" (a phrase applied by some later writers to the cell). The crystallization of animal matter took place, in accordance with certain laws of growth, around something that Reil called a *Kern* (basis or nucleus). Unlike von Haller, who had, by limiting irritability to muscle fibers, virtually identified "irritability" with the power to contract in response to a stimulus,[12] Reil defined irritability as the power possessed by all animal "organs" or living units to change their state in a particular way in response to particular external causes, e.g. muscles contracted, a stimulated optic nerve aroused visual impressions, a stimulated acoustic nerve those of sound.[13] Every "complete" organ, not necessarily every "simplest" organ, had its own innate *vita propria,* its peculiar forms of life and disease.[14]

We know that the doctrine of the fiber as the ultimate structural and functional unit was replaced in the second quarter of the nineteenth century by the doctrine of the cell, and that the observations on which the cell theory was based have their own history, dating back to the seventeenth century.[15] But the replacement of the fiber by the cell was an affair of gradual change rather than revolutionary overthrow. The story is too long to recount here in detail, but in brief a series of observations on plant and animal tissues, on infusoria and animalcules, sometimes complicated by optical artifacts arising from the use of uncorrected lenses, led by way of the globule theory of the structure of fibers[16] and similar false paths to the beginnings of cell theory in a form recognizable to the modern biologist. Schwann's book on the correspondence of structure and growth in plants and animals[17] appeared in 1839, when cells of some kinds had already been accurately described and were in general a subject of lively discussion. Schwann's contribution to the discussion is more difficult to grasp than appears at first sight, but at least he presented and backed up the claim that all structural constituents of the body were cells or derived from cells. Furthermore, he offered a theory of cell genesis, the final overthrow of which was accomplished by Virchow in the 1850's. This theory of cell genesis, in effect, substitutes the cell for the fiber in Reil's theory of fiber genesis. For this reason the Schwannian theory of cells and cell genesis could be, and was, rapidly inserted into variants of the prevailing humoralism without causing any disturbance, as we can see from the books of the pathologists Lotze[18] and Rokitansky,[19] which were published only a few years after the appearance of Schwann's work.

Leaving to one side the mass of evidence presented by Schwann to support his thesis that bodily structures were derived from cells, we shall examine only his conception of the origin of cells, which he attributed to a kind of organic crystallization out of a structureless fluid *Zellenkeimstoff* or "cytoblastema." The sequence of events, he said, was for a nucleus or *Kern* to crystallize out as a rounded sac-like structure, followed by the laying down of a second envelope about the first, with the space between usually filled by fluid. Alternatively, a smaller body, the *Kernkörperchen* or nucleolus, formed first and around it in succession formed the envelopes of the nucleus and cell proper. He grants on the one hand that crystals are angular whereas cells are rounded, that they are solid bodies whereas cells are concentrically arranged, fluid-containing vesicles, that they grow by apposition whereas cells grow by intussusception, but points out on the other that cells, like crystals, form from a fluid matrix in accordance with certain laws, and that they, again like crystals, have the power to attract from appropriate solutions the substances needed to further their growth. He suggests that organic crystals occupy a mid-position between solids and fluids, admitting that the notion of an organism as a kind of composite crystal involves much that is paradoxical and uncertain.[20]

It would be a considerable oversimplification to describe the complicated interchange that took place during the half century after Reil's essay of 1795 as a transfer to the "cell" of the properties accumulated by the "fiber." A distinction between the general idea of the cell (including the "vesicles," "globules" and "spherules" mentioned in the literature of the period) and Schwann's cell theory would have to be made in order to describe these events properly. Furthermore, Schwann always stated his "cell theory" as (1) cells arise from the cytoblastema around a nucleus, and (2) all structures in the body arise from transformed or combined cells. The first half of the theory was based, as Schwann tells us in his book, partly on the findings of Schleiden, and the second on embryological studies of his own and others. He sharply separated the admittedly hypothetical remarks on the crystallization of cells (which I have matched here with some equally speculative remarks by Reil) under the heading of "theory of the cell." If we bear these reservations in mind it is evident that a transfer of sorts did take place. It was in fact under way before the appearance of Schwann's book. But to understand just how it came about a detailed examination of Vogel's article on the formation of pathological tissues and Valentin's article on the formation of physiological tissues in Wagner's *Handwörterbuch der Physiologie,*[21] as well as of the works on pathology written by Lotze, Lebert, Vogel, Rokitansky and Wedl already referred to, would have to be compared with presentations of a decade earlier by Mueller[22] and Andral,[23] and that task will not be attempted here. Looking back on this period in 1877 Virchow wrote:

Nothing was simpler, nothing more logical, nothing more closely in correspondence with the generality of natural-scientific views, than the doctrine of the origin of tissue com-

ponents from chemical substances, from the so-called blastemas or histogenetic materials. . . . The new "cell theory"
was the old doctrine of *generatio equivoca* applied to formative processes within plant and animal organisms. The field
for this theory was nowhere more favorable than in pathology. Every day brought a new confirmation of this theory
in the form of seemingly quite factual observations on the
organization of exudates and the primitive blastema. Appearances were so convincing that one could only wonder
why all this had not been recognized long before. And yet all
this has been proved false.[24]

V

How had it been proved false? By the studies of Virchow and
many others pointing to the conclusion that the formation of new
cells by division of the old, heretofore recognized to a very limited
extent, was the rule rather than the exception. As early as 1852
Remak made the general claim that neither normal nor abnormal
tissues were formed from extracellular cytoblastemas.[25] Virchow
stated in 1877 that the "heretical thought of the continual reproduction of cells" gradually germinated in his mind in the late forties
and became the basis of his cellular pathology, but that he did not
make the first "hesitant attempts" to proclaim his views publicly
until 1852.[26] The publication of 1852 to which he refers here seems
to be the one entitled "Nutritional Units and Centers of Disease."[27]
In this essay Virchow gave considerable weight to the views of the
Scot John Goodsir, to whom also *Cellular Pathology* is dedicated.
Goodsir is the author of a book published in 1845 in which cells are
held to constitute centers of nutrition and secretion, and to be
arranged in territories populated by the descendants of a single
"mother" cell. In Goodsir's own words: "A nutritive center, anatomically considered, is merely a cell, the nucleus of which is the
permanent source of successive broods of young cells, which from
time to time fill the cavity of their parent, and carrying with them
the cell wall of the parent, pass off in certain directions, and under
various forms, according to the texture or organ of which their
parent forms a part."[28] Virchow did not subscribe to all of Goodsir's
statements but some of them were clearly important in the genesis
of his own ideas. Finally, Virchow said, he expressed himself freely.

He did this in an essay, published in 1855, bearing the same title as his book of three years later.[29] There the hypotheses on which his cellular pathology rests are stated more plainly than in the book. They are as follows: (1) all diseases are reducible to active or passive disturbances of living cells, (2) all cells arise from other cells, *omnis cellula a cellula,* (3) the functional capacities of cells depend on intracellular physical and chemical processes and may to some extent be inferred from structural changes of cells, (4) all abnormalities of structure are degenerations, transformations or repetitions of normal structure. Unlike the "cellular" pathology, if so we may call it, of the writers mentioned above, Virchow's cellular pathology required a radical departure from Schwann's theory of the free formation of cells, and from blastemas and plastic exudates generally, which was part of a general "flight out of Egypt" of medical theory, as he put it in his essay of 1855.

Virchow appears to have wanted to forget his own commitment to the blastema hypothesis as quickly as possible. However there is little doubt but that he was the first to break away from it entirely, and none at all that his book on cellular pathology was the first to be based entirely on the new theory of cell formation. An excellent summary of the events associated with the gradual abandonment of blastemas and plastic exudates was given by Foerster in the first volume of his work on general pathological anatomy, published in 1855 (apparently before Virchow's essay of the same year). In discussing these events Foerster credits Virchow with formulations (2) and (4), as given in the previous paragraph, and calls him the man who brought the old theory to its highest point of development but became the first to turn his back on it without compromise. Foerster mentions that Virchow's views have found many adherents and that he himself, on the basis of the available evidence and his own experience, intends to accept them in the course of his book, but that he will do so tentatively and without completely ruling out other views.[30]

(Of course Virchow had done something more than merely to reject the blastema hypothesis and Schwann's theory of cell formation. He had transferred the locus of life and disease to the cell. In his essay of 1855 he admitted freely the justice of the remark made by his critic Spiess[31] that he had placed in the cell that irritability, or capability of response to stimulation, formerly located by Reil in the individual constituents of the body (perhaps in his "simplest organs"). The neural pathologist Spiess wished to seat life and irritability in the nervous system, said Virchow, but he himself seated it in the cell and he predicted that it would remain there:

> No matter how we twist and turn we shall always come back to the cell. The eternal merit of Schwann does not lie in his cell theory that has occupied the foreground for so long, and perhaps will soon be given up, but in his description of the development of the various tissues, and in his demonstration that this development (hence all physiological activity) is in the end traceable back to the cell. Now if pathology is nothing but physiology with obstacles, and diseased life nothing but healthy life interfered with by all manner of external and internal influences then pathology too must be referred back to the cell. This is the task that we have undertaken . . . .[32]

VI

In order to give substance to the foregoing remarks on Virchow's new theory of disease it will be useful to examine a crucial part of that theory bearing on the topic of inflammation, and to show how sharply Virchow diverged here from his contemporaries and immediate predecessors. Before doing so the reader should recall again that Virchow's *Cellular Pathology* was not, as he himself is at pains to point out in the preface to the first edition and insists on again in the preface to the second, intended to represent a complete and systematic treatment of its own subject (given in the title) and still less of the whole field of pathology in the traditional sense of that term. It was a survey of normal and abnormal (physiological and pathological) histology carried out in the spirit of Virchow's commitment to the new theory of cell genesis, *omnis cellula a cellula,* and to his tenet that disease processes were ultimately cell processes. While the discussion of inflammation, scattered through Lectures VII, XIV, XVII–XX, covers the chief features of Virchow's new view of this ancient problem, it is far from complete. The reader who wishes a more extended discussion will turn to

Virchow's study of inflammation (including remarks on therapy), a contribution to the six volumes of the *Handbuch der speciellen Pathologie und Therapie* which he edited between 1854 and 1876.[33]

For comparison with Virchow's views we may take Vogel's article of 1842 on inflammation in Wagner's *Handwörterbuch*,[34] with the understanding that Vogel's interpretation, while generally acceptable to pathologists (except to the relatively few "neural" pathologists, perhaps), has its own stance on many contended points. We find that Vogel gives the usual description of the sequence of changes observable in the microvasculature in inflammation: transitory narrowing of lumina and acceleration of flow, prolonged dilatation and slowing, margination of cells and disappearance of the clear zone between the wall of the vessel and the axial stream, oscillation and, finally, stasis. (The investigation of these changes had been proceeding at a lively rate since the turn of the century; an extensive review may be found in C. F. Koch's article of 1832.)[35] Then came the stage of exudation. A plastic exudate or "blastema" passed through the intact walls of small vessels, and the subsequent fate of the lesion was determined by the development of this exudate. Like embryonic blastemas it carried within itself certain developmental potentialities, although their unfolding was dependent on local factors. From the blastema cells were formed, more or less as described by Schwann, and thus came into being pus cells, fibrous tissue cells and replacements for lost or damaged tissues. We shall pass over Vogel's remarks on the external and internal causes of inflammation, on the role of irritation, on pyemia and the metastatic spread of abscesses, and broadly summarize his view of inflammation as follows: It is a functional disturbance of the microvasculature culminating in stasis and followed by a nutritive and formative disturbance dependent on the outpouring of a plastic exudate or blastema in which cells subsequently develop under the influence of local factors and the inherent potentialities of the blastema. A quite similar treatment of the subject may be found in Lotze.[36]

Virchow describes the microcirculatory changes of inflammation in great detail in the *Handbuch* article referred to above, although only cursorily in his *Cellular Pathology*. The primary event of inflammation, as he sees it, is a cellular change: Inflammation remains a local disturbance of nutritive relationships between the blood and the tissues, but the sequence is reversed. That is, the altered function of the tissue cells acts on the vasculature to bring more nutriment into the involved zone, rather than the sequence of irritation, vascular disturbance, stasis and exudation. Further, the blastema or exudate drops out of Virchow's scheme entirely and the nutritive disturbance becomes a disturbance of cell nutrition. For the cell *is* the primary nutritive center (Virchow's debt to Goodsir). The agents causative of inflammation (called *irritantia* or *Reizenden*) effect a passive derangement (called *irritamentum* or *Reiz*) of individual cells or groups of cells, and this in turn arouses a set of active or reactive changes (called *irritatio* or *Reizung*). As for the "teleological interpretation" of that reaction as a defense against noxious agencies of external or internal origin, Virchow regarded it as problematical, overstated, yet containing a germ of truth, since some of these changes did indeed, in his opinion, represent a restoration of equilibrium.[37] The immediate effects of irritants on cell structure are set forth in *Cellular Pathology*. Virchow first gave emphasis to these "degenerative" changes in his study of 1852 on parenchymatous inflammation, where he gave special attention to the cell changes observable in parenchymatous nephritis, or Bright's disease.[38] To sum up, Virchow regarded the difference between inflammation and irritation as merely quantitative. The transient, functional changes, most prominently those of the microvasculature, were merely irritative; the lasting nutritive and formative changes were the peculiar feature of inflammation. Inflammation was also marked out from other nutritive disturbances by its rapidity of course and dangerous character (*Charakter der Gefahr*.)[39]

We come now to the matter of the pus corpuscles and their relation to the white blood cells. The account given by Vogel—that the pus corpuscles were secondary formations, like other cells, in the exuded blastema—had replaced an older account of pus as a "secretion" of the blood, in which it was already supposed to exist in a pre-formed state. The older account had been displaced by a new view of the vascular system as a closed circuit of tubes with walls impermeable to particles as large as pus corpuscles, a view that took form once the open-ended capillary "exhalant" and "secretory" vessels had been generally discarded. Virchow believed, on the basis of his cytological observations, that pus corpuscles arose locally, not of course by free formation from a "blastema" but by multiplication and transformation of pre-existing cells in the connective tissue. It was on this point that Cohnheim, his former pupil, was soon to differ with him.

Virchow had carefully distinguished and named leukemia and leucocytosis (including splenic and lymphatic leukemia, physiological leucocytosis and the leucocytosis of pregnancy). He had rejected the old notion of "pyemia" as a condition due to the resorption into the blood stream of pus contained in abscesses. The walls of even the tiniest capillary vessels were, he said, as impermeable to bodies the size of pus corpuscles or white blood cells as would be a collodion membrane. On the other hand he was perfectly well aware that pus corpuscles and certain of the white cells of the blood were morphologically indistinguishable and that Addison and Zimmerman (cf. pp. 155, 482 of London 1860 edition of *Cellular Pathology;* pp. 188, 527 of New York 1863 edition) claimed that pus cells were actually white cells that had passed out of the blood stream. In fact, he discussed this subject in 1847,[40] two years before the appearance of Addison's book of 1849[41] and apparently before he knew of Waller's actual experimental observations made in 1846.[42] Judging from Virchow's publication of 1847 just referred to, the claim must have been fairly widespread, for he writes: "In recent times some have even fallen from one extreme into the other, and while for a time they regarded all colorless corpuscles in the blood as resorbed pus corpuscles, now they want to interpret all cells turning up in pus as extravasated colorless blood corpuscles." But the evidence was far from convincing (it can seem convincing to us only if we have accepted the conclusion in advance), as he rightly concluded after examining it, and furthermore the whole notion of "exudates" and "extravasates" had for him an outmoded look, more suited to the attire of a humoral than a cellular pathologist.

Cohnheim's first description of the migration of the leucocytes appeared in *Virchows Archiv* in 1867,[43] five years after the publication of the third edition of *Cellular Pathology*. Cohnheim admitted that the reason why the white blood corpuscles moved out of the vessels at sites of irritation escaped him. It was not until eleven years later that he set forth a new theory of inflammation, according to which it was considered to be a "disease," a "molecular lesion" of the vascular wall and its subsequent consequences, rather than a reaction of any kind, protective or otherwise.[44] The findings of Cohnheim made their mark in the fourth edition (1871) of *Cellular Pathology*, where we find Virchow rather plaintively noting that the work of Waller and Cohnheim had made the study of new formations more difficult, since it was now hard to decide which cells had moved out of the blood vessels into a given lesion and which had multiplied on the spot. It turned out also that the extravasated leucocytes were being assigned, by Cohnheim's followers and others, all formative potentialities once ascribed to the exudate.[45] The extent to which this was true will be seen by anyone who cares to read Arnold Heller's monograph of 1869,[46] but the perspicacious reader of Virchow's *Cellular Pathology* will also find that Virchow himself endowed his connective tissue cells with the generative capabilities formerly assigned to the blastema, including the power to generate inflammatory cells and the cells of benign and malignant tumors (including those of epithelial origin). Since Virchow did not revise his *Cellular Pathology* after the edition of 1871 the work of Metschnikov, which did not begin to appear until the '80's, was never incorporated into it. Metschnikov's elaboration of what he called a biological or comparative theory of inflammation, founded on his studies of cellular phagocytosis throughout the animal kingdom,[47] Virchow's encouragement of his work on the occasion of a chance meeting in Messina in Sicily, where Metschnikov had withdrawn in 1882 after the assassination of Tsar Alexander the Second, and the subsequent publication of Metschnikov's papers on phagocytosis in *Virchow's Archiv* form an interesting chapter in the history of medicine. It is obvious that Virchow could see in Metschnikov's findings the possibility for a return of the cell to the center of the stage and a vindication, in a roundabout way, of his own cellular theory of inflammation.[48]

Virchow's interest in inflammation continued and his last paper on the subject appeared in 1900.[49]

VII

One of the less fortunate effects of the triumph of Virchow's cellular pathology, the "pathology of the future," as he called it, was predicted by Spiess, when he wrote in 1855 that in spite of the wishes and professions of its founder cellular pathology ran a great danger of developing into nothing more than a new form of pathological anatomy:

> Insofar as cellular pathology deals only with changes of the form and mixture of the living body it remains merely pathological anatomy, i.e. not pathological physiology, and insofar as it seeks to raise itself to the latter we must, in accordance with all that has been said before, call it a decisive step backward to a past stage of development . . . pathological anatomy is only one of the pillars, even if perhaps the strongest and most important, on which the rich structure of pathological physiology, the real pathology of the future, has to rest. And not only pathological anatomists, but also physicians, physiologists, chemists and physicists, and even psychologists and philosophers must unite all their best efforts in order to procure, prepare and insert in the proper place the materials for this structure.[50]

These objections to a purely pathological anatomical approach to pathology were no news to Virchow, for he had made similar remarks himself in 1846 in his review of Rokitansky's handbook of pathological anatomy,[51] again in 1847,[52] and even more eloquently in 1854.[53] Doubtless he had reason for believing that cellular pathology could avoid this pitfall. But in fact it did not, as Virchow himself tacitly admitted in 1898 at a session of the German Society of Pathology when he reminded the members that their task was to become pathologists and not remain anatomists, and to elucidate pathological processes rather than merely anatomical states. He even went so far as to claim that the distinction between process and state was becoming blurred.[54]

And this in fact had happened, if only to a limited degree. The morphological imprint stamped on "pathology" by cellular path-ology was so deep that it has not yet worn off. The stamp blurred the distinctions hitherto made between pathology and pathological anatomy. Cellular pathology itself became confused with patho-logical anatomy, as both Bier[55] and Aschoff[56] were to complain in the nineteen thirties. The lines of distinction between pathology, pathological anatomy and cellular pathology (as Virchow envi-sioned it) became so blurred that many pathologists were unaware of their existence. But the eminent German pathologist Robert Rössle asked in 1930, with a backward look at Virchow's words of 1898:

> . . . as against the usual study of cells in dead tissue, where has the necessary pathological physiology remained? Has not pathology in our hands, under the pressure of our object, the dead body, and in accordance with the law that scientific developments, too, progress along the line of least resistance, developed one-sidedly in the morphological direction?[57]

In the United States "pathology" became practically synonymous with pathological anatomy, and textbooks of pathology adopted the structure and range of topics of older works on pathological anatomy. Even in the rare instances where a variation on this pat-tern was attempted, e.g. in MacCallum's textbook, the morpho-logical bias remained strong.[58] There resulted some undesirable consequences, including the dissatisfaction of clinicians with what was taught as "pathology" by pathologists (who were for the most part pathological anatomists), and the difficulty experienced by pathologists themselves, especially in the United States, in defining their identity by any other than purely pragmatic means.

VIII

A concluding word on the volume the reader now has in his hands: Chance's translation of the second edition of Virchow's *Cellular Pathology* contains numerous footnotes and an index, neither available in the four German editions (1858, 1859, 1862, 1871). The notes were contributed by Virchow, under whose close supervision the translation seems to have been carried out. (There is an amusing footnote on p. 387 [p. 430 of the American edition] that may perhaps indicate Virchow's notion of what was suited to the Anglo-Saxon mentality.) The excellent index is the work of the translator. Finally, for those who read the language, a reprint of the German edition of 1858 was made available in 1966 by the Georg Olms publishing house in Hildesheim.

BIBLIOGRAPHY AND NOTES

1. Ackerknecht, Erwin. *Rudolf Virchow. Doctor, Statesman, Anthropologist* (Madison, 1953).
2. Lebert, Hermann. *Physiologie pathologique* (3 vols., Paris, 1845).
3. Vogel, Julius. *Pathologische Anatomie des menschlichen Körpers* (Leipzig, 1845).
4. Wedl, Carl. *Grundzüge der pathologischen Anatomie* (Vienna, 1854).
5. Fernel, Jean. *Universa medicina* (6th ed., Frankfurt, 1607).
6. Cullen, William. *First lines of the Practice of Physic* (Edinburgh, 1784), p. XIX. For translations of pertinent works by Unzer and Prochaska see *The Principles of Physiology,* by John August Unzer; and *A Dissertation on the Functions of the Nervous System,* by Georg Prochaska (London, 1851). For a general review see Gernot Rath's "Neural Pathology; A Pathogenetic Concept of the 18th and 19th Centuries," *Bull. Hist. Med.* **33**:526, 1959.
7. Henle, Jacob. *Handbuch der rationellen Pathologie* (2 vols., Braunschweig, 1846–53).
8. Spiess, Gustav. *Die Lehre von der Entzündung* (Frankfurt, 1854).
9. For translations of pertinent works see Laënnec's *Treatise on the Diseases of the Chest* (New York, 1962), Corvisart's *An Essay on The Organic Diseases and Lesions of the Heart and Great Vessels* (New York, 1962), and Morgagni's *The Seats and Causes of Diseases Investigated by Anatomy* (New York, 1960), all reprints in the History of Medicine Series of the New York Academy of Medicine.
10. Berg, Alexander. "Die Lehre von der Faser als Form- und Funktionselement des Organismus," *Virchows Archiv* **309**:333, 1942.

11. Reil, Johann. "Von der Lebenskraft" (1795), reprinted in *Klassiker der Medizin* (Leipzig, 1910).

12. Haller, Albrecht von. *A Dissertation on the Sensible and Irritable Parts of Animals* (reprinted, Baltimore, 1936).

13. Reil, Johann, *op. cit.*, p. 46.

14. *Ibid.*, p. 59.

15. Baker, John R. "The Cell-theory: A Restatement, History and Critique," *Quarterly Journal of Microscopical Science* **89**:103, 1948; **90**:87, 1949; **93**:157, 1952.

16. Edwards, H. Milne. *Mémoire sur la structure élémentaire des principaux tissus organiques des animaux* (thesis, Paris, 1823).

17. Schwann, Theodor. *Mikroscopische Untersuchungen über die Übereinstimmungen der Structur und dem Wachstum der Thiere und Pflanzen* (Berlin, 1839).

18. Lotze, R. Hermann. *Allgemeine Pathologie und Therapie als mechanische Naturwissenschaften* (Leipzig, 1842).

19. Rokitansky, Carl von. *A Manual of Pathological Anatomy.* Translated by W. E. Swain (4 vols., London 1849–54), Vol. 1.

20. Schwann, *op. cit.*, p. 257.

21. Wagner, Rudolf. *Handwörterbuch der Physiologie, mit Rücksicht auf physiologische Pathologie* (vol. 1, Braunschweig, 1842), pp. 617–698 (Valentin) and 797–859 (Vogel).

22. Mueller, Johannes. *Handbuch der Physiologie des Menschen* (Coblenz, 1835), vol. 1, pp. 389–406. In the 2nd ed. of the *Handbuch* Mueller adopts Schwannian views.

23. Andral, Gabriel. *Précis d'anatomie pathologique* (Paris, 1829).

24. Virchow, Rudolf. "Über die Standpunkte in der wissenschaftlichen Medicin," *Virchows Archiv* **70**:1, 1877. Translated in *Disease, Life and Man: Selected Essays by Rudolf Virchow* (Stanford, 1958).

25. Remak, Robert. "Über extracellularer Entstehung thierischer Zellen und über Vermehrung derselben durch Theilung," *Archiv für Anatomie, Physiologie und wissenschaftlichen Medicin,* 1852, p. 57.

26. Virchow, *loc. cit.*, #24.

27. Virchow, Rudolf. "Ernährungseinheiten und Krankheitsherde," *Virchows Archiv* **4**:375, 1852.

28. Goodsir, John. *Anatomical and Pathological Observations*

(Edinburgh, 1845), p. 2.

29. Virchow, Rudolf. "Cellular-Pathologie," *Virchows Archiv* **8**:3, 1855. Translated in *Disease, Life and Man.*

30. Foerster, August. *Handbuch der allgemeinen pathologischen Anatomie* (Leipzig, 1855), vol. 1, p. 78. Virchow had this to say in 1847: "All organic formation takes place from an amorphous material . . . new formation, embryonal or pathologic, consists in the differentiation of formless matter. . . . The formless blastema comes as a fluid from the blood; it is a more or less unchanged part of the blood plasma" ("On the Developmental History of Cancer," *Virchow's Archiv* **1**:110, 1847).

31. Spiess, *op. cit.,* #8, p. 154.

32. Virchow, *loc. cit.,* #29.

33. Virchow, Rudolf, ed. *Handbuch der speciellen Pathologie und Therapie* (6 vols., Erlangen, 1854–76), vol. 1, especially pp. 46–94 and 326–355.

34. Vogel, Julius. In Wagner, *op. cit.,* pp. 311–367.

35. Koch, C. F. "Über die Entzündung nach mikroskopischen Versuchen," *Archiv für Anatomie und Physiologie* **6**:121, 1832.

36. Lotze, *op. cit.,* pp. 354–370.

37. Virchow, *Handbuch,* #33, vol. 1, p. 63.

38. Virchow, Rudolf. "Über parenchymatöse Entzündung," *Virchows Archiv* **4**:261, 1852.

39. Virchow, *Handbuch,* #33, vol. 1, p. 76.

40. Virchow, Rudolf. "Über die Reform der pathologischen und therapeutischen Anschauungen durch die mikroskopischen Untersuchungen," *Virchows Archiv* **1**:207, 1847.

41. Addison's book, *On Healthy and Diseased Structure,* was published in London in 1849. It summarized his investigations into the physiological and pathological roles of the white or colorless blood corpuscles, which he regarded as multipotent embryonic cells capable of participating in a wide range of extravascular formative processes. Virchow may have been familiar with some of Addison's ten communications on these topics to the *London Medical Gazette* between 1841 and 1845, or with Wharton Jones's harsh criticism in the *British and Foreign Medical Review* (**14**:585, 1842). Jones was equally harsh in his criticism of Cohnheim thirty-two years later (*Lancet,* 11 Oct. 1884, p. 630).

42. Waller, Augustus. "Microscopic observations on the perforation of the capillaries by the corpuscles of the blood, and on the origin of mucus and pus globules," *Philosophical Magazine* **29**:397, 1846. This journal was devoted to the physical rather than the medical sciences. In his paper Waller acknowledged a debt to Addison but considered, correctly enough, that he himself was for the first time offering a description of the actual mode of passage of blood corpuscles through capillary walls.

43. Cohnheim, Julius. "Über Entzündung und Eiterung," *Virchows Archiv* **40**:1, 1867.

44. Cohnheim, Julius. *Vorlesungen über allgemeine Pathologie* (2nd ed., Berlin, 1882). For a translation of the 2nd edition see *Cohnheim's lectures on General Pathology* (3 vols., London, 1889–90).

45. Virchow, Rudolf. *Die Cellularpathologie in ihrer Begründung auf physiologische und pathologische Gewebelehre* (4th ed., Berlin, 1871), pp. 390, 530–537.

46. Heller, Arnold. *Untersuchungen über die feineren Vorgänge bei der Entzündung* (Erlanger, 1869).

47. Metchnikoff, Elie. *Lectures on the Comparative Pathology of Inflammation; Delivered at the Pasteur Institute in 1891.* Translated by F. A. and E. H. Starling. Dover Reprint, 1968.

48. Rather, L. J. "Virchow und die Entwicklung der Entzündungsfrage im neunzehnten Jahrhundert," in the *Verhandlungen des XX. Internationalen Kongresses für Geschichte der Medizin, Berlin, 22–27 August 1966* (Hildesheim, 1968), pp. 161–177.

49. Virchow, Rudolf. "Zum neuen Jahrhundert. Ein Gruss," *Virchows Archiv* **159**:1, 1900.

50. Spiess, Gustav. "Die Cellular-Pathologie im Gegensatz zur Humoral- und Solidarpathologie," *Virchows Archiv* **8**:303, 1855. See also L. J. Rather, "Virchow's Review of Rokitansky's *Handbuch* in the *Preussische Medicinal-Zeitung,* Dec. 1846" (*Clio Medica,* **4**:127–140, 1969).

51. Virchow, Rudolf. "Rokitansky, Handbuch der allgemeinen pathologischen Anatomie, *Preussische Medicinal-Zeitung* **49**, pp. 237–238; **50**, pp. 243–244, Dec. 1846.

52. Virchow, Rudolf. "Über die Standpunke in der wissenschaft-

lichen Medicin," *Virchows Archiv* **1**:3, 1847. Translated in *Disease, Life and Man.*

53. Virchow, Rudolf. "Specifiker und Specifisches," *Virchows Archiv* **6**:1, 1854.

54. Virchow, Rudolf. "Über die Stellung der pathologischen Anatomie zu den klinischen Disciplinen," *Verhandlungen der deutschen pathologischen Gesellschaft* **1**:6, 1898.

55. Bier, August. "Rudolf Virchow als Systematiker und Philosoph," *Virchows Archiv* **300**:517, 1937.

56. Aschoff, Ludwig. *Virchows Cellularpathologie.* Protoplasma Monographien (Berlin, 1938).

57. Rather, L. J. Rudolf Virchow's Views on Pathology, Pathological Anatomy, and Cellular Pathology," *A.M.A. Arch. Path.* **82**:197, 1966.

58. MacCallum, W. G. *A Text-Book of Pathology* (1st ed., Philadelphia, 1916).

CELLULAR PATHOLOGY

As Based upon Physiological and
Pathological Histology

TO

JOHN GOODSIR, F.R.S., Etc.,

PROFESSOR OF ANATOMY IN THE UNIVERSITY OF EDINBURGH,

AS ONE OF THE EARLIEST AND MOST ACUTE OBSERVERS OF

CELL-LIFE,

BOTH PHYSIOLOGICAL AND PATHOLOGICAL,

THIS WORK ON

CELLULAR PATHOLOGY

𝕴𝔰 𝔇𝔢𝔡𝔦𝔠𝔞𝔱𝔢𝔡

AS A SLIGHT TESTIMONY OF HIS DEEP RESPECT

AND SINCERE ADMIRATION,

BY

THE AUTHOR.

AUTHOR'S PREFACE

———•◦•———

THE lectures which I herewith lay before the medical public at large were delivered in the early part of this year, in the new Pathological Institute of the University of Berlin, in the presence of a somewhat numerous assembly of medical men, for the most part physicians practising in the town. The object chiefly aimed at in them, illustrated as they were by as extensive a series of microscopical preparations as it was in my power to supply, was to furnish a clear and connected explanation of those facts upon which, according to my ideas, the theory of life must now be based, and out of which also the science of pathology has now to be constructed. They were more particularly intended as an attempt to offer in a better arranged form than had hitherto been done, a view of the cellular nature of all vital processes, both physiological and pathological, animal and vegetable, so as distinctly to set forth what even the people have long been dimly conscious of, namely, the unity of life* in all organized beings, in opposition to the one-sided humoral and neuristical (solidistic) tendencies which have been transmitted from the mythical days of antiquity to our own times, and at the same time to contrast with the equally one-sided interpretations of a grossly mechanical and chemical bias—the more delicate mechanism and chemistry of the cell.

In consequence of the great advances that have been made in the details of science, it has been becoming continually more and more

* See Lect. I., p. 40 and Lect. XIV., pp. 322–324.—TRANS.

difficult to the majority of those who are engaged in practice, to obtain in the subjects treated on in these lectures that amount of personal experience which alone can guarantee a certain degree of accuracy of judgment. Day by day do those who are obliged to consume their best energies in the frequently so toilsome and so exhausting routine of practice find it becoming less and less possible for them, not only to closely examine, but even to understand the more recent medical works. For even the language of medicine is gradually assuming another appearance; well-known processes to which the prevailing system had assigned a certain place and name in the circle of our thoughts, change with the dissolution of the system their position and their denomination. When a certain action is transferred from the nerves, blood, or vessels to the tissues, when a passive process is recognized to be an active one, an exudation to be a proliferation, then it becomes absolutely necessary to choose other expressions whereby these actions, processes, and products shall be designated; and in proportion as our knowledge of the more delicate modes, in which the processes of life are carried on, becomes more perfect, just in that proportion must the new denominations also be adapted to this more delicate ground-work of our knowledge.

It would not be easy for any one to attempt to carry out the necessary reform in medical opinion with more respect for tradition than I have made it my endeavour to observe. Still my own experience has taught me that even in this there is a certain limit. Too great respect is a real fault, for it favours confusion; a well-selected expression renders at once accessible to the understanding of all, what, without it, efforts prolonged for years would be able to render intelligible at most only to a few. As examples I will cite the terms, parenchymatous inflammation, thrombosis and embolia, leukæmia and ichorrhæmia, osteoid and mucous tissue, cheesy and amyloid metamorphosis, and substitution of tissues. New names cannot be avoided, where actual additions to experimental (empirical) knowledge are being treated of.

On the other hand, I have already often been reproached with endeavouring to rehabilitate antiquated views in modern science. In respect to this I can, I think, say with a safe conscience that I am just as little inclined to restore Galen and Paracelsus to the position they formerly held, as I am afraid openly to acknowledge whatever truth there is in their views and observations. In fact, I find not only that the physicians of antiquity and the middle ages had not in all cases their senses shackled by traditional prejudices, but more than this, that among the people common sense has clung to certain truths, notwithstanding the criticism of the learned had pronounced them overthrown. What should hinder me from avowing that the criticism of the learned has not always proved correct, that system has not always been nature, and that a false interpretation does not impair the correctness of the fact? Why should I not retain good expressions, or restore them, even though false ideas have been attached to them? My experience constrains me to regard the term fluxion (active congestion—Wallung)* as preferable to that of congestion; I cannot help allowing inflammation to be a definite form in which pathological processes display themselves, although I am unable to admit its claims to be regarded as an entity; and I must needs, in spite of the decided counter-statements of many investigators, maintain tubercle to be a miliary granule, and epithelioma a heteroplastic, malignant new-formation (cancroid).

Perhaps it is now-a-days a merit to recognise historic rights, for it is indeed astonishing with what levity those very men, who herald forth every trifle, which they have stumbled upon, as a discovery, pass their judgment upon their predecessors. I uphold my own rights, and therefore I also recognize the rights of others. This is the principle I act upon in life, in politics and in science. We owe it to ourselves to defend our rights, for it is the only guarantee for our individual development, and for our influence upon the community at large. Such a defence is no act of vain ambition, and it involves no renunciation of purely scientific aims. For, if we would serve science, we must extend her limits, not only as far as our own knowledge is concerned, but in the estimation of others. Now this estimation depends in a great measure upon the acknowledgment accorded to our rights, upon the confidence placed in our investigations, by others; and this is the reason why I uphold my rights.

In a science so directly practical as that of medicine, and at a time

* See the Author's 'Handbuch der speciellen Path. und Therapie,' Vol. I. p. 141.

when such a rapid accumulation of facts is taking place, as there is in ours, we are doubly bound to render our knowledge accessible to the whole body of our professional brethren. We would have reform, and not revolution: we would preserve the old, and add the new. But our contemporaries have a confused idea of the results of our activity. For only too much it is apt to appear as though nought but a confused and motley mass of old and new would thereby be obtained; and the necessity of combatting rather the false or exclusive doctrines of the more modern, than those of the older writers, produces the impression that our endeavours savour more of revolution than reformation. It is, no doubt, much more agreeable to confine oneself to the investigation and simple publication of what one discovers, and to leave to others to "take it to market" (verwerthen—exploiter), but experience teaches us that this is extremely dangerous, and in the end only turns out to the advantage of those who have the least tenderness of conscience. Let us undertake, therefore, every one of us to fulfil the duties both of an observer and of an instructor.

The lectures, which I here publish with the view of accomplishing this double purpose, have found such very patient auditors, that they may perhaps venture to hope for indulgent readers likewise. How greatly they stand in need of indulgence, I myself feel very strongly. Every kind of lecture can only satisfy the actual hearers; and especially when it is chiefly intended to serve as an explanation of drawings on a board, and microscopical preparations, it must necessarily appear heterogeneous and defective to the reader. When the intention is to give a concise view of a comprehensive subject, it necessarily becomes impossible to bring forward all the arguments that could be advanced, and to support them by the requisite quotations. In lectures such as these too the personal views of the lecturer may seem to be brought forward with undue exclusiveness, but as it is his business to give a clear exposition of the actual state of the science of which he treats, he is obliged to define with precision the principles, the correctness of which he has proved by his own experience.

I trust therefore that what I offer may not be taken for more than it is intended to be. Those, who have found leisure enough to keep up their knowledge by reading the current medical literature, will find but little that is new in these lectures. The rest will not, by reading them, be spared the trouble of being obliged to study the subjects, which are here only briefly touched upon, more closely in the histological, physiological and pathological works. But they will at least be in possession of a summary of the discoveries which are the most important as far as the cellular theory is concerned, and they will easily be able to add their more accurate study of the in dividual subjects to the connected exposition which I here give them of the whole. Nay, this very exposition may perhaps afford a direct stimulus for such more accurate study; and if it do but this, it will have done enough.

The time at my disposal was not sufficient to enable me to write out and revise a work like this. I was therefore constrained to have the lectures taken down in short-hand, just as they were delivered, and to publish them with but slight alterations. Herr Langenhaun has executed his stenographical task with great care. As far as the shortness of the time permitted, and wherever the text would other-wise have been difficult of apprehension to the inexperienced, I have had woodcuts made from the drawings on the board, and more par-ticularly from the microscopical preparations which were sent round. Completeness in this respect could not be attained, seeing that, even as it is, the publication of the work has been delayed some months in consequence of the preparation of the woodcuts.

RUD. VIRCHOW.

MISDROY, *August 20th*, 1858.

AUTHOR'S PREFACE
to the Second Edition

———•••———

THE present attempt to bring the results of my experience, which are at variance with what is ordinarily taught, before the notice of the medical public at large, in a connected form, has produced unexpected results; it has found many friends and vigorous opponents. Both of these results are certainly very desirable; for my friends will find in this book no arbitrary settlement of questions, nothing systematical or dogmatical, and my opponents will be compelled at length to abandon their fine phrases and to set to work and examine the matters for themselves. Both can only contribute to the impulsion and advancement of medical science.

But still both have also their depressing point of view. When one has laboured for ten years with all the energy and zeal of which he was capable, and has laid the results of his investigations before the judgment of his contemporaries, one is only too apt to imagine that a considerable part, that perhaps the greater and more important portion of them, would be pretty generally known. This was, as I have learned by experience, not the case with my labours. One of my critics attributes it to my bringing forward too many arguments and lengthy cases in support of my views. It may be so, but then I might perhaps have been allowed to expect that other critics would have sought for the proofs, which they did not find here in

sufficient abundance, in the original works.   For I had in the preface
to the first edition expressly pointed out that those who had kept up
their knowledge, by reading the current medical literature, would
here find but little that was new to them.

In this new edition I have contented myself with improving the
language, with expressing in more precise terms what was liable to
be misunderstood, and with expunging repetitions.   There no doubt,
still even now, remains a great deal requiring correction; but it
seemed to me that the whole ought as far as possible to preserve the
fresher impress of oral discourse, and of the unshackled range of
thought which there prevails, if it were for the future still to serve
as an active ferment to the labourers in the so very various fields
of medical science and practice.   For the book will have fulfilled its
object, if it assists in the propagation, not of cellular pathology, but
in general only of independent thought and investigation.

RUD. VIRCHOW.

BERLIN, *June 7th*, 1859.

TRANSLATOR'S PREFACE

— •••—

Professor Virchow and his works are so well known wherever the science of medicine is studied, that I think it quite unnecessary to give any account of them here.

When I arrived in Berlin in March, 1858, these lectures were in the course of delivery, and I was present at a few of the concluding ones. Subsequently, whilst attending the lectures, classes, and post-mortem examinations* which are held in the Pathological Institute by Professor Virchow, I had ample opportunities for seeing practical illustrations of most of the doctrines advocated in this book. It was natural, therefore, that I should feel a desire to translate these lectures, the more especially as I had every reason to suppose that the views put forward in them still remained unknown—in consequence, no doubt, of their German dress—to a large proportion of the English medical public, although they had already, many of them several years previously, appeared in Professor Virchow's larger works.

The translation will in many instances be found to differ somewhat from the original, for numerous additions, subtractions, and substitutions have been made, many of them at the suggestion of the Author, many at my own, but all with the Author's sanction.

A few notes will be found, especially in the later lectures. Of these some are literal, some free translations of, or are based upon, answers I received from Professor Virchow to questions I had put to him, whilst others (pp. 352, 406, 415-416) were made entirely at

* From 700 to 800 bodies are examined annually in the Institute.

his own suggestion, and are literal translations of his words.   In all cases, however, the notes have been submitted to the Author, and approved by him.

An index too, I thought might be of service, and I have therefore added a tolerably full one.

I cannot sufficiently thank Professor Virchow for the very great trouble—a trouble of which nobody but myself can have any idea— which he has taken in revising this translation, nor for the exceeding courtesy and kindness with which he has replied to the very numerous questions—many of them put for my own private information— which I have plagued him with.   He has written me fully fifty letters, most of them very long ones; and when I reflect that he daily passes eight or nine hours at the Charité, that he reads all the more important German, French, and English medical works which appear, and is besides constantly engaged in publishing something fresh, I can scarcely conceive how he has managed to find time to write these letters, of which a large proportion reached me by return of post.

To Dr. Harris I must return my best thanks for the assistance he has rendered me in reading the proof-sheets, and correcting any errors of language into which I might have fallen, and also for kindly permitting me to consult him whenever I met with any difficulty—a permission of which I have availed myself most freely.

The engravings will, I think, be found to be pretty faithful copies of the original woodcuts.

51 WIMPOLE STREET, *August* 10*th*, 1860.

LIST OF ENGRAVINGS

—•••—

CONTENTS

———•••———

Introduction and object. Importance of anatomical discoveries in the history of medicine. Slight influence of the cell-theory upon pathology. Cells as the ultimate active elements of the living body. Their nature more accurately defined. Vegetable cells; membrane, contents, nucleus. Animal cells; capsulated (cartilage) and simple. Nuclei of. Nucleoli of. Theory of the formation of cells out of free cytoblastema. Constancy of nucleus and its importance in the maintenance of the living cell. Diversity of cell-contents and their importance as regards the functions of parts. Cells as vital unities. The body as a social organization. Cellular in contradistinction to humoral and solidistic, pathology.—Explanation of some of the preparations. Young shoots of plants. Growth of plants. Growth of cartilage. Young ova. Young cells in sputa.

Falsity of the view that tissues and fibres are made up of globules (elementary granules). The investment theory (Umhüllungstheorie). Equivocal [spontaneous] generation of cells. The law of continuous development.—General classification of the tissues. The three categories of General Histology. Special tissues. Organs and systems, or apparatuses.—The EPITHELIAL TISSUES. Squamous, cylindrical, and transitional epithelium. Epidermis and rete Malpighii. Nails, and their diseases. Crystalline lens. Pigment. Gland-cells.—The CONNECTIVE TISSUES. The theories of Schwann, Henle, and Reichert. My theory. Connective tissue as intercellular substance. Cartilage (hyaline, fibro- and reticular). Mucous tissue. Adipose tissue. Anastomosis of cells; juice-conveying system of tubes or canals.

LECTURE I.

FEBRUARY 10, 1858.

CELLS AND THE CELLULAR THEORY.

Introduction and object—Importance of anatomical discoveries in the history **of** medicine—Slight influence of the cell-theory upon pathology—Cells as the ultimate active elements of the living body—Their nature more accurately defined —Vegetable cells; membrane, contents, nucleus—Animal cells; capsulated (cartilage) and simple—Nuclei of—Nucleoli of—Theory of the formation of cells out of free cytoblastema—Constancy of nucleus and its importance in **the** maintenance of the living cell—Diversity of cell-contents and their importance as regards the functions of parts—Cells as vital unities—The body as a **social** organization—Cellular, in contradistinction to humoral and solidistic, pathology. Explanation of some of the preparations—Young shoots of plants—Growth of **plants** —Growth of cartilage—Young ova—Young cells in sputa.

GENTLEMEN,—Whilst bidding you heartily welcome to benches which must have long since ceased to be familiar to you, I must begin by reminding you, that it is not my want of modesty which has summoned you hither, but that I have only yielded to the repeatedly manifested wishes of many among you. Nor should I have ventured either to offer you lectures after the same fashion in which I am accustomed to deliver them in my regular courses. On the contrary, I will make the attempt to lay before you in a more succinct manner the development which I myself, and, I think, medical science also, have passed through in the course of the last fifteen years. In my announcement of these lectures, I described the subject of them in such a way as to couple histology with pathology ; and for this reason, that I thought I must take it for granted that many busily occupied physicians were not quite familiar with the most recent histological changes, and did not enjoy sufficiently frequent opportunities of examining microscopical objects for themselves. Inasmuch as, however, it is upon such examinations that the most important conclusions are grounded which we now draw, you will pardon me if, disregarding those among you who have a perfect acquaintance with the subject, I behave just as if you all were not completely familiar with the requisite preliminary knowledge.

The present reform in medicine, of which you have all been witnesses, essentially had its rise in new anatomical observations, and the exposition also, which I have to make to you, will therefore principally be based upon anatomical demonstrations. But for me it would not be sufficient to take, as has been the custom during the last ten years, pathological anatomy alone as the groundwork of my views ; we must add thereto those facts of general anatomy also, to which the actual state of medical science is due. The history of medicine teaches us, if we will only take a somewhat comprehensive survey of it, that at all times permanent advances have been marked by anatomical innovations, and that every more important epoch has been directly ushered in by a series of important discoveries concerning the structure of the body. So it was in those old times, when the observations of the Alexandrian school, based for the first time upon the anatomy of man, prepared the way for the system of Galen ; so it was, too, in the Middle Ages, when Vesalius laid the foundations of anatomy, and therewith began the real reformation of medicine ; so, lastly, was it at the commencement of this century, when Bichat developed the principles of general anatomy. What Schwann, however, has done for histology, has as yet been but in a very slight degree built up and developed for pathology, and it may be said that nothing has penetrated less deeply into the minds of all than the cell-theory in its intimate connection with pathology.

If we consider the extraordinary influence which Bichat in his time exercised upon the state of medical opinion, it is indeed astonishing that such a relatively long period should have elapsed since Schwann made his great discoveries, without the real importance of the new facts having been duly appreciated. This has certainly been essentially due to the great incompleteness of our knowledge with regard to the intimate structure of our tissues which has continued to exist until quite recently, and, as we are sorry to be obliged to confess, still even now prevails with regard to many points of histology to such a degree, that we scarcely know in favour of what view to decide.

Especial difficulty has been found in answering the question, from what parts of the body action really proceeds—what parts are active, what passive ; and yet it is already quite possible to come to a definitive conclusion upon this point, even in the case of parts the structure of which is still disputed. The chief point in this application of histology to pathology is to obtain a recognition of the fact, that the cell is really the ultimate morphological element in which there is any manifestation of life, and that we must not transfer the seat of real action to any point beyond the cell. Before you, I shall have no particular reason to justify myself, if in this respect I make quite a special reservation in favour of life. In the course of these lectures you will be able to convince yourselves that it is almost impossible for any one to entertain more mechanical ideas in particular instances than I am wont to do, when called upon to interpret the individual processes of life. But I think that we must look upon this as certain, that, however much of the more delicate interchange of matter, which takes place within a cell, may not concern the material structure as a whole, yet the real action does proceed from the structure as such, and that the living element only maintains its activity as long as it really presents itself to us as an independent whole.

In this question it is of primary importance (and you will excuse my dwelling a little upon this point, as it is one which is still a matter of dispute) that we should determine what is really to be understood by the term cell. Quite at the beginning of the latest phase of histological development, great difficulties sprang up in crowds with regard to this matter. Schwann, as you no doubt recollect, following immediately in the footsteps of Schleiden, interpreted his observations according to botanical standards, so that all the doctrines of vegetable physiology were invoked, in a greater or less degree, to decide questions relating to the physiology of animal bodies. Vegetable cells, however, in the light in which they were at that time universally, and as they are even now also frequently regarded, are structures, whose identity with what we call animal cells cannot be admitted without reserve.

When we speak of ordinary vegetable cellular tissue, we generally understand thereby a tissue, which, in its most simple and regular form is, in a transverse section, seen to be composed of nothing but four- or six-sided, or, if somewhat looser in texture, of roundish or polygonal bodies, in which a tolerably thick, tough wall (*membrane*) is always to be distinguished. If now a single one of these bodies be isolated, a cavity is found, enclosed by this tough, angular, or round wall, in the interior of which very different substances, varying according to circumstances, may be deposited, *e. g.* fat, starch, pigment, albumen (*cell-contents*). But also, quite independently of these local varieties in the contents, we are enabled, by means of chemical investigation, to detect the presence of several different substances in the essential constituents of the cells.

The substance which forms the external membrane, and is known under the name of cellulose, is generally found to be destitute of nitrogen, and yields, on the addition of iodine and sulphuric acid, a peculiar, very characteristic, beautiful

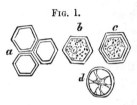

FIG. 1.

blue tint. Iodine alone produces no colour ; sulphuric acid by itself chars. The contents of simple cells, on the other hand, do not turn blue ; when the cell is quite a simple one, there appears, on the contrary, after the addition of iodine and sulphuric acid, a brownish or yellowish mass, isolated in the interior of the cell-cavity as a special body (*protoplasma*), around which can be recognised a special, plicated, frequently shrivelled membrane (*primordial utricle*) (fig. 1, *c*). Even rough chemical analysis generally detects in the simplest cells, in addition to the non-nitrogenized (external) substance, a nitrogenized internal mass ; and vegetable physiology seems, therefore, to have been justified in concluding, that what really constitutes a cell is the presence within a non-nitro-

Fig. 1. Vegetable cells from the centre of the young shoot of a tuber of *Solanum tuberosum*. *a*. The ordinary appearance of the regularly polygonal, thick-walled cellular tissue. *b*. An isolated cell with finely granular-looking cavity, in which a nucleus with nucleolus is to be seen. *c*. The same cell after the addition of water; the contents (protoplasma) have receded from the wall (membrane, capsule). Investing them a peculiar, delicate membrane (primordial utricle) has become visible. *d*. The same cell after a more lengthened exposure to the action of water ; the interior cell (protoplasma with the primordial utricle and nucleus) has become quite contracted, and remains attached to the cell-wall (capsule) merely by the means of fine, some of them branching, threads.

genized membrane of nitrogenized contents differing from it.

It had indeed already long been known, that other things besides existed in the interior of cells, and it was one of the most fruitful of discoveries when Robert Brown detected the *nucleus* in the vegetable cell. But this body was considered to have a more important share in the formation than in the maintenance of cells, because in very many vegetable cells the nucleus becomes extremely indistinct, and in many altogether disappears, whilst the form of the cell is preserved.

These observations were then applied to the consideration of animal tissues, the correspondence of which with those of vegetables Schwann endeavoured to demonstrate. The interpretation, which we have just mentioned as having been put upon the ordinary forms of vegetable cells, served as the starting-point. In this, however, as after-experience proved, an error was committed. Vegetable cells cannot, viewed in their entirety, be compared with all animal cells. In animal cells, we find no such distinctions between nitrogenized and non-nitrogenized layers; in all the essential constituents of the cells nitrogenized matters are met with. But there are undoubtedly certain forms in the animal body which immediately recall these forms of vegetable cells, and among them there are none so characteristic as the cells of cartilage, which is, in all its features, extremely different from the other tissues of the animal body, and which, especially on account of its non-vascularity, occupies quite a peculiar position. Cartilage in every respect stands in the closest relation to vegetable tissue. In a well-developed cartilage-cell we can distinguish a relatively thick external layer, within which, upon very close inspection, a delicate membrane, contents, and a nucleus are also to be found. Here, therefore, we have a structure which entirely corresponds with a vegetable cell.

It has, however, been customary with authors, when describing cartilage, to call the whole of the structure of which I have just given you a sketch (fig. 2, *a—d*) a cartilage-corpuscle, and in consequence of this having been viewed as analogous to the cells in other parts of animals, difficulties have arisen by which the knowledge of the true state of the case has been exceedingly obscured. A cartilage-corpuscle, namely, is not, as a whole, a cell, but the external layer, the *capsule*, is the product of a later development (secretion, excretion). In young cartilage it is very thin, whilst the cell also is generally smaller. If we trace the development still farther back, we find in cartilage, also, nothing but simple cells, identical in structure with those which are seen in other animal tissues, and not yet possessing that external secreted layer.

Fig. 2.

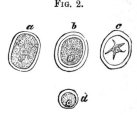

You see from this, gentlemen, that the comparison between animal and vegetable cells, which we certainly cannot avoid making, is in general inadmissible, because in most animal tissues no formed elements are found which can be considered as the full equivalents of vegetable cells in the old signification of the word ; and because in particular, the cellulose membrane of vegetable cells does not correspond to the membrane of animal ones, and between this, as containing nitrogen, and the former, as destitute of it, no typical distinction is presented. On the contrary, in both cases we meet with a

Fig. 2. Cartilage-cells as they occur at the margin of ossification in growing cartilage, quite analogous to vegetable cells (cf. the explanation to fig. 1). *a—c.* In a more advanced stage of development. *d.* Younger form.

body essentially of a nitrogenous nature, and, on the whole, similar in composition. The so-called membrane of the vegetable cell is only met with in a few animal tissues, as, for example, in cartilage ; the ordinary membrane of the animal cell corresponds, as I showed as far back as 1847, to the primordial utricle of the vegetable cell. It is only when we adhere to this view of the matter, when we separate from the cell all that has been added to it by an after-development, that we obtain a simple, homogeneous, extremely monotonous structure, recurring with extraordinary constancy in living organisms. But just this very constancy forms the best criterion of our having before us in this structure one of those really elementary bodies, to be built up of which is eminently characteristic of every living thing—without the pre-existence of which no living forms arise, and to which the continuance and the maintenance of life is intimately attached. Only since our idea of a cell has assumed this severe form—and I am somewhat proud of having always, in spite of the reproach of pedantry, firmly adhered to it—only since that time can it be said that a simple form has been obtained which we can everywhere again expect to find, and which, though different in size and external shape, is yet always identical in its essential constituents.

In such a simple cell we can distinguish dissimilar constituents, and it is important that we should accurately define their nature also.

In the first place, we expect to find a *nucleus* within the cell ; and with regard to this nucleus, which has usually a round or oval form, we know that, particularly in the case of young cells, it offers greater resistance to the action of chemical agents than do the external parts of the cell, and that, in spite of the greatest variations in the external form of the cell, it generally maintains its form. The nucleus is accordingly, in cells of all shapes, that part which is the most constantly found unchanged. There are indeed isolated cases, which lie scattered throughout the whole series of facts in comparative anatomy and pathology, in which the nucleus also has a stellate or angular appearance ; but these are extremely rare exceptions, and dependent upon peculiar changes which the element has undergone. Generally, it may be said that, as long as the life of the cell has not been

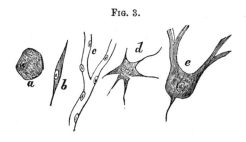

brought to a close, as long as cells behave as elements still endowed with vital power, the nucleus maintains a very nearly constant form.

The nucleus, in its turn, in completely developed cells, very constantly encloses another structure within itself —the so-called *nucleolus*. With regard to the question of vital form, it cannot be said of the nucleolus that it appears to be an absolute requisite ; and, in a considerable number of young cells, it has as yet escaped detection. On the other hand, we regularly meet with it in fully developed, older forms ; and it, therefore, seems to mark a higher degree of development in the cell. According to the view which was put forward in the first instance by Schleiden, and accepted by Schwann, the

Fig. 3. *a.* Hepatic cell. *b.* Spindle-shaped cell from connective tissue. *c.* Capillary vessel. *d.* Somewhat large stellate cell from a lymphatic gland. *e.* Ganglion-cell from the cerebellum. The nuclei in every instance similar.

connection between the three coexistent cell-constituents
was long thought to be on this wise : that the nucleolus
was the first to shew itself in the development of tissues,
by separating out of a formative fluid (*blastema, cyto-blastema*), that it quickly attained a certain size, that then
fine granules were precipitated out of the blastema and
settled around it, and that about these there condensed
a membrane.   That in this way a nucleus was completed,
about which new matter gradually gathered, and in due
time produced a little membrane (the celebrated watch-
glass form, fig. 4, *d'*).   This description of the first development of cells
out of free blastema, according to
which the nucleus was regarded as
preceding the formation of the cell,
and playing the part of a real cell-
former (*cytoblast*), is the one which is usually concisely
designated by the name of the *cell-theory* (more accurately, theory of *free* cell-formation),—a theory of development which has now been almost entirely abandoned,
and in support of the correctness of which not one single fact can with certainty be adduced.   With respect to
the nucleolus, all that we can for the present regard as
certain, is, that where we have to deal with large and
fully developed cells, we almost constantly see a nucleolus in them ; but that, on the contrary, in the case of
many young cells it is wanting.

Fig. 4.

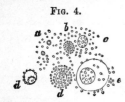

You will hereafter be made acquainted with a series

Fig. 4. From Schleiden, ' Grundzüge der wiss. Botanik,' I, fig. 1.   " Contents of
the embryo-sac of *Vicia faba* soon after impregnation.   In the clear fluid, consisting of gum and sugar, granules of protein-compounds are seen swimming about
(*a*), among which a few larger ones are strikingly conspicuous.   Around these latter the former are seen conglomerated into the form of a small disc (*b, c*).   Around
other discs a clear, sharply defined border may be distinguished, which gradually
recedes farther and farther from the disc (the cytoblast), and, finally, can be distinctly recognised to be a young cell (*d, e*)."

of facts in the history of pathological and physiological development, which render it in a high degree probable that the nucleus plays an extremely important part within the cell—a part, I will here at once remark, less connected with the function and specific office of the cell, than with its maintenance and multiplication as a living part. The specific (in a narrower sense, animal) function is most distinctly manifested in muscles, nerves, and gland-cells; the peculiar actions of which—contraction, sensation, and secretion—appear to be connected in no direct manner with the nuclei. But that, whilst fulfilling all its functions, the element remains an element, that it is not annihilated nor destroyed by its continual activity—this seems essentially to depend upon the action of the nucleus. All those cellular formations which lose their nucleus, have a more transitory existence; they perish, they disappear, they die away or break up. A human blood-corpuscle, for example, is a cell without a nucleus; it possesses an external membrane and red contents; but herewith the tale of its constituents, so far as we can make them out, is told, and whatever has been recounted concerning a nucleus in blood-cells, has had its foundation in delusive appearances, which certainly very easily can be, and frequently are, occasioned by the production of little irregularities upon the surface (Fig. 52). We should not be able to say, therefore, that blood-corpuscles were cells, if we did not know that there is a certain period during which human blood-corpuscles also have nuclei; the period, namely, embraced by the first months of intra-uterine life. Then circulate also in the human body nucleated blood-cells, like those which we see in frogs, birds, and fish throughout the whole of their lives. In mammalia, however, this is restricted to a certain period of their development, so that at a later stage the red blood-cells no longer exhibit all the characteristics of a cell, but have lost an important constituent in their composition. But we are also all agreed upon this point, that the blood is one of those changeable constituents of the body, whose cellular elements possess no durability, and with regard to which everybody assumes that they perish, and are replaced by new ones, which in their turn are doomed to annihilation, and everywhere (like the uppermost cells in the cuticle, in which we also can discover no nuclei, as soon as they begin to desquamate) have already reached a stage in their development, when they no longer require that durability in their more intimate composition for which we must regard the nucleus as the guarantee.

On the other hand, notwithstanding the manifold investigations to which the tissues are at present subjected, we are acquainted with no part which grows or multiplies, either in a physiological or pathological manner, in which nucleated elements cannot invariably be demonstrated as the starting-points of the change, and in which the first decisive alterations which display themselves, do not involve the nucleus itself, so that we often can determine from its condition what would possibly have become of the elements.

You see from this description that, at least, two different things are of necessity required for the composition of a cellular element; the membrane, whether round, jagged or stellate, and the nucleus, which from the outset differs in chemical constitution from the membrane. Herewith, however, we are far from having enumerated all the essential constituents of the cell, for, in addition to the nucleus, it is filled with a relatively greater or less quantity of *contents*, as is likewise commonly, it seems, the nucleus itself, the contents of which are also wont to differ from those of the cell. Within the cell, for example, we see pigment, without the nucleus containing any. Within a smooth muscular fibre-cell, the contractile sub-stance is deposited, which appears to be the seat of the contractile force of mus-cle ; the nucleus, however, remains a nucleus. The cell may develop itself into a nerve-fibre, but the nucleus remains, lying on the outside of the medullary [white[1]] substance, a constant constituent. Hence it follows, that the special peculiar-ities which individual cells exhibit in particular places, under particular circum-stances, are in general dependent upon the varying properties of the cell-contents, and that it is not the constituents which we have hitherto considered (membrane and nucleus), but the contents (or else the masses of matter deposited without the cell, *intercellular*), which give rise to the functional (physiological) dif-ferences of tissues. For us it is essential to know that in the most various tissues these constituents, which, in some measure, represent the cell in its abstract form, the nucleus and membrane, recur with great con-stancy, and that by their combination a simple element is obtained, which, throughout the whole series of living vegetable and animal forms, however different they may be externally, however much their internal composition may be subjected to change, presents us with a structure

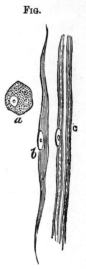

FIG.

Fig. 5. *a.* Pigment-cell from the choroid membrane of the eye. *b.* Smooth mus-cular fibre-cell from the intestines. *c.* Portion of a nerve-fibre with a double con-tour, axis-cylinder, medullary sheath and parietal, nucleolated nucleus.

[1] All words included in square brackets have been inserted by the Translator, and are intended to be explanatory.

of quite a peculiar conformation, as a definite basis for all the phenomena of life.

According to my ideas, this is the only possible starting-point for all biological doctrines. If a definite correspondence in elementary form pervades the whole series of all living things, and if in this series something else which might be placed in the stead of the cell be in vain sought for, then must every more highly developed organism, whether vegetable or animal, necessarily, above all, be regarded as a progressive total, made up of larger or smaller number of similar or dissimilar cells. Just as a tree constitutes a mass arranged in a definite manner, in which, in every single part, in the leaves as in the root, in the trunk as in the blossom, cells are discovered to be the ultimate elements, so is it also with the forms of animal life. *Every animal presents itself as a sum of vital unities*, every one of which manifests all the characteristics of life. The characteristics and unity of life cannot be limited to any one particular spot in a highly developed organism (for example, to the brain of man), but are to be found only in the definite, constantly recurring structure, which every individual element displays. Hence it follows that the structural composition of a body of considerable size, a so-called individual, always represents a kind of social arrangement of parts, an arrangement of a social kind, in which a number of individual existences are mutually dependent, but in such a way, that every element has its own special action, and, even though it derive its stimulus to activity from other parts, yet alone effects the actual performance of its duties.

I have therefore considered it necessary, and I believe you will derive benefit from the conception, to portion out the body into *cell-territories* (Zellenterritorien). I say territories, because we find in the organization of animals a peculiarity which in vegetables is scarcely at all to be witnessed, namely, the development of large masses of so-called *intercellular substance.* Whilst vegetable cells are usually in immediate contact with one another by their external secreted layers, although in such a manner that the old boundaries can still always

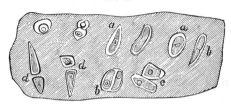

FIG 6.

be distinguished, we find in animal tissues that this species of arrangement is the more rare one. In the often very abundant mass of matter which lies between the cells (*intermediate, intercellular substance*), we are seldom able to perceive at a glance, how far a given part of it belongs to one or another cell ; it presents the aspect of a homogeneous intermediate substance.

According to Schwann, the intercellular substance was the cytoblastema, destined for the development of new cells. This I do not consider to be correct, but, on the contrary, I have, by means of a series of pathological observations, arrived at the conclusion that the intercellular substance is dependent in a certain definite manner upon the cells, and that it is necessary to draw bounda-

Fig. 6. Cartilage from the epiphysis of the lower end of the humerus of a child. The object was treated first with chromate of potash, and then with acetic acid. In the homogeneous mass (intercellular substance) are seen, at *a*, cartilage-cavities (Knorpelhöhlen) with walls still thin (capsules), from which the cartilage-cells, provided with a nucleus and nucleolus, are separated by a distinct limiting membrane. *b.* Capsules (cavities) with two cells produced by the division of previously simple ones. *c.* Division of the capsules following the division of the cells. *d.* Separation of the divided capsules by the deposition between them of intercellular substance—Growth of cartilage.

ries in it also, so that certain districts belong to one cell,
and certain others to another. Yow will see how sharply
these boundaries are defined by pathological processes
(Fig. 129), and how direct evidence is afforded, that any
given district of intercellular substance is ruled over by
the cell, which lies in the middle of it and exercises
influence upon the neighbouring parts.

It must now be evident to you, I think, what I understand by the territories of cells. But there are simple
tissues which are composed entirely of cells, cell lying
close to cell. In these there can be no difficulty with
regard to the boundaries of the individual cells, yet it is
necessary that I should call your attention to the fact
that, in this case, too, every individual cell may run its
own peculiar course, may undergo its own peculiar
changes, without the fate of the cell lying next it being
necessarily linked with its own. In other tissues, on the
contrary, in which we find intermediate substance, every
cell, in addition to its own contents, has the superin-
tendence of a certain quantity of matter external to it,
and this shares in its changes, nay, is frequently affected
even earlier than the interior of the cell, which is rendered more secure by its situation than the external
intercellular matter. Finally, there is a third series of
tissues, in which the elements are more intimately connected with one another. A stellate cell, for example,
may anastomose with a similar one, and in this way a
reticular arrangement may be produced, similar to that
which we see in capillary vessels and other analogous
structures. In this case it might be supposed that the
whole series was ruled by something which lay who
knows how far off ; but upon more accurate investigation, it turns out that even in this chainwork of cells a
certain independence of the individual members prevails,
and that this independence evinces itself by single cells

undergoing, in consequence of certain external or internal influences, certain changes confined to their own limits, and not necessarily participated in by the cells immediately adjoining.

That which I have now laid before you will be sufficient to show you in what way I consider it necessary to trace pathological facts to their origin in known histological elements ; why, for example, I am not satisfied with talking about an action of the vessels, or an action of the nerves, but why I consider it necessary to bestow attention upon the great number of minute parts which really constitute the chief mass of the substance of the body, as well as upon the vessels and nerves. It is not enough that, as has for a long time been the case, the muscles should be singled out as being the only active elements ; within the great remainder, which is generally regarded as an *inert mass*, there is in addition an enormous number of active parts to be met with.

Amid the development which medicine has undergone up to the present time, we find the dispute between the humoral and solidistic schools of olden times still maintained. The humoral schools have generally had the greatest success, because they have offered the most convenient explanation, and, in fact, the most plausible interpretation of morbid processes. We may say that nearly all successful practical, and noted hospital, physicians have had more or less humoro-pathological tendencies ; aye, and these have become so popular, that it is extremely difficult for any physician to free himself from them. The solido-pathological views have been rather the hobby of speculative inquirers, and have had their origin not so much in the immediate requirements of pathology, as in physiological and philosophical, and even in religious speculations. They have been forced to do violence to facts, both in anatomy and physiology, and have therefore never become very widely diffused. According to my notions, the basis of both doctrines is an incomplete one ; I do not say a false one, because it is really only false in its exclusiveness ; it must be reduced within certain limits, and we must remember that, besides vessels and blood, besides nerves and nervous centres, other things exist, which are not a mere theatre (Substrat) for the action of the nerves and blood, upon which these play their pranks.

Now, if it be demanded of medical men that they give their earnest consideration to these things also ; if, on the other hand, it be required that, even among those who maintain the humoral and neuro-pathological doctrines, attention at last be paid to the fact, that the blood is composed of many single, independent parts, and that the nervous system is made up of many active individual constituents—this is, indeed, a requirement which at the first glance certainly offers several difficulties. But if you will call to mind that for years, not only in lectures, but also at the bedside, the activity of the capillaries was talked about—an activity which no one has ever seen, and which has only been assumed to exist in compliance with certain theories—you will not find it unreasonable, that things which are really to be seen, nay are, not unfrequently, after practice, accessible even to the unaided eye, should likewise be admitted into the sphere of medical knowledge and thought. Nerves have not only been talked about where they had never been demonstrated ; their existence has been simply assumed, even in parts in which, after the most careful investigations, no trace of them could be discovered, and activity has been attributed to them in parts where they absolutely do not penetrate. It is therefore certainly not unreasonable to demand, that the greater part of the body be no longer entirely ignored ; and if no longer ignored, that we no longer content ourselves with merely regarding the nerves as so many wholes, as a simple, indivisible apparatus, or the blood as a merely fluid material, but that we also recognise the presence within the blood and within the nervous system of the enormous mass of minute centres of action.

In conclusion, I have still some preparations to explain, and will begin with a very common object (Fig. 7). It has been taken from the tuber of a potato, at a spot where you can view in its pefection the structure of a vegetable cell, where the tuber, namely, is beginning to put forth a new shoot, and there is, consequently, a probability of young cells being found, at least, if we suppose that all growth consists in the development of new cells. In the interior of the tuber all the cells are, as is well known, stuffed full with granules of starch; in the young shoot, on the other hand, the starch is used up, in proportion to the growth, and the cell is again exhibited in its more simple form. In a transverse section of a young sprout near its exit from the tuber, about four different layers may be distinguished—the cortical layer, next a layer of larger, then a layer of smaller, cells, and lastly, quite on the inside, a second layer of larger cells. Here we see nothing but regular structures; thick capsules of hex-

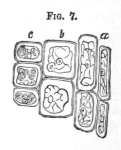

FIG. 7.

Fig. 7. From the cortical layer of a tuber of solanum tuberosum, after treatment with iodine and sulphuric acid. *a.* Flat cortical cells, surrounded by their capsule (cell-wall, membrane). *b.* Larger, four-sided cells of the same kind from the cambium; the real cell (primordial utricle), shrunken and wrinkled, within the capsule. *c.* Cells with starch-granules lying within the primordial utricle.

agonal form, and within them one or two nuclei (Fig. 1). Towards the cortex (corky layer) the cells are four-sided, and the farther one proceeds outwards, the flatter do they become ; still, nuclei may be distinctly recognised in them also. Wherever the so-called cells come in contact, a boundary line may be recognised between them ; then comes the thick layer of cellulose, in which fine streaks may be observed ; and in the interior of the capsular cavity you see a compound mass, in which a nucleus and nucleolus may be easily distinguished, and after the application of reagents the primordial utricle also makes its appearance as a plicated, wrinkled membrane. This is the perfect form of a vegetable cell. In the neighbouring cells lie a few larger, dimly lustrous, laminated bodies, the remains of starch (Fig. 7, c). The next object is of importance in my eyes, because I shall afterwards have to refer to it when instituting a comparison with new formations in animals. It is a longitudinal section of a young lilac bud, developed by the warm days we have had this month (February). In the bud a number of young leaves have already begun to develop themselves, each composed of numerous young cells. In these, the youngest parts, the external layers, are composed of tolerably regular layers of cells, which have a rather flat, four-sided appearance, whilst in the internal layers the cells are more elongated, and in a few parts spiral vessels show themselves. Especially would I call your attention to the little out-growths (leaf-hairs—Blatthaare), which protrude everywhere along the border, and very much resemble certain animal excrescences, e. g., in the villi of the chorion, where they mark the spots at which young, secondary villi will shoot out. In our preparation, you see the little club-shaped protuberances, which are repeated at certain intervals and are connected internally with the rows of cells in the cambium. They are structures in which the more delicate forms of cells can best be distinguished, and, at the same time the peculiar mode of growth be discovered. This growth is effected thus: a division takes place in some of the cells, and a transverse septum is formed; the newly-formed parts continue to grow as independent elements, and gradually increase in size. Not unfrequently divisions take place also longitudinally, so that the parts become thicker (Fig. 8, *c*). Every protuberance is therefore originally a single cell, which, by continual subdivison in a transverse direction (Fig. 8, *a, b*), pushes its divisions forwards, and then, when occasion offers, spreads out also in a lateral direction. In this way the hairs shoot out, and this is in general the mode of growth, not only in vegetables, but also in the physiological and pathological formations of the animal body.

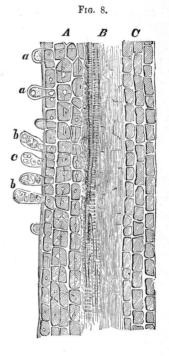

FIG. 8.

Fig. 8. Longitudinal section of a young February-shoot from the branch of a syringa. *A.* The cortical layer and cambium; beneath a layer of very flat cells are seen larger, four-sided, nucleated ones, from which, by successive transverse division, little hairs (*a*) shoot out, which grow longer and longer (*b*), and, by division in a longitudinal direction (*c*), thicker. *B.* The vascular layer, with spiral vessels. *C.* Simple, four-sided, oblong, cortical cells.—Growth of Plants.

In the following preparation—a piece of costal cartilage, in a state of morbid growth—changes are evident
even to the naked eye, namely, little protuberances upon

FIG. 9.

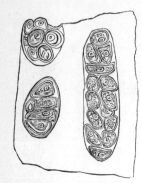

the surface of the cartilage. Corresponding to these the microscope
shows a proliferation of cartilage-
cells, and we find the same forms
as in the vegetable cells; large
groups of cellular elements, each
of which has proceeded from a
single previously existing cell,
arranged in several rows, and differing from proliferating vegetable
cells only in this—that there is
intercellular substance between the individual groups.
In the cells we can as before distinguish the external
capsule, which, indeed, in the case of many cells, is composed of two, three, or more layers, and within them
only does the real cell come with its membrane, contents,
nucleus, and nucleolus.

In the following object you see the young ova of a
frog, before the secretion of the yolk-granules has begun.
The very large ovum (Eizelle) (Fig. 10, *C*) contains a
nucleus likewise very large, in which a number of little
vesicles are dispersed—and tolerably thick, opaque contents, beginning, at a certain spot, to become granular
and brown. Around the cell may be remarked the relatively thin, connective tissue of the Graafian vesicle,
with a hardly visible layer of epithelium. In the neigh-

Fig. 9. Proliferation of cartilage; from the costal cartilage of an adult. Large
groups of cartilage-cells within a common envelope (wrongly so-called parent-
cells), produced from single cells by successive subdivisions. At the edge, one of
these groups has been cut through, and in it is seen a cartilage-cell invested by a
number of capsular layers (external secreted masses). 300 diameters.

bourhood are lying several smaller ova, which show the gradual progress of their growth.

Fig. 10.

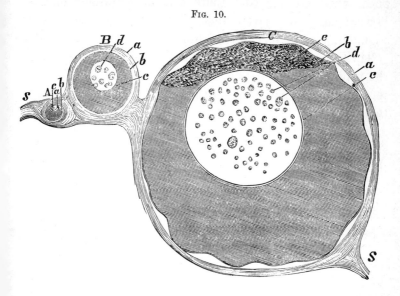

As a contrast to these gigantic cells, I place before you an object from the bed-side ; cells from fresh catarrhal sputa. You see cells in comparison very small, which with a higher power, prove to be of a perfectly globular shape, and, in which, after the addition of water and reagents, a membrane, nuclei, and, when fresh, cloudy contents can clearly be distinguished. Most of

Fig. 11.

Fig. 10. Young ova from the ovary of a frog. *A*. A very young ovum. *B*. A larger one. *C*. A still larger one, with commencing secretion of brown granules at one pole (*e*), and shrunken condition of the vitelline membrane from the imbibition of water. *a*. Membrane of the follicle. *b*. Vitelline membrane. *c*. Membrane of the nucleus. *d*. Nucleolus. *S*. Ovary. 150 diameters.

Fig. 11. Cells from from fresh catarrhal sputa. *A*. Pus-corpuscles. *a*. Quite fresh. *b*. When treated with acetic acid. Within the membrane the contents have cleared up, and three little nuclei are seen. *B*. Mucus-corpuscles. *a*. A simple one. *b*. Containing pigment granules. 300 diameters.

the small cells belong, according to the prevailing terminology, to the category of pus-corpuscles ; the larger
ones, which we may designate mucus-corpuscles or catarrhal cells, are partly filled with fat or greyish-black
pigment, in the form of granules.

These structures, however small their size, possess all
the typical peculiarities of the large ones ; all the characters of a cell displayed by the large ones again present
themselves in them. But this is, in my opinion, the
most essential point—that, whether we compare large or
small, pathological or physiological, cells, we always find
this correspondence between them.

LECTURE II.

FEBRUARY 17, 1858.

PHYSIOLOGICAL TISSUES.

Falsity of the view that tissues and fibres are made up of globules (elementary granules)—The investment theory (Umhüllungstheorie)—Equivocal [spontaneous] generation of cells—The law of continuous development.

General classification of the tissues—The three categories of General Histology—Special tissues—Organs and systems, or apparatuses.

The EPITHELIAL TISSUES—Squamous, cylindrical, and transitional epithelium—Epidermis and rete Malpıghii—Nails, and their diseases—Crystalline lens—Pigment—Gland-cells.

The CONNECTIVE TISSUES—The theories of Schwann, Henle, and Reichert—My theory—Connective tissue as intercellular substance—Cartilage (hyaline, fibro- and reticular)—Mucous tissue—Adipose tissue—Anastomosis of cells; juice-conveying system of tubes or canals.

IN my first lecture, gentlemen, I laid before you the general points to be noted with regard to the nature and origin of cells and their constituents. Allow me now to preface our further considerations with a review of the animal tissues in general, and this both in their physiological and pathological relations.

The most important obstacles which, until quite recently, existed in this quarter, were by no means chiefly of a pathological nature. I am convinced that pathological conditions would have been mastered with far less difficulty if it had not, until quite lately, been utterly impossible to give a simple and comprehensive sketch of the physiological tissues. The old views, which have in part come down to us from the last century, have exercised such a preponderating influence upon that part of histology which is, in a pathological point of view, the most important, that not even yet has unanimity been arrived at, and you will therefore be constrained, after you have inspected the preparations I shall lay before you, to come to your own conclusions as to how far that which I have to communicate to you is founded upon real observation.

If you read the ' Elementa Physiologiæ ' of Haller, you will find, where the elements of the body are treated of, the most prominent position in the whole work assigned to *fibres*, the very characteristic expression being there made use of, that the fibre (fibra) is to the physiologist what the line is to the geometrician.

This conception was soon still further expanded, and the doctrine that fibres serve as the groundwork of nearly all the parts of the body, and that the most various tissues are reducible to fibres as their ultimate constituents, was longest maintained in the case of the very tissue in which, as it has turned out, the pathological difficulties were the greatest—in the so-called cellular tissue.

In the course of the last ten years of the last century there arose, however, a certain degree of reaction against this fibre-theory, and in the school of natural philosophers another element soon attained to honour, though it had its origin in far more speculative views than the former, namely, the *globule*. Whilst some still clung to their fibres, others, as in more recent times Milne Edwards, thought fit to go so far as to suppose the fibres, in their turn, to be made up of globules ranged in lines. This view was in part attributable to optical illusions in microscopical observation. The objectionable method which prevailed during the whole of the last and a part of the present century—of making observations (with but indifferent instruments) in the full glare of the sun—caused a certain amount of dispersion of light in nearly all microscopical objects, and the impression communicated to the observer was, that he saw nothing else than globules. On the other hand, however, this view corresponded with the ideas common amongst natural philosophers as to the primary origin of everything endowed with form.

These globules (granules, molecules) have, curiously enough, maintained their ground, even in modern histology, and there are but few histological works which do not begin with the consideration of elementary granules. In a few instances, these views as to the globular nature of elementary parts have, even not very long ago, acquired such ascendancy, that the composition, both of the primary tissues in the embryo and also of the later ones, was based upon them. A cell was considered to be produced by the globules arranging themselves in a spherical form, so as to constitute a membrane, within which other globules remained, and formed the contents. In this way did even Baumgärtner and Arnold contend against the cell theory.

FIG. 12.

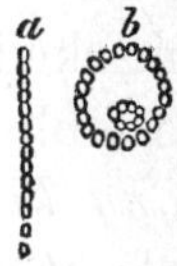

This view has, in a certain manner, found support even in the history of development—in the so-called *investment-theory* (Umhüllungstheorie)—a doctrine which for a time occupied a very prominent position. The upholders of this theory imagined, that originally a number of elementary globules existed scattered through

FIG. 13.

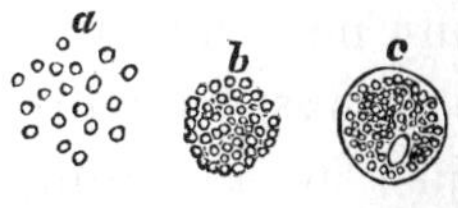

Fig. 12. Diagram of the globular theory. *a.* Fibre composed of elementary granules (molecular granules) drawn up in a line. *b.* Cell with nucleus and spherically arranged granules.

Fig. 13. Diagram of the investment- (cluster-) theory. *a.* Separate elementary

a fluid, but that, under certain circumstances, they gathered together, not in the form of vesicular membranes, but so as to constitute a compact heap, a globe (mass, cluster—Klümpchen), and that this globe was the starting point of all further development, a membrane being formed outside and a nucleus inside, by the differentiation of the mass, by apposition, or intussusception.

At the present time, neither fibres, nor globules, nor elementary granules, can be looked upon as histological starting-points. As long as living elements were conceived to be produced out of parts previously destitute of shape, such as formative fluids, or matters (*plastic matter*, *blastema*, *cytoblastema*), any one of the above views could of course be entertained, but it is in this very particular that the revolution which the last few years have brought with them has been the most marked. Even in pathology we can now go so far as to establish, as a general principle, *that no development of any kind begins* de novo, *and consequently as to reject the theory of equivocal* [spontaneous] *generation just as much in the history of the development of individual parts as we do in that of entire organisms.* Just as little as we can now admit that a tænia can arise out of saburral mucus, or that out of the residue of the decomposition of animal or vegetable matter an infusorial animalcule, a fungus, or an alga, can be formed, equally little are we disposed to concede either in physiological or pathological histology, that a new cell can build itself up out of any non-cellular substance. Where a cell arises, there a cell must have previously existed (*omnis cellula e cellula*), just as an animal can spring only from an animal, a plant only from a plant. In this manner, although there

---

granules. *b*. Heap of granules (cluster). *c*. Granule-cell, with membrane and nucleus.

are still a few spots in the body where absolute demonstration has not yet been afforded, the principle is nevertheless established, that in the whole series of living things, whether they be entire plants or animal organisms, or essential constituents of the same, an eternal law of *continuous development* prevails. There is no discontinuity of development of such a kind that a new generation can of itself give rise to a new series of developmental forms. No developed tissues can be traced back either to any large or small simple element, unless it be unto a cell. In what manner this continuous *proliferation of cells* (Zellenwucherung), for so we may designate the process, is carried on, we will consider hereafter ; to-day, my especial object only was to deter you from assuming as the groundwork of any views you might entertain with regard to the composition of the tissues, these theories of simple fibres or simple globules (elementary fibres or elementary globules).—

If it be wished to classify the normal tissues, a very simple point of view, founded upon marked characteristics, offers itself, upon which their division into three categories may be based.

We either have tissues which consist exclusively of cells, where cell lies close to cell—in fact, cellular tissue in the modern sense of the word—or we find tissues, in which one cell is regularly separated from the other by a certain amount of intermediate matter (intercellular substance), and, therefore, a kind of uniting medium exists, which, while it visibly connects the individual elements, yet holds them separate. To this class belong the tissues which are now-a-days generally comprehended under the name of connective tissues (Gewebe der Bindesubstanz), and of which what was formerly universally called cellular tissue constitutes the chief portion. Finally, there is a third group of tissues, in which the cells have attained specific, higher forms of development, by means of which their constitution has acquired a type entirely peculiar ; indeed, in part so peculiar, as to appertain exclusively to the animal economy. These are the tissues which are really characteristic of animals, although a few among them exhibit transitions of vegetable forms. To this class belong the nervous and muscular systems, the vessels and the blood. Herewith is the list of tissues concluded.

You must now proceed to consider, in what respect, in this summary of the result of histological researches, a contrast is afforded to what was formerly, chiefly in imitation of Bichat, regarded as constituting a tissue. Bichat's tissues would, for the most part, not so much represent what we now regard as the subjects of General Histology, as what we must rather designate as belonging to Special Histology. For, if we regard the tissues in the light they were formerly regarded ; if we, for example, separate tendons, bones, and faciæ, from one another, we then obtain an extraordinary variety of categories (Bichat had twenty-one), but there are not quite as many simple forms of tissue to correspond to them.

In accordance with modern notions, the whole domain of anatomy should first be divided into the categories of General Histology (*tissues* properly so called). Special Histology, then, takes up the instances, in which a combination of tissues, sometimes very different, into a single whole (*organ*) takes place. Thus we speak, for example, of osseous tissue ; but this tissue, the tela ossea of general histology, does not of itself form bone, for no bone consists entirely of tela ossea, but it has necessarily superadded at least periosteum and vessels. Nay, and from this simple conception of a bone, every bone of considerable size, for example, a long bone.

differs ; for that is a real organ, in which we can distinguish at least four different tissues. We have in it the tela ossea properly so called, the cartilaginous layer, the stratum of connective tissue belonging to the periosteum, and the peculiar medullary tissue. These several parts again are exceedingly heterogeneous in their nature, inasmuch as, for example, vessels and nerves enter into the composition of the marrow, the periosteum, etc. All these must be taken together to constitute the entire organism of a bone. Before we come, therefore, to *systems* or *apparatuses*, properly so called, the special subject of descriptive anatomy, a long series of gradations must be traversed, and in discussions we must always begin by having a clear idea of what the question is. When bone and osseous tissue are confounded together, the extremest confusion is occasioned, and so also when it is sought to identify nervous with cerebral matter. The brain contains many things which are not of a nervous nature, and its physiological and pathological conditions cannot be comprehended if they are regarded as occurring in an aggregation of purely nervous parts, and no consideration is paid to the membranes, the interstitial substance, and the vessels, as well as the nerves.

If, now, we consider the first of the classes into which we have divided General Histology, namely, the simple cellular tissues, a little more attentively, we find that those of which we can best obtain a general idea are unquestionably the *epithelial formations*, such as we meet with in the epidermis and the rete Malpighii, upon the external surface of the body, and in the cylindrical and scaly epithelium of mucous and serous membranes. Their general plan is, that cell lies close to cell, so that in the most favorable specimens, as in plants, four- or six-sided cells lie in immediate apposition one to the

other, and nothing at all is found between them. The
same is the case in many places with the scaly or pave-
ment-epithelium (Fig. 16). These forms are evidently
in a great measure due to pressure. For all the elements
of a cellular tissue to possess perfect regularity of form, it
is requisite that they should all grow in a perfectly uniform manner, and simultaneously. If their development
takes place under circumstances such that less resistance
is offered in one direction, it then may come to pass
that, as in the case of columnar or cylindrical epithelium,
the cells will shoot out in this one direction and become
very long, whilst in the other direction they remain very

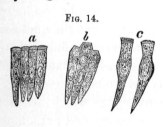

Fig. 14.

a   *b*   *c*

narrow. But even one of
these cells, when seen in
transverse section, will present an hexagonal shape,
and if we look down upon
the free surface of cylindrical epithelium, we see in it,
too, regularly polygonal forms (Fig. 14, *b*).

Contrasting with these, singularly irregular forms are
met with in places where the cells shoot up in an irregular manner, and accordingly they are found with remarkable constancy on the surface of the urinary passages, in
their whole extent from the calyces of the kidneys down
to the urethra. In all these parts it is very common to
meet with instances in which a cell is round at one end,
whilst at the other it terminates in a point, or where it
exhibits the appearance of a somewhat thick spindle, or is

Fig. 14. Columnar or cylindrical epithelium from the gall-bladder. *a.* Four contiguous cells seen in profile, each with a nucleus and nucleolus, their contents
slightly marked with longitudinal striæ; along the free (upper) edge, a thickish
border, marked with fine, radiated lines. *b.* Similar cells, with their free (upper,
outer) surface seen obliquely, so as to show the hexagonal form of a transverse
section, and their thick border. *c.* Cells altered by imbibition, somewhat swollen
up and with the upper border split into fibrils.

slightly rounded on one side and excavated on the other,
or where a cell is so thrust in between others as to assume
a clubbed or jagged form.
But in these cases also the
one cell always corresponds
with the other in form, and
it is not any peculiarity in
the cell which gives rise to
its shape, but the way in
which it lies, its relations
to the neighbouring cells,
and its having to adapt
itself to the arrangement of the parts next to it.   In
the direction of the least resistance the cells acquire
points, jaggs and projections of the most manifold description.   As they did not well admit of classification, Henle
gave them the name, which has since been adopted, of
transitional epithelium, to express their gradual transition into distinct scaly and cylindrical epithelium. Sometimes, however, this is not the case, and another name
for them might just as well have been adopted.

FIG. 15.

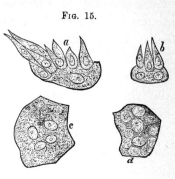

On account of the importance of the subject, I will
just add a few words with regard to the cuticle (epidermis).   In this it fortunately happens that, what is not
the case in many mucous membranes, many layers of
cells lie one above the other, and that the young layers
(the *rete Malpighii* [mucosum]) can easily and conveniently be separated from the older ones (the *epidermis proper*).

Fig. 15. Transitional epithelium from the urinary bladder. *a.* A large cell, with
excavations along its border, into which more delicate club- and spindle-shaped
cells fit. *b.* The same; the larger cell with two nuclei. *c.* A larger, irregularly
angular cell, with four nuclei. *d.* A similar cell, with two nuclei and nine depressions, as seen from above, corresponding to the excavations of the border. (Comp.
' Archiv. für path. Anat. und Phys.,' vol iii., plate i., fig. 8.)

On examining a perpendicular section of the surface of the skin, we for the most part see externally a very dense stratum, of variable thickness, which at the first glance is discovered to consist of nothing but flattened cells, that, when viewed edgeways, look like lines. They might be taken for fibres, piled up one above the other, and with slight differences of level making up the the whole external layer. Beneath these layers we find, differing in thickness and substance, the so-called rete Malpighii, and next to this, in a downward direction, the papillæ of the skin. If, now, we examine the boundary between the epidermis and the rete, the result we obtain by nearly every method of examination is,

FIG. 16.

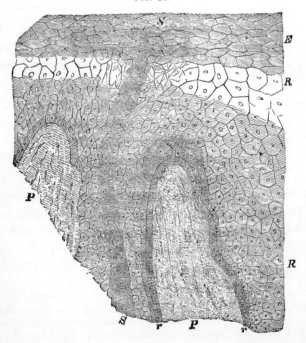

Fig. 16. Perpendicular section through the surface of the skin of a toe, treated with acetic acid. *P. P.* Extremities of cut papillæ, in each of which a vascular loop,

that to the innermost layer of the epidermis, very closely and almost abruptly, there succeed cells, which at first are also flattened, but in a less degree, and within which very distinct nuclei may be distinguished. These tolerably large cells mark the transition from the oldest layers of the rete Malpighii to the youngest of the epidermis. This is the point from which proceeds the regeneration of the epidermis, in itself an inert mass, which is gradually removed from the surface. And here is also generally the boundary, at which pathological processes set in. The farther we advance inwards, the smaller do the cells become ; the last of them standing in the form of little cylinders upon the surface of the papillæ (Fig. 16 *r, r*).

On the whole, the relations of the individual parts throughout the whole surface of the skin are everywhere the same, however manifold the peculiarities of detail may be, which the individual layers offer in respect to thickness, position, firmness, and connection. A section of a nail, for example, which in its external appearance certainly widely differs from ordinary epidermis, presents, nevertheless, on the whole, the same conformation, and has only one essentially distinctive feature, that, namely, in it two different epidermoidal structures are thrust, the one over the other, and thus a complication arises, which, if not duly attended to, may lead to the assumption of certain specific differences between it and other parts of the epidermis, whilst it really consists only in a peculiar change in the position of certain layers of

and near it little spindle-shaped, connective-tissue corpuscles, displaying at the base a reticulated arrangement, may be observed; to the left, a bulging out of the papillæ, corresponding to a tactile corpuscle, no longer visible, and situated at a deeper level. *R. R.* The rete Malpighii; immediately around the papilla a very dense layer of small, cylindrical cells (*r, r*); more externally, polygonal cells, gradually increasing in size. *E.* Epidermis, consisting of flat and more closely packed layers of cells. *S S.* Duct of a sweat gland passing through. 300 diameters.

the epidermis with regard to one another. The extremely dense and hard scales, which constitute the uppermost part, the so-called *body of the nail* (Nagelblatt), may, by different methods, be restored to forms in which they present the ordinary appearances of cells , and this is best seen after treatment with an alkali, when every scale swells up into a large, broadly oval, cell.

In the uppermost layers of the epidermis the cells become everywhere flatter, and towards the external surface no more nuclei at all can be discovered in them. Still there is no original difference between the epidermis and the rete Malpighii ; the latter is only the matrix of the epidermis, or indeed its youngest layer, inasmuch as from it there is a constant apposition of new parts taking place, which gradually become flatter and flatter, and move upward as fast as the scales on the outside disappear through friction of the surface, washing, or rubbing. But between the lowest layer of the rete and the surface of the cutis vera there are no intervening layers ; there is no amorphous fluid or blastema to be found there in which the cells could be generated, but they lie in direct contact with the papillæ of connective tissue of the cutis. There is therefore nowhere any space here, as there was thought to be even a short time ago, into which fluid transudes from the papillæ and the vessels contained therein, in order that new cells may arise and develop themselves out of it. Of such a fluid there is absolutely nothing discernible, but throughout the whole series of the layers of cells of the rete and epidermis the same relations exist that we are familiar with in the bark of a tree. The cortical layer of a potato (Fig. 7) exhibits in a similar manner, externally, corky, epidermoidal cells, and underneath, as in the rete Malpighii, a layer of nucleated cells, the cambium, constituting the matrix for the subsequent growth of the cortex.

Very much the same is the case with the nails. On examining the section of a nail, made transversely to the long axis of the finger, we see virtually the same structure as in ordinary skin, only every single indentation of the inferior surface does not correspond to a conical prolongation of the cutis, or papilla, but to a ridge which runs along the entire length of the bed of the nail, and may be compared with the ridges which are to be seen upon the palmar surface of the fingers. Upon these ridges of the bed of the nail are dwarfish, stunted papillæ, and upon them rests the rather cylindrically shaped youngest layer of the rete Malpighii ; then follow cells continually increasing in size, until at last the really hard substance comes, which corresponds to the epidermis.

Nevertheless—to discuss the subject at once, seeing that I shall not again have occasion to mention it—the structure of the nails has been difficult to make out, because they were conceived to be a simple formation. Nearly all the discussions, therefore, which have taken place, have turned upon the question where the matrix of the nail was, and whether the growth of the latter took place from the whole surface or from the little fold into which it is received behind. If we consider the nail with respect to its proper firm substance, its compact *body* (Nagelblatt), this only grows from behind, and is pushed forwards over the surface of the so-called *bed of the nail* (Nagelbett), but this in its turn also produces a definite quantity of cellular elements, which are to be regarded as the equivalents of an epidermic layer. On making a section through the middle of a nail, we come, most externally, to the layer of nail which has grown from behind, next to the substance which has been secreted by the bed of the nail, then to the rete Malpighii, and lastly to the ridges upon which the nail rests.

Thus the nail lies in a certain measure loose, and can easily move forwards, pushing itself over a moveable substratum, while it is kept in place by the ridges with which its bed is beset. When a section is made transversely through a nail, we see, as already mentioned, essentially the same appearance presented as that offered by the skin, only that a long ridge corresponds to every single papilla seen in ordinary sections of the skin; the undermost part of the nail has slight indentations corresponding to these ridges, so that, while gliding along over them, it can execute lateral movements only within certain limits. In this manner, the body of the nail which grows from behind moves forwards over a *cushion* of loose epidermic substance (Fig. 17, *a*) in grooves which are provided by the ridges and furrows of the bed of the nail. The uppermost part of the nail, if examined when fresh, is composed of so dense a substance that it is scarcely possible to distinguish individual cells in it without applying reagents, and at many points an appearance is presented like that which we see in cartilage. But by treating it with potash, we can convince ourselves that this substance is composed of nothing but epidermis-cells. From this mode of development you will see how easily intelligible distinctions may be drawn between the different diseases of the nails.

There are diseases of the bed of the nail which do not affect the growth of its body, but may give rise to changes in its position. When there is a very abundant development of cells in the bed of the nail, the body may be pushed upwards (Fig. 17, *b*); nay, it sometimes happens that the nail, instead of growing horizontally, shoots perpendicularly upwards, the space underneath being filled with a thick accumulation of the loose cushiony substance (Polstermasse) (Fig. 17, *c*). Thus suppuration may take place in the bed of the nail without the development of its body being thereby impeded. The most singular changes occur in small pox. When a pock forms upon the bed of the nail, there is nothing to be seen but a yellowish, somewhat uneven, spot ; but if, on the other hand, it is developed upon the fold, then its traces are left in the shape of a circularly depressed, and, as it were, excavated spot in the body of the nail as it gradually advances, a proof of a loss of substance precisely similar to that which takes place in the epidermis.

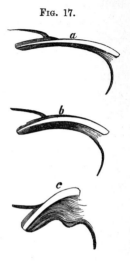

FIG. 17.

I will not to-day, gentlemen, enter more particularly into the special history of the formation of epidermis and epithelium, although it is of great importance for the right comprehension of many pathological processes, but content myself with calling your attention to the fact, that, under particular circumstances epithelial cells may undergo a series of transformations, through which they become extremely unlike what they originally were, and gradually assume appearances which render it impossible for those who are unacquainted with the history of their development to realize their original epidermic nature. The greatest abnormity of the kind is met with in the *crystalline lens* of the eye, which is originally a mere

Fig. 17. Diagrammatic representation of a longitudinal section of a nail. *a.* The normal condition ; a gently curved, horizontal nail, implanted in its fold, and separated from its bed by a thin cushion. *b.* A more markedly curved and somewhat thicker nail, with great thickening of the cushion, and much increased curvation of the bed, the fold being shorter and wider. *c.* Onychogryphosis; the nail, short and thick, reared up at a considerable angle, the fold short and wide, the bed furrowed on its surface, the cushion very thick and composed of layers of loose cells, piled up one above the other.

accumulation of epidermis. It has its origin, as is well
known, in a saccular involution of the external skin. At
first its connection with the external parts continues to
be maintained by means of a delicate membrane, the
membrana capsulo-pupillaris; afterwards this atrophies
and leaves the lens isolated in the interior of the eye.
The fibres of the lens are therefore, as C. Vogt has
shown, nothing more than epidermoidal cells which have
been developed in a peculiar manner, and their regeneration, after the extraction of a cataract for example, is
only possible as long as there still remains epithelium in
the capsule to undertake the new formation, and to
represent, as it were, a thin layer of rete Malpighii.
This reproduces the lens in the same way that the ordinary rete Malpighii of the external surface does the
cuticle. Amongst the other changes of epithelial structures we shall in due time revert to the peculiar pigment cells that are produced in the most different parts
by the direct transformation of epidermic cells, the contents of which either become coloured by imbibition, or
have pigment engendered in them by a (metabolic)
transposition of their elements.

With the history of epithelial elements properly so
called is immediately connected that of a peculiar class
of structures which play a very important part in the
accomplishment of the functions of an animal, namely
the *glands.* The really active elements of these organs
are essentially of an epithelial nature. One of Remak's
greatest merits consists in his having shown that in the
normal development of the embryo the outer and inner
of the well-known three layers of the germinal membrane chiefly produce epithelial structures, from a gradual proliferation of the elements of which glandular
structures arise. Other observers, for example, Kölliker,
had indeed before him made similar observations, but by

Remak was first established the law that the formation of glands in general must be regarded as consequent upon a direct process of proliferation on the part of epithelial structures. Previously large quantities of cytoblastema had been conceived to exist, in which, spontaneously, glandular substance took its rise; but, with the exception of the lymphatic glands, and perhaps those belonging to the sexual organs, their mode of origin is everywhere this—that at a certain point, in a manner very similar to that which I described to you in the foregoing lecture, when speaking of the excrescences of plants, an epithelial cell begins to divide, and goes on dividing again and again, until by degrees a little process composed of cells grows inwards, and, spreading out laterally, gives rise to the development of a gland, which thus straightway consitutes a body continuous with layers of cells originally external. Thus arise the glands of the surface of the body (the sudoriferous and sebaceous glands of the skin and the mammary gland), and thus also arise the internal glands of the digestive tract (the stomach glands and liver.) The most simple forms which glands can present do not occur at all in man. In inferior animals, however, *uni-cellular glands* have recently been discovered. The glands of the human body are invariably made up of a number of elements, which can, however, ultimately be traced back to a nearly simple type. Besides, in our own glands, in consequence of their size and complicated structure, other necessary constituents generally enter into their composition, so that, regarded as organs, they certainly do not consist of gland-cells only. But all parties are now pretty well agreed that the gland-cells are the really essential elements, just as the primitive bundles are in muscle, and that the specific action of a gland is dependent upon the properties and peculiar arrangement of these elements.

Generally speaking, therefore, glands consist of accumulations of cells, which usually form open canals. With

FIG. 18.

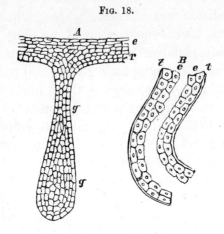

the exception of the glands, whose functions are uncertain, such as the thyroid body and supra-renal capsules, there are in the human body only the ovaries which form an exception to this rule, inasmuch as their follicles are only open at times ; yet they too must be open when the specific secretion of the ova has to take place. In most glands there is found indeed besides a certain quantity of transuded fluid, but this only constitutes the vehicle which floats off either the cells themselves, or their specific products. Suppose, for example, that in one of the ducts of the testicle a cell, in which there is a production of spermatozoa, becomes detached, then there transudes at the same time a certain quantity of fluid, which carries them away ; but what makes the semen, semen, and constitutes the specific character of the action

Fig. 18. *A*. Development of sweat-glands by means of the proliferation of the cells of the rete Malpighii in an inward direction. *e*. Epidermis. *r*. Rete Malpighii. *g g*. Solid process, constituting the first rudiments of a gland. After Kölliker.

B. Portion of the duct of the sweat-gland in a state of complete development. *t t*. Tunica propria. *e e*. Layers of epithelium.

is the peculiar power of the cell; the mere transudation from vessels is no doubt a means of conveyance onwards, but does not constitute the specific action of the gland nor the real secretion. In an analogous manner, in all the glands of which we can follow the action in all its details with precision, the essential peculiarities of their energy are derived from the development and transformation of epithelial cells.

The second histological group is formed by the *connective* tissues (Gewebe der Bindesubstanz). This is the subject in which I take the most interest, because it was here that my own observations, which have led to the result to which I directed your attention at the beginning of these lectures, originated. The alterations which I have succeeded in introducing in the views of histologists with regard to the whole group have, at the same time, enabled me to give a certain degree of roundness and completeness to the cellular theory.

Previously, connective tissue had nearly universally been regarded as essentially composed of fibres. On examining loose connective tissue in different regions, as, for example, beneath the corium, in the pia mater, subserous and submucous cellular tissue, we find wavy bundles of fibres, the so-called *wavy connective tissue* (Fig. 19, *A*). This wavy character, which is interrupted at certain intervals, so as to give rise to a kind of fasciculation, could, it was thought, with the less hesitation be attributed to the presence of separate fibres, because at the end of each bundle isolated filaments could in reality be seen to protrude. In spite of this, however, an attack was made upon this very hypothesis, somewhat more than ten years ago, and has proved of very great importance, though in a manner different to to that which was intended. Reichert endeavoured, namely, to show that the fibres were only an optical illusion produced by folds, and that connective tissue in all parts formed a homogeneous mass, endowed with a great tendency to the formation of folds.

Fig. 19.

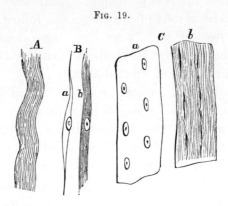

Schwann had, in reference to the formation of connective tissue, assumed that there originally existed spindle-shaped cells, the *caudate corpuscles* (geschwänzte Körperchen) (fibro-plastic corpuscles of Lebert), which afterwards became so famous ; and that out of these cells fasciculi of connective tissue were directly developed by the splitting up of the body of the cell into distinct fibrils, whilst the nucleus remained as such (Fig. 19, *B*). Henle, on the other hand, thought the only conclusion his observations would warrant was, that there were originally no cells at all, but that nuclei only were formed in the blastema at certain intervals ; whilst the

Fig. 19. *A.* Bundle of common, wavy, connective tissue (intercellular substance), splitting at its end into fine fibrils.

B. Diagram of the development of connective tissue according to Schwann. *a.* Spindle-shaped cell (caudate corpuscle, fibro-plastic corpuscle of Lebert), with nucleus and nucleolus. *b.* Cleavage of the body of the cell into fibrils.

C. Diagram of the development of connective tissue, according to Henle. *a.* Hyaline matrix (blastema), with nucleolated nuclei regularly distributed through it. *b.* Fibrillation of the blastema (direct formation of fibrils), and transformation of the nuclei into nucleus-fibres.

fibres, which afterwards appeared, were produced by a direct fibrillation of the blastema ; and that, whilst the intermediate substance was thus being differentiated into fibres, the nuclei gradually became elongated, so as at length to run into one another, and thus give rise to peculiar longitudinal fibres, *nucleus-fibres* (Kernfasern) (Fig. 19, *C*). Reichert took an extremely important step in opposition to these views. He showed, namely, that originally there were only cells, and those in great abundance, between which intercellular substance was deposited. But the membrane of the cells became, he thought, at a certain period, blended with the intercellular tissue, and then a stage was reached analogous to that described by Henle, in which there no longer existed any boundary between the original cells and the intermediate substance. And, finally, he imagined that the nuclei, too, entirely disappeared in some instances, whilst they were preserved in others. On the other hand, he positively denied the occurrence of the spindle-shaped cells of Schwann, and declared all such, as well as the caudate and jagged cells, to be just as much artificial products as the fibres, which were said to be seen in the intervening substance, were a false interpretation of an optical image.

Now, my own investigations have shown, that both Schwann's and Reichert's observations, up to a certain point, have some foundation in truth. That, in the first place, in opposition to Reichert, spindle-shaped and stellate cells indisputably do exist (Fig. 20) ; and secondly, in opposition to Schwann, and with Reichert, that a direct splitting up of the cells into fibres does not take place, but that on the contrary, what is afterwards presented to our sight as connective tissue has really taken the place of the previously homogeneous intercellular substance. I have found, moreover, that Reichert,

Henle, and Schwann, were wrong in maintaining that
ultimately at best only nuclei or nucleus-fibres remained ;

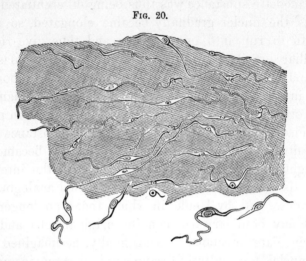

FIG. 20.

and that, on the contrary, in most cases the cells themselves preserve their integrity. The connective tissue
of a later period is therefore not distinguished in its
general structure and disposition in any respect from
that of an earlier date. There is not an embryonic connective tissue with spindle-shaped cells and a perfectly
developed one without them, but the cells remain the
same, although they are often not easy to see.

Essentially, therefore, this whole series of lower tissues may be reduced to one simple plan. Usually, the
greater part of the tissue is composed of intercellular
substance, in which, at certain intervals, cells lie imbedded, which in their turn present the most manifold forms.
But these tissues cannot be distinguished by one's con-

Fig. 20. Connective tissue from the embryo of a pig, after long-continued boiling. Large spindle-shaped cells (connective-tissue corpuscles (Bindegewebskörper-
chen)), some isolated, some still imbedded in the basis-substance, and anastomosing
one with the other. Large nuclei, with their membrane detached; cell-contents in
some cases shrunken. 350 diameters.

taining only round, another's, on the contrary, only caudate or stellate, cells. but in all connective tissues

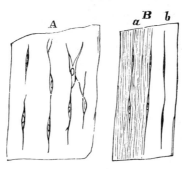

Fig. 21.

round, long and angular cells may occur. The simplest case is where round cells lie at certain intervals, and intercellular substance appears between them. This is the form which we see most beautifully shown in hyaline cartilage, as in that lining the joints, for example, in which the intercellular matter is perfectly homogeneous, and we see nothing but a substance which, though, perhaps, slightly granulated here and there, is on the whole quite as clear as water, so that as long as we do not see the edges of the preparation, doubt may arise as to whether anything at all exists between the cells.

This substance is characteristic of *hyaline cartilage*. Now we find that, under certain circumstances, the round cells became even in cartilage transformed into oblong

Fig. 21. Diagram of the development of connective-tissue, according to my investigations. *A*. Earliest stage. Hyaline basis- (intercellular) substance, with largish cells (connective-tissue corpuscles); the latter drawn up in rows at regular intervals; at first separated, spindle-shaped, and simple; at a later period anastomosing and branched. *B*. More advanced stage; at *a*, the basis-substance which has become striated (fibrillated), presents a fasciculated appearance on account of the cells imbedded in it in rows, the cells becoming narrower and smaller; at *b*, the striation of the basis-substance has disappeared under the influence of acetic acid, and the fine and long anastomosing fibre-cells (connective-tissue corpuscles), still retaining their nuclei, are seen.

spindle-shaped ones, as, for example, with great regularity in the immediate neighbourhood of the articular

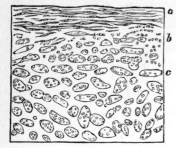

surfaces. The nearer, in the examination of articular cartilage, we approach to the free surface (Fig. 22, *a*,) the smaller do the cells become; and, at last, nothing more is seen but small, flatly lenticular bodies, the substance intervening between which sometimes presents a slightly striated appearance. Here, therefore, without the tissue's having ceased to be cartilage, a new type displays itself, which we much more regularly meet with in pure connective tissue, and hence the idea might easily arise that articular cartilage is invested with a special membrane. This is, however, not the case, for there is no synovial membrane spread over the cartilage, but its boundary towards the cavity of the joint is everywhere formed of cartilage itself. The synovial membrane only begins where the cartilage ceases—at the edge of the bone. On the other hand, we see that at certain points the cartilage passes directly into forms in which the cells become stellate, and the way is paved for their final anastomosis; ultimately, spots are met with at which it is no longer possible to say where the one cell ends and the other begins, inasmuch as they communicate so directly one with another that it is impossible to detect a line of separation between their membranes. When

Fig. 22. Perpendicular section through the growing cartilage of a patella. *a.* The articular surface, with spindle-shaped cells (cartilage-corpuscles) disposed in layers parallel to it. *b.* Incipient proliferation of the cells. *c.* Advanced proliferation; large, roundish groups—within the enlarged capsules a continually increasing number of round cells. 50 diameters.

such a case occurs, the cartilage, which up to that time had remained hyaline and homogeneous, becomes hete-rogeneous and striated, and has long since been called *fibro-cartilage*.

From these forms a third has been distinguished, the so-called *reticular* [yellow or spongy] *cartilage*, as seen in the ear and nose, in which the cells are round, but encircled by a peculiar kind of thick, stiff fibres, whose mode of production has not yet been thoroughly made out, but they are, perhaps, derived from the metamor-phosis of the intercellular substance.

Under these different types, presented by cartilage in its different localities, all the different aspects which the other connective tissues offer are included. There is also true connective tissue with round, long, and stellate cells. Just in the same manner we find, for example, in the peculiar tissue which I have named *mucous tissue* (Schleimgewebe), round cells in a hyaline, or spindle-shaped ones in a striated, or reticular ones in a meshy, basis-substance. The only criterion we possess for dis-tinguishing them consists in the determination of the chemical constitution of the intercellular substance. Every tissue is called connective tissue whose basis-substance yields gelatine when boiled ; the intercellular substance of cartilage produces chondrine ; mucous tis-sue, on expression, a substance, mucin, precipitable by acetic acid, and insoluble in an excess of it, though dis-solving in muriatic acid when added in considerable quantity.

Besides these, a few solitary points of difference in regard to peculiarity of form and contents may be pre-sented by individual cells at some later period of their existence. What we concisely designate *fat* is a tissue which is intimately connected with those of which we have been treating, and is distinguished from the rest by

the fact that some of the cells enlarge and become stuffed
full of fat, the nucleus being thereby thrust to one side.
In itself, however, the structure of adipose tissue is precisely the same as that of connective tissue, and, under
certain circumstances, the fat may so completely disappear that the adipose tissue is once more reduced to the
state of simple, gelatinous connective, or mucous tissue.

Amongst these different species of connective tissue
the most important for our present pathological views,
are, generally speaking, those in which a reticular arrangement of the cells exists, or, in other words, in which
they anastomose with one another.   Wherever, namely,
such anastomoses take place, wherever one cell is connected with another, it may with some degree of certainty be demonstrated that these anastomoses constitute
a peculiar system of tubes or canals which must be
classed with the great canalicular system of the body,
and which particularly, forming as they do a supplement
to the blood- and lymphatic vessels, must be regarded as
a new acquisition to our knowledge, and as in some sort
filling up the vacancy left by the old vasa serosa which
do not exist.   This reticular arrangement is possible in
cartilage, connective tissue, bone and mucous tissue in
the most different parts ; but in all cases those tissues
which possess anastomoses of this description may be
distinguished from those whose elements are isolated, by
the greater energy with which they are capable of con-
ducting different morbid processes.

LECTURE III.

FEBRUARY 20, 1858.

PHYSIOLOGICAL AND PATHOLOGICAL TISSUES.

The higher animal tissues : muscles, nerves, vessels, blood.
    Muscles—Striped and smooth—Atrophy of—The contractile substance and con·
        tractility in general—Cutis anserina and arrectores pili.
    Vessels—Capillaries—Contractile vessels—Nerves.
Pathological tissues (Neoplasms), and their classification—Import of vascularity—
    Doctrine of specific elements—Physiological types (reproduction)—Heterology
    (heterotopy), heterochrony (heterometry), and malignity—Hypertrophy and
    hyperplasy—Degeneration—Criteria for prognosis.
Law of continuity—Histological substitution and equivalents—Physiological and
    pathological substitution.

In my last lecture I portrayed to you the first two groups of tissues, the one embracing epithelium or epidermis, and the other the different kinds of connective tissue. What still remains forms a somewhat heterogeneous group, the individual members of which do not, indeed, in the degree that is the case with epithelium and connective tissue, bear a real relationship to one another, yet, on the whole, present a certain correspondence, in that they constitute the higher animal structures, and are distinguished by their specific mode of development from the less highly organized epithelial and connective tissues. Moreover, most of them appear under the form of connected, more or less tubular, structures. If a comparison be instituted between muscles, nerves, and vessels, the idea very readily suggests itself that we have in all three structures to deal with real tubes, filled with now more, now less, moveable contents. But this notion, however well it may accord with a superficial view of the matter, does not express the whole truth, inasmuch as we cannot compare the contents of the different tubes.

The blood which is contained in the vessels, cannot, at least at present, be regarded as analogous to the axis-cylinder, or the medullary [white] substance of a nerve-tube, or to the contractile substance of a primitive muscular fasciculus (Muskelprimitivbündel [muscular fibre]). I must, indeed, here remark, that the original development of all the structures which may be included in this group is still a subject of great controversy, and that the view maintaining the simply cellular structure of most of these elements is by no means completely established. This much, however, appears to be certain, that, at any rate in fœtal parts, the blood-corpuscles are just as much cells as the individual constituents of the walls of the vessels within which the blood flows ; and that the vessel cannot be designated as a tube which invests the blood-corpuscles, as the cell-membrane does its contents. It is therefore necessary in the case of the vessels to draw a line between their contents and proper walls, and to repudiate the seeming resemblance between the vessels, and the nerves and muscular fibres. Again, if we wished to adopt the mode of origin of the several tissues as the basis of our classification, we should, in accordance with prevailing views, have to associate the lymphatic glands also with the blood, and might be rather reminded of a connection such as we have seen to exist in the relations between the epidermis and the rete mucosum. But here I must once more impress upon you that the lymphatic glands are distinguished from glands properly so called, not only by their not possessing any excretory duct in the ordinary sense of the word, but also because from the mode of their development they by no means occupy the same position as ordinary glands, but are on the contrary at every period of their existence nearly allied to the connective tissues, and that, therefore, the temptation would rather be to class them with the tissues which we see produced by the transformation of the connective tissues. Yet this would at the present moment be still rather a venturous undertaking.

Amongst all the forms of which we have here to treat, the *elements of muscle* have generally been regarded as the most simple. If we examine an ordinary red muscle (I do not say a voluntary one, inasmuch as in the heart also we meet with fibres of the same form) we find it to be essentially composed of a number of cylinders, for the most part of equal thickness (primitive fasciculi [fibres]), which on a transverse section are seen to have a cylindrical form, and on which we at once perceive the well-known transverse striæ, that is, broad

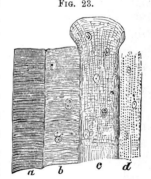

FIG. 23.

lines which generally run transversely through the fasciculus with a somewhat wavy outline, and are almost as broad as the intervals that separate them. In addition to this transverse striation we also see, especially when certain modes of preparation have been adopted, striæ fol-

Fig. 23. A group of primitive muscular fasciculi [fibres]. *a.* The natural appearance of a fresh primitive fasciculus, with its transverse striæ (bands or discs). *b.* A fasciculus gently acted upon by acetic acid; the nuclei stand out distinctly, and in one of them two nucleoli are visible, whilst in another the division is complete. *c.* A fibre acted upon more strongly by acetic acid; the contents are swollen up at the end, so as to protrude from the sheath (sarcolemma). *d.* Fatty atrophy. 300 diameters.

lowing a longitudinal direction, and these, indeed, in
some preparations preponderate to such a degree, that the
muscular fasciculus appears to be striated almost exclusively in this direction.   If now we add acetic acid, there
are forthwith disclosed immediately beneath the sheath,
and now and then also more towards the centre, nuclei
which are tolerably large, and mostly contain large nucleoli in greater or less number.   In this manner, therefore,
after we have cleared up the internal substance by the
application of acetic acid, we again obtain an appearance
which reminds us of the original cell-form ; and there
has been the greater tendency to regard the whole of a
primitive fasciculus as having sprung from a single cell,
because according to the view which was formerly
entertained, the individual primitive fasciculi of every
muscle were thought to extend from the point of origin
to that of insertion, and were therefore held to be
as long as the muscle itself.   This latter supposition
has, however, been shaken by investigations which
were set on foot in Vienna, under Brücke's direction
by Rollet, for he demonstrated that in the course of
muscles the ends of primitive fasciculi are to be seen
running into points, so that a primitive muscular fasciculus would comport itself like a large fibre-cell (Fig.
105, A).   These ends fit one into the other, and, according to this, the length of a primitive fasciculus would by
no means correspond to the whole extent of the muscle.

On the other hand, I must remark, that observations
have been made in different quarters quite recently,
which are rather of a nature to throw doubts upon the
uni-cellular nature of these elements.   Leydig regards
them as rather containing a series of cells of a smaller
kind, between which the contractile substance is lodged,
his idea being based upon the circumstance that every
nucleus (Figs. 23, b, c ; 24, B) is enclosed in a special

elongated cavity.[1] In discussions respecting these ultimate elements of muscle, extremely difficult relations
are involved, and I for my own part must confess that,
however much I am inclined to admit the uni-cellular
nature of the primitive fasciculi, I am still too familiar
with the peculiar appearances in their interior not to be
obliged to allow that another
view may be advanced. For
the present, however, we
must bear in mind that we
have to do with a structure
in which an external mem-
branous sheath (sarcolem-
ma) and contents are to be
distinguished. In the latter, acetic acid causes nuclei
to show themselves, and, when they (the contents) are
in their natural condition, the peculiar transverse and
longitudinal striation may be recognised in them. This

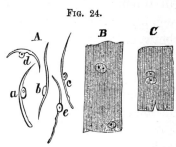

FIG. 24.

Fig. 24. Muscular elements from the heart of a puerperal woman. *A*. Peculiar
spindle-shaped cells precisely like the fibre-cells of the pulp of the spleen, probably
belonging to the sarcolemma and set free in teasing out the preparation. *a*. Cres-
centically curved cell, somewhat flat at one end, viewed on its surface. *b*. A
similar one, seen in profile, with flat nucleus. *c*, *d*. Cells, the nuclei of which lie
in a hernial protrusion of the membrane. *e*. A similar cell, viewed on its surface, with its nucleus, as it were, lying upon it. *B*. A primitive fasciculus, without
its sheath (sarcolemma), with distinct longitudinal fibrils and large, roundish nuclei,
of which one contains two nucleoli (incipient partition). *C*. A primitive fasciculus,
which has been teased asunder and slightly cleared up by acetic acid ; besides a
divided nucleus, fine, awl-shaped, nucleus-like bodies are seen imbedded between
the longitudinal fibrils. 300 diameters.

[1] This cavity Leydig supposes to be lined by a membrane, and therefore really
to constitute a cell (connective-tissue corpuscle). The nuclei of every primitive
fasciculus would, therefore, according to this view, be the nuclei of connective-
tissue corpuscles, and the contractile substance, lying between these, would be
equivalent to the intercellular substance of ordinary connective tissue. The nuclei
here alluded to are the ordinary nuclei of muscle, as seen in the figs. quoted above
and must not be confounded with the awl-shaped bodies represented in fig. 24, *C*,
lying between the fibrils ; for, though these bodies look like nuclei, they are really,
according to Leydig, portions of the divided processes of some of his connective-
tissue corpuscles.—*From a MS. note by the Author.*

striation is altogether internal and not external. The
membrane in itself is perfectly smooth and even ; the
transverse striation belongs to the contents, which, when
seen in a mass, form the red substance of the muscle.

Now it is this substance which has the property of
contractility indubitably inherent in it, and even varies
in appearance according to its state of contraction, becoming broader when contracted, whilst the intervals
between the individual transverse bands become somewhat narrower, so that a change in the arrangement of
its minutest constituents takes place, and this, as seems
probable from the investigations of Brücke, not merely
in the case of its physical molecules, but also in that of
its visible anatomical constituents. Brücke, namely,
by examining muscle by polarized light, has discovered
different optical properties in the individual layers of
substance—in those which compose the transverse striæ
and those which form the intervening mass. On the
adoption of certain methods of preparation, every primitive muscular fasciculus appears to be made up of
plates or discs of a different nature, piled up one above
another, and these in their turn to be entirely composed
of minute granules (Bowman's sarcous elements). In
reality, however, the contents of a primitive fasciculus
consist of a certain number of fine, longitudinal fibrils,
every one of which contains minute granules corresponding in position to the transverse striæ or apparent discs
of the primitive fasciculus, and held together by a pale,
intervening substance. Now, since a considerable number of primitive fibrils lie in apposition side by side,
there arises, in consequence of the symmetrical position
of the little granules, this very appearance of discs which
really do not exist. In proportion to the activity of the
muscle these parts assume an altered position with regard to one another ; during contraction the granules

are approximated, whilst the intervening substance becomes shorter and, at the same time, broader.

Compared with this, the structure of the *smooth, organic,* or, although this is a less expressive term, *involuntary muscular fibres,* appears much more simple. On examining any part of those organs in which smooth muscular fibres are contained, we find in the majority of cases, first of all, just as was the case with the transversely striated muscles, little fasciculi—as, for example, in the muscular coat of the urinary bladder. Within these fasciculi, upon further investigation, a series of distinct elements can be distinguished, of which a certain number, six, ten, twenty, or more, are held together by a common connective substance. According to the notion which universally prevailed until quite recently, every one of these elements was analogous to the primitive fasciculus of striped muscle. For as soon as we succeed in separating these fasciculi of smooth muscle into their more minute constituents, we find their ultimate elements to consist of long, spindle-shaped cells, which usually contain a nucleus in their centre (Fig. 5, *b*). According to the view on the contrary, which, especially in consequence of the impulsion given by Leydig's investigations, has quite lately

Fig. 25.

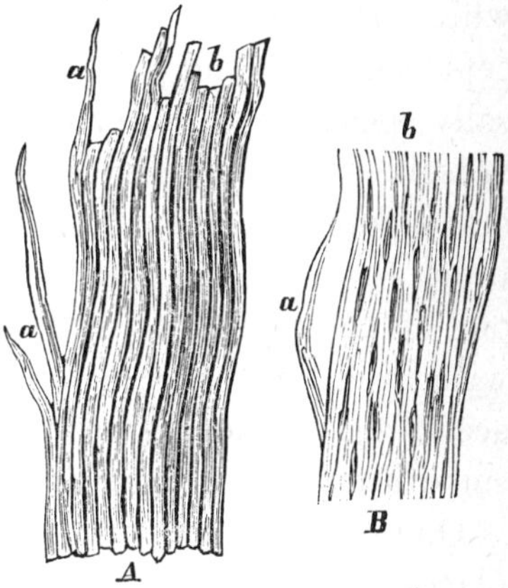

Fig. 25. Smooth muscular fibres from the parietes of the urinary bladder. *A.* Fasciculus still coherent, out of which at *a, a* single isolated fibre-cells protrude, whilst at *b* their simple divided ends appear. *B.* A similar fasciculus after being treated with acetic acid, whereby the long and narrow nuclei have become evident. *a.* and *b,* as above. 300 diameters.

begun to be mooted in various quarters, we should have to regard the bundle, in which a whole series of fibre-cells is contained, rather as analogous to a transversely striated primitive fasciculus. Until, however, this point has been satisfactorily settled, I consider it advisable and more in accordance with known facts to regard each fibre-cell as the equivalent of a primitive fasciculus. Should, however, any change of opinion shortly occur, you will now at any rate be prepared for it.

In one of these spindle-shaped or fibre-cells it is difficult to distinguish anything particular. In very large cells of this kind, and with a high magnifying power, we can certainly frequently distinguish a fine longitudinal striation (Fig. 5, *b*), so that it looks as if here, too, fibrils of some sort were disposed lengthways in the interior, whilst ordinarily no trace of any transverse striæ is perceptible. Yet the pale, smooth muscles exhibit, chemically speaking, a pretty close agreement with the transversely striped ones, since a similar substance (the so-called Syntonian of Lehmann) can, by the help of diluted hydrochloric acid, be extracted from both ; and one of the most characteristic substances which is met with in red muscles, namely Creatine, is met with also, according to the investigations of G. Siegmund, in the smooth muscular fibres of the uterus.

One of the preparations of red muscle which I have placed before you exhibits an appearance which is also pathologically interesting ; among the fasciculi, namely, is one which presents the condition of the so-called *progressive* (fatty) *atrophy.* The degenerated fasciculus is smaller and narrower, and at the same time little fat-globules are seen arranged in rows between the longitudinal fibrils (Fig 23, *d*). Atrophy in muscles is chiefly characterized by a diminution in the diameter of the primitive fasciculi affected ; in fatty atrophy the more palpable change is added, that little rows of fat-globules appear in the interior of the primitive fasciculus, during the accumulation of which the proper contractile substance decreases in bulk. The more fat there is, the less contractile substance ; or, in other words, the muscle becomes less capable of performing its functions in proportion as the normal contents of its fibres diminish. Pathological experience, therefore, also designates as the seat of the contractile power a definite substance, the occurrence of which, as especially the important investigations of Kölliker have taught us, is connected with certain histological elements. Whilst formerly many other things besides the substance of muscle, as for example, certain forms of connective tissue, were assumed to be contractile, lately the whole theory of contractility in the human body has been withdrawn within the limits of that substance, and observers have succeeded in tracing back nearly all the peculiar phenomena of motion to the existence of minute parts of a really muscular nature. Thus, in the human skin there lie little muscles about as large as the smallest fasciculi in the parietes of the urinarybladder, bundles consisting of diminutive fibre-cells, which run from the base of the hair-follicles towards the surface of the skin, and, when they contract, approximate the two. The result of this is naturally that the skin becomes uneven, and we get what is called a goose-skin. This singular phenomenon, which was previously regarded as inexplicable, has been simply explained by the demonstration of these purely microscopical muscles, the *arrectores pilorum*.

So also we now know that the greater part of the muscular layers in vessels is composed of elements of this kind, and that the phenomena of contraction exhibited by the vessels must be referred solely and exclusively to the action of muscular fibres, which are contained in them in the form of circular or longitudinal layers. A small vein or a small artery can contract only in proportion to the quantity of muscle with which it is provided, and they are only distinguished by the circumstance that either the longitudinal or the transverse muscular layers are the more strongly developed.

I have called your attention to this point because you

FIG. 26.

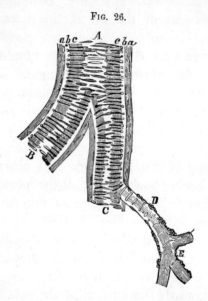

can see from it, how a simple anatomical discovery may supply the most important information with regard to

Fig. 26. Small artery from the base of the cerebrum after the application of acetic acid. *A.* Small trunk; *B* and *C*, larger branches; *D* and *E*, branches of the smallest size (capillary arteries). *a, a.* External coat, with nuclei, which run in the direction of the length of the vessel, and are seen first in a double and afterwards in a single layer, with a striated basis-substance; at *D* and *E* the coat is reduced to a single layer, with longitudinal nuclei, which here and there have been replaced by masses of fat-granules (fatty degeneration). *b, b.* Middle coat (circular fibrous, or muscular, coat), with long, cylindrical nuclei, which run transversely around the vessel, and at its borders (where they look as though they had been cut across) present the appearance of round bodies; at *D* and *E* transverse nuclei of the middle coat becoming continually scarcer. *c, c.* Internal coat, at *D* and *E* with longitudinal nuclei. 300 diameters.

physiological facts, which are widely separated from one another, and how the demonstration of definite morphological elements may at once most essentially contribute to the elucidation of functions, which, without any such data, would be utterly incomprehensible.

I will omit to speak here of the more intimate structure of the nervous system, because I shall have occasion hereafter to consider it in a more connected form, else this would be the subject which would most suitably come next, seeing that there exist many points of resemblance in the structure of muscular and nerve-fibres. But in the nervous system we find, in addition, nerve-cells (Ganglienzellen), which connect the individual fibres with one another, and must be regarded as the most important storehouses for all nervous energy.

Concerning the structure of the vascular system also I will not here treat in detail, but will only say as much as is necessary to give a cursory view of the matter.

A capillary vessel is a simple tube (Fig. 3, *c*), in which we have, with the aid of our present appliances, hitherto only been able to discover a simple membrane, beset at intervals with flattened nuclei, which, when seen in the middle of the surface of the vessel, present the same appearance as in the elements of muscle, only that they usually lie more at the sides, and therefore frequently have an awl-shaped appearance, from their sharp border alone being perceived. It is this, the most simple class of vessels, which we now-a-days solely and exclusively call capillaries, and with regard to them we cannot say that they become wider or narrower by means of any action of their own, but at most that their elasticity renders a certain degree of contraction possible. Nowhere are there to be witnessed in them genuine processes of contraction or relaxation succeeding it. The discussions which formerly took place with regard to the contracti-

lity of the capillaries really had reference to small arteries and veins, the calibre of which grows narrower
through the contraction of their muscular coats, or wider
upon the occurrence of relaxation in consequence of the
pressure of the blood. This is one of the first facts, and
an important one it is, which have resulted from the
more accurate histological knowledge of the smaller and
larger vessels, and it shows us that we cannot speak of
the general properties of vessels, inasmuch as the capillaries differ essentially in structure from the small arteries and veins. These are composite structures, partak-
ing of the nature of organs, whilst a capillary vessel is
rather a simple *histological* element.

Now that we have, gentlemen, completed a very
general survey of the physiological tissues, the question
arises, how the pathological ones in their turn comport
themselves. By pathological tissues, of course, those
only can be meant which really constitute pathological
new formations, and not physiological parts which have
simply undergone alteration in consequence of some
deviation from the normal processes of nutrition. We
have in them to deal with genuine *neoplasms,* with the
additional matter furnished by the growth of new tissues
in the course of pathological processes, and the question
is, whether the general types which we have established
for the physiological tissues will also be found to hold
good in the case of the pathological ones. To this I un-
reservedly reply, yes ; and however much I herein differ
from many of my living contemporaries, however positively the peculiar (specific) nature of many pathological
tissues has been insisted upon during the last few years,
I will nevertheless endeavour in the course of these lectures to furnish you with proofs that every pathological
structure has a physiological prototype, and that no
form of morbid growth arises which cannot in its ele-

ments be traced back to some model which had previously maintained an independent existence in the economy.

The classification of pathological new formations, of genuine neoplasms, was formerly by most observers attempted to be based upon their different degrees of *vascularity*. If you examine the different treatises which appeared upon this subject up to the time of the cell-theory, you will find that the question of organization was always decided by that of vascularity. Every part which contained vessels was regarded as organized, and every part as unorganized which was destitute of vessels. But this, according to present notions, is an incorrect view of the matter, inasmuch as we have also physiological tissues without vessels, as for example, cartilage.

But at a time when the more minute elements of tissues were at most only known as globules, and when very different virtues were attributed to these globules, it was quite excusable that everything should be referred to the vessels, particularly after the comparison John Hunter made between pathological new formations and the development of the chick in the egg, when he endeavoured to show that, just as the punctum saliens in the hen's egg constitutes the first phenomenon of life, the vessels also where the first things to show themselves in pathological formations. You no doubt still remember how several "parasitical" new formations were described by Rust and Kluge as provided with an independent vascular system, which without having any connection with the old vessels, developed itself quite independently, as is the case in the chick. Many attempts had indeed been made even before this to refer the apparently so irregular forms of new formations to physiological paradigms, and herein essential service has been rendered by natural philosophers. At the time when theromorphism played a conspicuous part, and many analogies were discovered between pathological processes and the normal states of inferior animals, comparisons also began to be instituted between new formations and familiar parts of the body. Thus, Johann Friedr. Meckel, the younger, spoke of mammary and pancreatic sarcoma. What has very recently been described in Paris as heteradenia (Heteradenie), or a heterologous formation of glandular substance, was in the school of the natural philosophers a pretty generally accepted fact.

Since the study of embryology has been prosecuted in a more histological manner, the conviction has gradually more and more been acquired, that most new formations contain parts which correspond to some physiological tissue, and in the micrographical schools of the west a certain number of observers have come to the conclusion, that in the whole series of new formations there is only one particular structure which is specifically different from natural formations, namely cancer. With regard to this, the most important points urged are, that it differs altogether from every other tissue, and that it contains elements *sui generis*, whilst, singularly enough, a second formation, between which and cancerous tissue the older writers were wont to draw parallels, namely tubercle, has—although to it too nothing strictly analogous could be discovered—been much neglected, owing to its having been regarded as an incomplete and somewhat crude product, and as a structure which had never become properly organized. Yet, upon a more careful examination of cancer or tubercle, we shall find that everything depends upon our searching for that stage in their development, in which they are exhibited in their perfect form. We must not examine at too early a period, when their development is incomplete, nor yet at too late a one, when it has proceeded beyond its highest point. If we restrict our observations to the time when development is really at its height, a physiological type may be found for every pathological formation, and it is just as possible to discover such types for the elements of cancer as to find them, for example, for pus, which, if it be sought to maintain the specific nature of certain formations, is just as much entitled to be regarded as something peculiar as cancer. Both of them stand upon precisely the same footing in this respect, and when the older writers spoke of cancer-pus they were in a certain measure right, inasmuch as cancer-juice is only distinguished from pus by the higher degree of development to which its individual elements have attained.

A classification of pathological structures also may be made upon exactly the same plan as that which we have already ventured upon in the case of the physiological tissues. In the first place, there are also among these structures some which, like the epithelial ones, are essentially composed of cellular elements, without the addition of anything else of consequence. In the second place, we meet with tissues which are allied to those called connective, inasmuch as in addition to the cells a certain quantity of intercellular substance is present. In the third and last place come those formations which are akin to the more highly organized structures, blood, muscles, nerves, etc. Now, a point to which I must at once direct your attention is, that in pathological formations those elements the more frequently exist, and the more decidedly prevail, which do not represent the higher grades of really animal development, and that, therefore, on the whole, those elements are most rarely imitated which belong to the more highly organized, and especially, to the muscular and nervous, systems. Still, these formations are by no means excluded; we find pathological new formations of every description, no matter to what tissue they may be analogous, provided it possesses distinctive features. It is only with regard to their frequency and importance that a difference prevails, and this is of such a nature that the great majority of pathological productions contain cells analogous to epithelial cells, or to the corpuscles of the connective tissues, and that of those structures which we have included in the last class of normal tissues, the vessels and parts which may be compared with lymph and lymphatic glands are the most frequently met with as new formations, whilst real blood, muscles, and nerves, are the most seldom found as such.

But, if we ultimately arrive at such a simple view of the matter, the question of course arises, what becomes of the doctrine of the *heterology* of morbid products, to the upholding of which we have long been accustomed, and to which the most simple reflection almost inevitably conducts us. Hereunto I can return no other answer than that there is no other kind of heterology in morbid structures than the abnormal manner in which they arise, and that this abnormity consists either in the production of a structure at a point where it has no business, or at a time when it ought not to be produced, or to an extent which is at variance with the typical formation of the body. So then, to speak with greater precision, there is either a *Heterotopia*, an aberratio loci, or an aberratio temporis, a *Heterochronia*, or lastly, a mere variation in quantity, *Heterometria*. But we must be very careful not to connect this kind of heterology in the more extended sense of the word with the notion of *malignity*. Heterology is a term that, in its histological meaning may be applied to a large proportion of pathological new formations, which, as far as the prognosis is concerned, may unquestionably be called benignant ; it is not rare for a new formation to occur at a point where it is certainly entirely misplaced, but at the same time does not occasion any considerable mischief. A lump of fat may very likely arise in a place where we should expect no fat, as, for example, in the submucous tissue of the small intestines, but, let the worst come to the worst, the result is only a polypus, which protrudes on the inner surface of the bowel, and may become tolerably large without giving rise to any symptoms of disease.

If we consider the structures which are called heterologous in the more restricted sense of the word, with reference, namely, to the points at which they arise, they may be easily separated from the homologous ones (homœoplastic ones of Lobstein), by their deviating from the type of the part in which they arise. When a fatty tumour arises in fatty tissue, or a connective tissue (fibrous) tumour Bindegewebs-Geschwulst) in connective tissue, the type followed in the formation of the new structure is homologous to the type followed in the formation of the old one. All such formations are, as usually designated, included under the term hypertrophy, or under that of *hyperplasia*, if we adopt the name I have proposed for the sake of more accurate distinction. Hypertrophy, according to the meaning which I attach to the word, designates those cases in which the individual elements af a structure take up a considerable amount of matter, and thereby become larger ; and in consequence of the simultaneous enlargement of a number of elements, at last the whole of an organ may become swollen. When a muscle becomes thicker, all its primitive fasciculi become thicker. A liver may become hypertrophied simply in consequence of a considerable

enlargement of its individual cells. In this case there
is real hypertrophy without, properly speaking, any

FIG. 27.

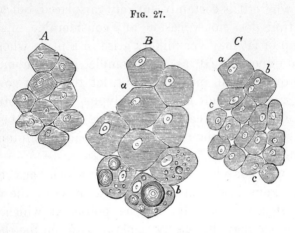

new formation. Essentially different from this process
are the cases in which an enlargement takes place in
consequence of an *increase in the number of the elements*.
A liver, namely, may also become enlarged by a very
abundant development of a series of small cells in the
place of the ordinary ones. Thus, when simply hypertrophied, we see the panniculus adiposus of the skin swell
up in consequence of every single fat-cell's absorbing a
larger quantity of fat than usual, and when this takes
place in thousands upon thousands, nay, we may say,
in hundreds of thousands and millions of cells, the result is very obvious and strikes the eye (polysarcia).
but it is just as possible for new cells to form in addition to the old ones, and for an increase of size to take
place without any enlargement of the individual cells.

Fig. 27. Diagrams of hepatic cells. *A*. Their simple physiological appearance.
B. Hypertrophy : *a*, simple; *b*, with accumulation of fat (fatty degeneration, fatty
liver). *C*. Hyperplasy (numerical or adjunctive hypertrophy). *a*. Cell with nucleus
and divided nucleolus. *b*. Divided nuclei. *c, c*. Divided cells.

These are essentially different processes, and may be styled *simple and numerical hypertrophy.*

Hyperplastic processes (numerical hypertrophy) in all cases produce a tissue similar to that of the original part ; hyperplasia of the liver gives rise to new hepatic cells ; that of a nerve to new nerve-substance ; that of the skin to a fresh production of the elements of the skin. A heteroplastic process, on the contrary, engenders histological elements which correspond, indeed, to natural forms, elements, for example, resembling in structure those peculiar to glands, nerve-substance, the connective and epithelial tissues, but these elements do not arise in consequence of a simple increase in the number of such as previously existed, but in consequence of a change in the original type of the parent tissue. When cerebral matter forms in the ovary, it does not arise out of pre-existing cerebral matter, nor through any act of simple cell-proliferation ; when epidermis springs up in the muscular substance of the heart, however much it may correspond to that on the external surface of the skin, it is, notwithstanding, a heteroplastic structure. When we find hairs quite natural in structure in the substance of the brain, however great the correspondence they exhibit with the hairs of the external surface, they will nevertheless be heteroplastic hairs. In like manner we see cartilaginous tissue arise, without the existence of any essential difference between it and ordinary, familiar cartilage, as, for example, an enchondromata. Still, an enchondroma is a heteroplastic tumour, even when occurring in bone, for perfect bone has no longer any cartilage in the parts where the enchondroma forms, and the term *cartilage* of bone (Knochenknorpel), as a designation for the organic basis of bone, is nothing but a term. It is either from osseous or medullary tissue that the enchondroma

springs, and at the very point where real cartilage exists, for example, at the articular ends of the bone, no
cartilaginous tumours, in the ordinary sense of the word,
arise. It is not, therefore, with an hypertrophy of pre-
existing cartilage that we have here to deal, but with a
genuine new formation, which begins with a change in
the local histological type. According to this manner
of viewing the subject which is essentially different from
that previously current, no attention is therefore paid,
in considering the question of the heterologous nature of
a new formation, to the composition of the structure as
such, but only to the relations which subsist between it
and the parent soil from which it springs. Heterology,
in this sense, designates the difference of development
in the new, as contrasted with the old, tissue, or, as we
are wont to say, a *degeneration*, a deviation from the
typical conformation.

This is, as you will see, also really the most important
point upon which we can ground our prognosis. We
find tumours, which present the most striking resemblance to the most familiar physiological tissues. An
epidermic [epithelial] tumour (Epidermis-Geschwulst)
may, as I have already pointed out, in its elementary
structure entirely correspond to ordinary epidermis, but
in spite of this it is not always a benignant tumour of
merely local import, which may be traced to a merely
hyperplastic increase in pre-existing tissues, for it sometimes arises in the midst of parts which are far from
containing epidermis or epithelium, as, for example, in
the interior of lymphatic glands, or in that of thick
layers of connective tissue, which are at a distance from
any surface, and even in bone. In these cases the formation of epidermis is certainly quite as heterologous as
it is possible to conceive anything to be. But practical
experience has shown us that it was altogether incorrect

to conclude from the mere correspondence of the pathological tissue with a physiological one, that the case would continue to follow a benignant course.

It has been, as I must remark with particular emphasis, one of the greatest, and at the same time best-founded, reproaches which have been levelled against the most recent micrographical doctrines, that, regarding the subject from the certainly excusable point of view, namely, the correspondence between many normal and abnormal structures, they have declared every pathological new formation to be innocuous which exhibits a reproduction of pre-existing and familiar tissues of the body. If what I have communicated to you as my view be correct, namely, that throughout the whole range of pathological growths no structure of an absolutely new form is to be found, but that we everywhere meet with structures which may in one way or another be regarded as the *reproduction of physiological tissues*, then this point of view falls to the ground. In support of my view, I can at least adduce the fact that I have, in all disputes concerning the innocent or malignant nature of definite forms of tumours, up to the present time always proved to be in the right.

Before we quit the consideration of General Histology, I would invite your attention for a few moments to a few points of primary importance which obtrude themselves upon us on nearly every occasion. Whilst, namely, the animal tissues were being studied in their affinities to one another, questions relating to these affinities were at different times stumbled upon, which gave rise to generalizations that were more of a physiological character.

When Reichert undertook to collect the connective tissues into one larger group, he set out with this position chiefly, that the demonstration of the *continuity of tis-*

sues must be regarded as a decisive proof of their intimate relationship. That as soon as one part could be made out to be continuously (by union, not mere juxtaposition) connected with another, both must be regarded as parts of a common whole. In this manner he sought to prove that cartilage, periosteum, bone, tendons, fasciæ, etc., really formed a continuous mass, a kind of basis-tissue (Grundgewebe) for the body, a *connective substance*, which had only experienced certain changes in these different localities, without their being, however, of such a nature as to destroy the character of the tissue as such. This so-called *law of continuity* soon suffered the most violent shocks, and quite recently such a terrible breach has been made in it, that it can scarcely any longer be possible to derive therefrom any general criterion for the determination of the nature of a tissue. On the other hand, namely, new facts have been continually brought forward in support of the continuity of such histological elements as, according to Reichert, would be separated *toto cœlo* from one another, as, for example, of epithelial and connective tissue ; and there has been a continually increasing mass of evidence in support of the assertion that cylindrical epithelium is capable of becoming elongated into fibres, which in the shape of filaments anastomose with connective-tissue corpuscles. Nay, it has been quite recently asserted by a whole series of observers that these superficial cells are prolonged inwardly, and then enter into direct connection with nerve-fibres. With regard to this last point, I must confess that I am not yet convinced of the correctness of the representation ; but with respect to the former one, that is a matter which will probably end in the demonstration of the real continuity of the elements. It would seem, therefore, that it is even now no longer possible to mark out the exact limits which divide every kind of epithelium from every kind of connective tissue, but only where scaly epithelium is met with, whilst the limits are doubtful wherever cylindrical epithelium exists.

Just in the same manner elsewhere also do the boundary lines become obliterated. Whilst formerly the limits which separate the elements of muscle from those of tendon were considered to be most distinctly defined, extremely decisive proofs have in this case also been afforded, and first by Hyde Salter and Huxley, that fibres proceed from connective-tissue corpuscles, which whilst pursuing their course in an inward direction, all at once assume the character of transversely striped muscle. So, then, in the case of connective tissue, it would seem there exists a continuous connection between the elements of the surface and the more highly developed ones of the deeper parts. Now if, on the other hand, it has turned out to be very probable that the corpuscles of connective tissue have definite relations to the vascular system, we are, as you see, almost justified in regarding this tissue as a kind of *neutral ground* for parts to *meet upon* (indifferenter Samelpunkt), as a peculiar arrangement for their intimate connection, an arrangement which, though certainly not exercising any great influence upon the higher functions of the animal, is yet of great importance as far as its nutrition is concerned.

In the place of the law of continuity, therefore, we must necessarily put something else. And here, I think, the doctrine which has the strongset claims to our attention is that of *histological substitution*. In the case of all tissues of a like nature it is quite possible, even whilst confining our attention to what occurs physiologically in the various classes of animals. to find one tissue at a certain fixed point of the body replaced by an analogous one belonging to the same group, or, in other words, by an *histological equivalent*.

A spot invested with cylindrical, may acquire scaly,

epithelium. A surface upon which cilia were originally seen, may afterwards be found to have ordinary epithelium. Thus, on the surface of the ventricles of the brain we meet at first with ciliated, and at a later period with simple scaly, epithelium. Thus, too, we see the mucous membrane of the uterus usually covered with ciliated epithelium, but during pregnancy we find the layer of ciliated cylinders replaced by one of squamous epithelium. Thus, also, in places where soft epithelium ordinarily is found, epidermis may, under particular circumstances, be generated, as, for example, in the prolapsed vagina. Thus, again, in the sclerotic coat of the eyes of fish, cartilage is found, whilst in man this tunic consists of dense connective tissue ; in many animals bone is found in parts of the skin, where in man there is only connective tissue ; but in man, too, in many places where there was original cartilage, osseous tissue is afterwards discovered. But the most striking instances of such substitutions are met with in muscles. One animal has transversely striped muscular fibres in the same place that another has smooth ones.

In diseased conditions *pathological substitutions* occur, in which a given tissue is replaced by another ; but even when this new tissue is produced from the previously existing one, the new formation may deviate more or less from the original type. There is therefore a great chasm between physiological and pathological substitution, or at least, between the physiological and certain forms of the pathological one.

Physiologically, the substitution is constantly effected by the introduction of another tissue of the same group (*homology*) ; pathologically, very frequently by the agency of a tissue belonging to another (*heterology*). To this we must reduce the whole doctrine of the specific elements of pathology which have played so conspicuous a part in the last twenty years.

LECTURE IV.

FEBRUARY 24, 1858.

NUTRITION AND ITS CHANNELS.

Action of the vessels—Relations between vessels and tissues—Liver—Brain—Muscular coat of the stomach—Cartilage—Bone.
Dependence of tissues upon vessels—Metastases—Vascular territories [Gefässterritorien] (vascular unities)—Conveyance of nutriment in the juice-conveying canals (Saftkanäle) of the tissues—Bone—Teeth—Fibro-cartilage—Cornea—Semilunar cartilages.

ACCORDING to the ideas usually entertained with regard to nutrition, the vessels are regarded as the canals by means of which not only the interchange of material (Stoffverkehr) is accomplished, but upon the assistance of which, sometimes actively and sometimes passively afforded, reliance is placed whenever it is required to control an individual part in its interchange of material. The regulating principle in the process of nutrition was long designated by an expression which has even crept into the language of the present day, namely, the "action of the vessels," as if they were endowed with a special power of actively influencing the condition of the neighbouring histological constituents.

As I pointed out to you the last time, when upon the subject of muscular fibres (p. 85), we can now-a-days only speak of action in the vessels as far as muscular fibres are present in them, and the vessels are thus enabled by the contraction of these fibres to grow narrower or shorter. This narrowing of their channel may have the effect of impeding transudation of fluids, whilst, on the contrary, in the case of the relaxation or paralysis of the muscular fibres, the widening of the vessel may favour such transudation. Let us admit this for the present, but allow me, before proceeding farther, to enter somewhat into the analysis of the mass of tissue which lies around the vessels, and is generally conceived to be of a very simple and uncomplicated nature.

If we select parts where the vessels lie very closely packed, and there is perhaps nearly as much vessel as tissue, as, for example, the *liver*, in which this condition really does occur (for a liver, when its vessels are full, contains nearly as large a volume of vessels as it does of proper hepatic substance), we see that the interstices which are left between the vessels are filled with quite a small number of cells.

If we examine a single acinus of the liver by itself, we find, when a very lucky transverse section has been obtained, in its centre the vena centralis or intralobularis, which runs into the hepatic vein, at the periphery branches of the portal vein, which send capillary twigs into the interior. These at once form a network, which at first has long, but afterwards more regularly shaped, meshes, and extends in the direction of the central (or hepatic) vein, and at last terminates in it. The blood, therefore, after it has en-

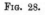

Fig. 28.

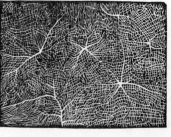

Fig. 28. Section from the periphery of the liver of a rabbit; the vessels completely injected. 11 diameters.

tered by the interlobular (or portal) vein, flows through
the capillary network into the intralobular vein, whence,
by means of the hepatic veins, it is conducted back again
to the heart. Now, in the case of an injected liver, this
network is seen to be so close that what interstices there
are left seem almost to occupy less room than the vessels themselves. We can thus easily imagine how the
older anatomists, such as Ruysch, came to be led by
their injections to the supposition that nearly everything
in the body was made up of vessels, and that the different organs were only distinguished by differences in the
arrangement of their vessels. But just the opposite to
what is observed in an injected preparation does the
proportion between vessel and tissue appear to be in an
ordinary specimen from a liver. In this the vessels are
scarcely perceptible. A similar network is indeed seen,
but it is the network formed by the hepatic-cells (Fig.
27), which, closely crowded, one against the other, fill
up all the inter-spaces of the vessels. It is plain, therefore, that the capillary and hepatic-cell networks are
interwoven in the most intricate manner, so that cells
belonging to the parenchyma of the liver everywhere lie in
almost immediate contact with the walls of the vessels,
there being at most a fine layer between the cells and
the walls, concerning which it is still a matter of dispute
amongst histologists whether it is to be regarded as a
peculiar coat, constituting the finest gall-ducts, or only
as a very small quantity of connective tissue accompanying the vessels.

In this extremely simple case, a tolerably simple relation may certainly be assumed to exist between the vessels and the cells ; it may be conceived that the blood
which flows through the vessels may, in proportion to
the degree in which they are contracted or dilated, and
to its own quantity, exercise a direct influence upon the

adjoining cells. It might indeed be objected, with regard to the conditions of nutrition, that we have here
to deal with quite a peculiar arrangement of the vessels,
which are essentially of a venous nature, as being composed of ramifications of the portal and hepatic veins, but
the hepatic artery also enters into the formation of this
capillary network, so that the blood in it cannot be
resolved into its individual arterial and venous constituents. Injections from each of the vessels named ultimately find their way into the same capillary network.

In most parts, however, the relations do not present
such a simple form as in the liver ; considerable interspaces often separate the individual cells, and no inconsiderable quantities of these elements are enclosed in
every capillary mesh. I show you here a second object
derived from a fresh human *brain*—from a lunatic who
died with his cerebrum in a highly hyperæmic state.

FIG. 29.

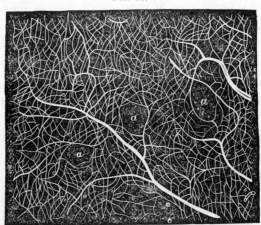

The section has been made through the corpus striatum,
which was of a deep red colour. You have a good view

Fig. 29. Natural injection of the corpus striatum of a lunatic. *a, a.* Gaps destitute of vessels, and corresponding to the strands of nervous fibres which traverse the
ganglion. 80 diameters.

of the naturally injected vessels ; and the width of the individual meshes of the capillary network may be clearly seen. The section has been carried transversely through the corpus striatum, and at certain intervals large, roundish spots may be distinguished, which appear dark by transmitted light (Fig. 29, *a, a, a*), but by reflected light and to the naked eye look white, and are formed by transverse sections of the nervous fibres which run in long strands towards the spinal marrow. The vessels scarcely penetrate into them. The rest of the mass, on the other hand, consists of the proper grey substance of the corpus striatum, within which a vascular network with very fine meshes is distributed, the grey substance of the nervous centres being everywhere, both in their interior and in their cortical substance, distinguished from the white by its greater vascularity. A few large vessels are observable in the object, giving off branches, the ramifications of which continually diminish in size, until at last they terminate in capillary networks with very fine meshes. Still, however close this network may be, every element of the substance of the brain by no means comes into immediate contact with a capillary vessel.

The third object is a very slightly magnified injected preparation from the *muscular coat of the stomach*, in which, with a high power, the direction of the muscular fibres is indicated by fine longitudinal striæ ; here the vessels form tolerably regular networks, connected with one another by

Fig. 30.

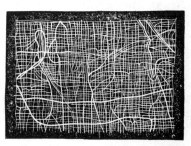

Fig. 30. Injected preparation from the muscular coat of the stomach of a rabbit, magnified 11 diameters.

transverse anastomoses, and splitting up into smaller
and smaller vessels, which form fine networks within
the tissue, so that the whole of it is by this means mapped out into a series of irregularly four-sided divisions.
To each of the ultimate intervascular spaces is allotted
a certain number of muscular elements, so that the vessels are in some parts in contact with the muscular
fibres, whilst in others they lie at a greater distance
from them.

If we go on in this way examining the structure of the
different organs and tissues, we pass from such as, when
injected, seem to consist almost entirely of vessels, in
time to those which contain scarcely any, and at last to
such as really have none at all.   This is most strikingly
the case with the connective tissues, and the most important amongst these are *bone* and *cartilage*. Perfectly
developed cartilage has no longer any vessels at all ;
perfectly developed bone certainly contains vessels, but
in a very variable degree.   That perfectly developed
cartilage contains no vessels, you will not, I suppose, call
upon me to convince you by any additional, special
proofs, inasmuch as you have seen various preparations of cartilage, in which not a trace of them was to
be observed.   (Figs. 6, 9, 22.)   I now place before you
a piece of young cartilage, because you can see in it
what the arrangement of the vessels in cartilage is at
an earlier period.   It is a section from the calcaneum of
a new-born child, and in it the vessels run up from the
already-formed central osseous mass into the cartilage
which still remains.   The preparation shows along the
outermost surface of the cartilage the transition from it
into the perichondrium, whilst the lower part of the section is taken from the border of the already-formed
bone.   From this part large vessels are seen running
up and terminating in the middle of the cartilage by

the formation of loops and plexuses, as it were a tree of villi (Zottenbaum) in the cartilage, and very much resembling a villus of the chorion of the ovum. In fact, the vessels mount up into the cartilage from the nutrient artery of the bone, but only to a certain height. There they form real loops, and at length break up into a fine

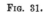

Fig. 31.

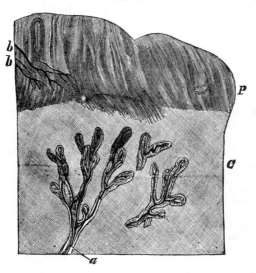

plexus of capillaries, out of which veins are ultimately formed, and run out again pretty near the spot where the artery entered. But the whole of the rest of the mass consists of non-vascular cartilage, the corpuscles of which, with a low power, look like fine points. Thus there is a whole host of cartilage-corpuscles lying between the terminal loops and the external surface, and the whole of this layer is therefore dependent for its

Fig. 31. Section of cartilage from the calcaneum of a new-born child. *C*. The cartilage, with its cells indicated by fine points. *P*. Perichondrium and adjoining fibrous tissue. *a*. Inferior border very near to the line of junction between the cartilage and the bone, with the vascular loops ascending from the nutrient artery. *b, b*. Vessels which make their way through the perichondrium in the direction of the cartilage. 11 diameters.

nutrition upon the juice which exudes from the terminal loops and permeates the tissue, though to a trifling extent also upon the materials which the scanty vessels of the perichondrium convey to it. The vessels which spring from the nutrient artery mark in all bones, at a tolerably early period, pretty exactly the limits to which the ossification subsequently proceeds, whilst the remnants of the cartilage which remain bordering upon the joint never contain vessels.

With regard to the *bones* themselves, the disposition of their blood-vessels is in itself tolerably simple, but at

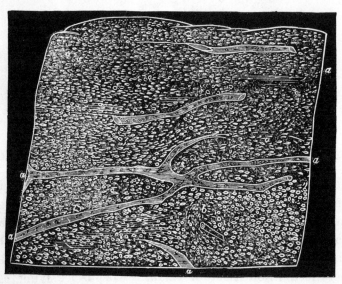

FIG. 32.

the same time very characteristic. If we examine the compact substance, we can usually, even with the naked eye, distinguish upon its surface small openings through which vessels enter from the periosteum. With a mode-

Fig. 32. Longitudinal section from the cortex of a sclerotic tibia. *a, a.* Medullary (vascular [Haversian]) canals, between them the bone-corpuscles for the most part parallel; but at *b* (in transverse section) concentrically arranged. 80 diameters.

rately high power we discover that these vessels (Fig.
32, *a*) immediately beneath the surface form a network
with somewhat long meshes, or a series of tubes anastomosing with one another and, generally speaking, running longitudinally, for though they sometimes take a
somewhat more oblique course inwardly, they still
essentially maintain a longitudinal direction. Between
these meshes there remain comparatively wide interspaces, within which, precisely as we before saw the
cartilage cells, we here see the bone-corpuscles, and
indeed also in a longitudinal direction, parallel to the
surface. If the same part be examined in transverse
section, we of course see, where the longitudinal canals
were previously observed, nothing but their transverse
sections here and there united by oblique communications! Between them lies the proper osseous tissue,
deposited in lamellar layers, some of them parallel to

FIG. 33.

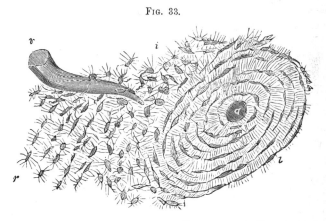

the surface, some concentrically arranged around the
vessels. In the deeper layers of the compact substance

Fig. 33. Section of bone. *a*. Transverse section of medullary (vascular [Haver-
sian]) canal, around which the concentric lamellæ, *l*, lie with bone-corpuscles and
anastomosing canaliculi. *r*. Lamellæ divided longitudinally and parallel. *i*. Irregular arrangement in the oldest layers of bone. *v*. Vascular canal. 280 diameters.

this concentric arrangement around the vessels constantly prevails.

Between these more lamellated parts is left a small quantity of osseous substance (Fig. 33, *i*) which does not present the same structure, but is arranged upon another, and independent, plan. Upon more accurate examination it is seen to be formed of little columns, which are generally perpendicular to the long axis of the bone, but sometimes curve round, and so become parallel to the long axis. These are the remains of the spicula first formed during the growth of the bone in thickness, and are therefore of older date.

As in the sections which are obtained by grinding down bone, the vessels themselves cannot for the most part any longer be distinguished, the cavities [Haversian

F𝙸𝙶. 34.

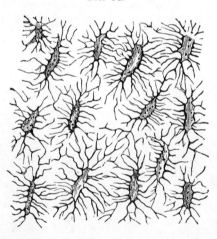

canals] (Fig. 32, *a*, 33, *a*, *v*,) in which they run have been named medullary canals, improperly, inasmuch as

Fig. 34. Bone-corpuscles from a morbid formation of bone in the dura mater of the brain. Their branching and anastomosing prolongations (canaliculi) are seen, as well us minute spots upon their walls, marking the funnel-shaped commencements of the canaliculi. 600 diameters.

there is usually no marrow contained in these narrow channels ; they should properly be called vascular canals ; still the other term is so universally received, that it is even employed in cases where the wall of the vessel is in immediate contact with the internal surface of the cavity. Immediately surrounding these canals we see a series of peculiar structures ; oblong or roundish bodies which usually appear black when the object is not fully brought into focus, and are provided with jaggs or processes. They used to be called bone-corpuscles, and their processes bone-canals (canaliculi ossei) ; and as the view was originally entertained that the calcareous matter was really deposited in them, and that the dark appearance which they usually present when viewed by transmitted light resulted from the presence of this matter, the canals were also termed canaliculi chalicophori, a name which has now been altogether abandoned, because convincing proofs have been obtained that, so far from being contained in them, the lime is, on the contrary, diffused throughout the homogeneous basis-substance which lies between them.

As soon as this discovery was made, that, namely, the distribution of the lime in the osseous tissue took place in a manner just the reverse of that in which it had been supposed it did, the other extreme was immediately run into, and for the name of bone-corpuscles that of bone-cavities (lacunæ) was substituted, and it was assumed that bone contained nothing but a series of empty cavities and canals, which were indeed penetrated by a fluid, but still were really nothing more than fissures in the bone. Some few observers indeed actually called them bone fissures Now I have endeavoured to demonstrate in various manners that they are real corpuscles, and not mere cavities in a dense basis-tissue, but structures provided with special walls and boundaries of their

own, which separate them from the intermediate substance. For by the help of chemical reagents (concentrated mineral acids, and particularly hydrochloric acid)
we are enabled, by dissolving the basis-substance,
namely, to disengage the corpuscles from it. In this way
we furnish, I think, the most complete demonstration
that they are really independent structures. Besides, a
nucleus may be distinguished within these bodies ; and,
even without entering into the history of their development, we discover that here too we have once more to
deal with cellular elements of a stellate form. Bone
therefore exhibits in its composition a tissue, containing,
in an apparently altogether homogeneous basis-substance,
peculiar, stellate bone-cells distributed in a very regular
manner.

The intervals which exist between every two of the
vessels in bone are often very considerable ; whole systems of lamellæ, beset with numerous bone-corpuscles,
thrust themselves in between the medullary canal. Here
it is certainly difficult to conceive the nutrition of so
complicated an apparatus to depend upon the action of
vessels some of them so remote, and especially so, to understand how every individual particle of this extensive
compound mass can manage to maintain a special relation of nutrition to the vessels. For experience shows
us that every single bone-corpuscle really possesses conditions of nutrition peculiar to itself.

I have laid these details before you, in order to point
out to you the gradual transition which takes place from
the vascular and abundantly vascular, to the scantily
vascular and non-vascular parts. If we would form a
simple conception of the conditions of nutrition, I think
we must lay it down as a logical principle, that whatever is enunciated with regard to the nutrition of very
vascular parts, must also hold good for that of scantily

and non-vascular parts ; and that, if the nutrition of individual parts is considered to be directly dependent upon the vessels or the blood, it must at all events be demonstrated that all the elements which stand in immediate connection with one and the same vessel, and are assigned to a single vessel for their support, present conditions of life essentially similar. In the case of bone it would be necessary to show that every system of lamellæ which has only one vessel for its nutrition, always exhibits a similar state of nutrition. For if that vessel, or the blood which circulates in it, be the active agent concerned in the nutrition, the utmost that can be admitted is, that one part of the elements may be more, another less, subjected to their influence ; but still it must essentially be a common and similar influence which they experience. That this is no unreasonable requirement, that a certain dependency of definite territories of tissue upon definite vessels must undoubtedly be admitted, the most beautiful illustrations are afforded us in the doctrine of metastases, in the study of the changes which are effected by the occlusion of single capillary vessels, and with which we have become acquainted from the history of capillary embolia. In such cases, in fact, we see that a whole portion of tissue, as far as its immediate connection with a vessel extends, in its pathological relations also constitutes a whole—a *vascular unity*. But this vascular unity to a finer apprehension still appears a compound, and it is not sufficient to split up the body into vessel-territories (Gefässterritorien) alone, but within them a further division must be made into cell-territories (Zellenterritorien).

This view has, I think, been essentially furthered by our having discovered, as I lately pointed out to you (p. 76), the existence of a special system of anastomosing elements in the connective-tissues, and by our having in this manner filled the place of the vasa serosa (which the older writers imagined as a complement to the capillaries for these ultimate purposes of nutrition) with something definite, by means of which the circulation of nutritive juices is rendered possible in parts which are in themselves poor in vessels.   To keep to *bone*, we should

Fig. 35.

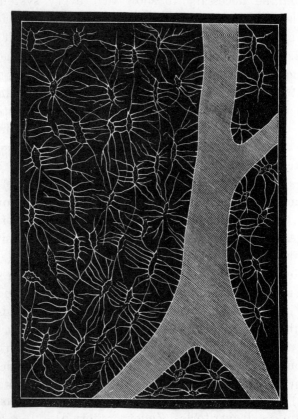

scarcely be justified in assuming the existence of vasa serosa in it.   The hard basis-substance is throughout

Fig. 35. Section of an osseous plate from the arachnoid of the cerebrum, but quite normal in its structure.   A branching vascular (medullary) canal is seen with canaliculi opening into it, and leading to the bone corpuscles.   350 diameters.

uniformly filled with calcareous salts, so uniformly indeed, that no interval can be perceived between the individual calcareous particles. Though some few writers have assumed that little granules can be distinguished in it, this is an error. The only differentiation which can be seen is caused by the prolongation into the basis-substance of the canaliculi, which all ultimately lead back to the bodies of the bone-cells (bone-corpuscles) and in their turn give out branches. The peripheral extremities of these little branches or processes extend right up to the surface of the vascular (medullary) canal. They are therefore inserted exactly where the membrane of the vessel begins (Fig. 35), for they can be distinctly perceived as very minute orifices upon the wall of the canal. Now since the different bone-corpuscles are in their turn distinctly connected with one another, means are afforded by which a certain quantity of juice taken up from the surface of the vascular canal is not diffused throughout the whole mass of tissue, but confined to these delicate, continuous, and specially provided channels, and forced to move onwards in canals which are inaccessible to injections from the vessel. For a time it was believed that the canaliculi could be injected from the vessel, but this is only possible when the vascular canal has become empty by maceration.

This is a condition precisely similar to what we observe in the *teeth*, in which the canaliculi can be injected from the pulp-cavity when empty. If a solution of carmine be injected into this cavity, the dental canaliculi are displayed in the form of numerous tubules running up to the surface side by side in a radiated manner. The substance of the teeth also forms a tolerably broad layer of non-vascular material. Vessels are found nowhere but in the pulp-cavity, in proceeding from which outwards we find nothing but the proper substance of the tooth (dentine) with its system of tubes, which extend nearly up to the surface, and in the root of the tooth are directly continuous with a layer of real bony substance (cement) the corpuscles of which are seated upon the ends of the tubes. A provision for the conveyance of the juices similar to that which in bone originates in the marrow, here takes its rise in the pulp, whence the nutritive fluid can be conveyed up to the surface by the means of tubes.

These systems of tubes which are found in such a very marked form in bone and the teeth, are to be seen with far less distinctness in the soft structures, and it is chiefly for this reason, I imagine, that the analogy which exists between the soft connective tissues and the hard texture of bone has not been clearly comprehended. These systems are most distinctly seen in parts which are more of a cartilaginous nature, as, for example, in fibro-cartilage. But it is a fact of great significance that we find a series of transitional forms between cartilage and the other connective tissues, in which the same conditions are constantly repeated. In the first place, parts which chemically belong to the class of cartilages, for example, the cornea, which yields chondrine when boiled, although nobody regards it as real cartilage. But more striking is the arrangement in those parts in which the external appearance speaks in favour of a cartilaginous nature, but the chemical properties do not correspond, as for example, in the semi-lunar cartilages (Bandscheiben) of the knee-joint, which are interposed between the femur and tibia for the purpose of protecting the articular cartilages from too violent contact. These parts, which even now are generally described as cartilage, yield no chondrine on boiling, but gelatine ; and yet, in this hard connective tissue, we meet with the same system of anastomosing corpuscles that prevails in the cornea and in

fibro-cartilage, and it is displayed with unusual distinctness and clearness.   Vessels are almost entirely wanting
in these cartilages, but in ex-
change they contain a system
of tubes of rare beauty.   On
making a section, we see that
the whole is in the first place
mapped out into large divisions, exactly like a tendon ;
these are subdivided into
smaller ones, and these are
pervaded by a fine, stellate
system of tubes, or, if you
will, of cells, inasmuch as the
notion of a tube and that of a
cell here quite coincide.   The
networks of cells which here

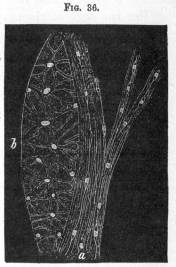

FIG. 36.

form the system of tubes, terminate externally in the septa
bounding the individual divisions, and we here see in close
proximity considerable collections of spindle-shaped cells.
In these cartilages, too, the whole mass of tissue is only
connected by its exterior with the circulatory system ;
everything that penetrates into the interior must pass
by a very circuitous route through a system of canals
with numerous anastomoses, and the nutrition of the internal parts is altogether dependent upon this mode of
conveyance.   The semi-lunar cartilages are structures of
considerable extent and great density, and as they are
entirely dependent for their nutrition upon this ultimate,
minute system of cells, we have in them, much more

Fig. 36. Section from the semi-lunar cartilage of the knee-joint of a child.   *a.*
Bands of fibres, with spindle-shaped, parallel and anastomosing cells (seen in longitudinal section).   *b.* Cells, forming a network, with broad, branching, and anastomosing canaliculi (seen in transverse section).   Treated with acetic acid.   350
diameters.

than in cartilage, to deal with such an arrangement for the supply of nutritive juices, as cannot be under the direct control of the vessels.

For the sake of elucidation, I will merely add that the ultimate elements are seen to consist of very delicate cells, which are prolonged into fine filaments, that in their turn ramify, and look, when cut across, like small points in which a clear centre can be recognised. The filaments can ultimately be very distinctly traced back to the common cell just as in bone. They are extremely fine tubes which are intimately connected with one another, only that here they are in certain spots collected into large groups, by means of which the conveyance of the nutritive juice is principally effected, and that the intercellular substance in no instance becomes infiltrated with lime, but always preserves its character as connective tissue.

LECTURE V.

FEBRUARY 27, 1858.

NUTRITION, AND CONVEYANCE OF THE NUTRITIVE JUICES.

Tendons—Cornea—Umbilical cord.
Elastic tissue—Corium.
Loose connective tissue—Tunica dartos.
Importance of cells in the special distribution of the nutritive juices.

ALLOW me, gentlemen, as a supplement to what we saw and discussed in the preceding lecture, to lay before you a few more preparations in illustration of that peculiar species of nutritive arrangement which we have already seen to exist in various tissues, and which, I hope, will appear to you of very great importance in pathological processes also.

You will remember that the last object of our consideration was a ligamentous disc (Bandscheibe), as it occurs in its most marked form in the knee-joint in the so-called semi-lunar cartilages, which are really no cartilages at all. On the contrary, they possess the qualities of a flat tendon, and the individual structural relations which we found in them, are repeated throughout the whole of the transverse section of a tendon.

We have to-day a series of objects from the tendo Achillis, both of the adult and the child, displaying the different stages of its development ; and as this is, more-

over a tendon which is of importance in more than one
way in an operative point of view, I may, I am sure, be
excused for speaking a little more at length concerning it.

On the surface of a tendon we see, as you well know,
with the naked eye, a series of parallel, whitish striæ
which run pretty close to one another in a longitudinal
direction, and give rise to the characteristic glossy appearance. In a microscopical longitudinal section these
striæ lie farther apart, so that the tendon presents a

FIG. 37.

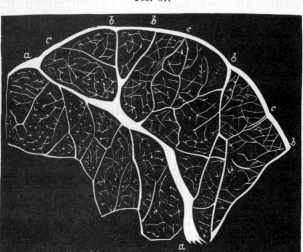

somewhat fasciculated appearance and looks less homogeneous than on the surface. This becomes much more
evident in a transverse section, in which a series of

Fig. 37. Transverse section from the tendo Achillis of an adult. From the sheath
of the tendon, septa are seen at a, b, and c, running inwardly, and uniting into a
network so as to form the boundaries of the primary and secondary fasciculi. The
larger ones (a and b) generally contain vessels, the smaller ones (c) do not. Within
the secondary fasciculi is seen the delicate network formed by the tendon-corpuscles (reticulating cells—Netzzellen), or the intermediate system of juice-conveying
canals (Saftkanalsystem). 80 diameters.

smaller and larger divisions (bundles, fasciculi) are offered to the view.

On magnifying the object, an internal arrangement is shown almost exactly corresponding to that which we have observed in the semi-lunar cartilages. Externally, the tendon is invested in its whole circumference by a fibrous mass, in which the vessels are contained, that are entwined around the tendon. From these at different points vessels proceed into the interior, where they are to be seen in the larger partitions which separate the fasciculi (Fig. 37, *a*) ; but into the interior of the fasciculi themselves no trace of a vessel enters, any more than it does into the interior of the semi-lunar cartilages ; there, on the contrary, we again meet with the network of cells we have been talking about, or, in other words, the peculiar system of juice-conveying canals of which we lately considered the import in bone.

Tendons may therefore in the first place be divided into larger (primary) bundles, and these in their turn into a certain number of smaller (secondary) fasciculi, which are separated by broadish bands of a fibrous substance containing vessels and fibre-cells, so that a transverse section of a tendon presents a meshed appearance. From this intervening substance, which must not, however, be regarded as a tissue of a peculiar description, there pass into the interior of the fasciculi stellate cells (*tendon-corpuscles*) which anastomose with another and establish a communication between the external vascular, and the internal non-vascular, parts of the fasciculi. This relation is, of course, much more evident in the tendons of children than in those of adults. The older the parts become, namely, the larger and finer do the processes of the cells in general become, so that in many sections we do not meet with the real bodies of the cells, but only see minute speck , which, by altering the focus, may be traced into filaments—or point-like orifices. The individual cells, therefore, come to be more widely

Fig. 38.

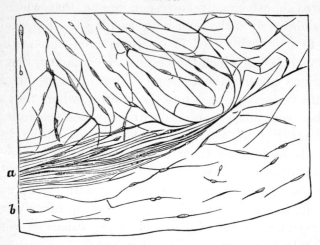

separated, and it becomes more and more difficult to obtain a view of the whole of a cell at once. Besides, we must first obtain a clear notion of the relation between a longitudinal and a transverse section. Where, namely, in a longitudinal section, there are spindle-shaped cells, in a transverse section will be seen stellate ones, and to the network of cells displayed in the transverse section corresponds the regular succession of spindle-shaped corpuscles, arranged in rows which we see in a longitudinal section, entirely in correspondence with the plan which we have shown to be followed in connective tissue. The cells, therefore, are here also only apparently simply spindle-shaped, when an exactly longitudinal section is examined; but if it has been

Fig. 38. Transverse section from the interior of the tendo Achillis of a new-born child. *a.* The intervening mass which separates the secondary fasciculi (corresponding to Fig. 37, *c*), and entirely composed of densely aggregated spindle-shaped cells. Directly anastomosing with these, we see on both sides at *b, b,* reticulating and spindle-shaped cells running into the interior of the fasciculi. 300 diameters.

made a little obliquely, the lateral processes are perceived, by means of which the cells of one row communicate with those of another.

FIG. 39.

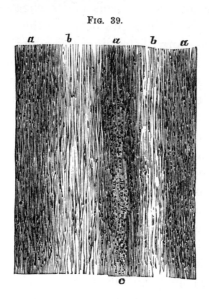

Up to the present moment the progress of the growth of tendons after birth has not been made the subject of a regular investigation, and it is unknown whether any further multiplication of the cells takes place in them ; this much, however, is certain, that the cells in many places afterwards become much elongated, and the intervals between the individual nuclei extremely great. The actual structural relations, however, do not thereby experience any change ; the original cells also continue members of the great system of tubes, which in the perfectly developed tendon pervades the whole tissue.

Fig. 39. Longitudinal section from the interior of the tendo Achillis of a newborn child. *a, a, a.* Intervening bands. *b, b.* Fasciculi. In both we see spindle-shaped, nucleated cells, partially anastomosing, with an inter-cellular substance slightly striated in a longitudinal direction, the cells being more crowded in the bands, and less numerous in the fasciculi. *c.* Section of an interstitial blood-vessel. 250 diameters.

Hence we see how, although the tendon contains no vessels in its most internal parts, and, as may be observed in every case of tenotomy, receives but little blood by the external vessels of its sheath, and by the internal vessels of the septa between the larger fasciculi, it is possible, notwithstanding, for a uniform nutrition of the parts to take place. This we cannot imagine to be effected in any other way than by the distribution of nutritive juices in a regular manner throughout the entire substance of the tendon by means of special canals distinguishable from the vessels. The natural divisions of the tendon are, however, nearly entirely symmetrical, so that an equally large quantity of intercellular substance falls to the share of every cellular element, and as the cell-networks in the interior can be directly traced into the dense bundles of cells of the septa, and these in their turn up to the vessels (Figs. 37, 38), we may, I think, unhesitatingly regard these reticulating cells as the channels for the transmission of this intermediate current of nutritive juice, which has no communication by means of orifices with the general circulation.

You have here a fresh instance in support of my view with regard to cell-territories. I would parcel out the whole tendon, not into primary and secondary fasciculi, but rather into certain series of cells connected in a retiform manner ; to each series, moreover, I would assign a certain district of tissue, so that in a longitudinal section, for example, about half of each band of basis-substance would belong to one, the other half to another series of cells. What is, therefore, regarded as constituting the proper fasciculi of the tendon, would, according to this view, have really to be split up, and the tendon portioned out into a great number of nutritive districts (Ernährungs-Territorien).

This is the condition which we everywhere find recurring in these tissues, and upon it will at the same time be found to depend, as I hope you will convince yourselves by direct observation, the size of the districts invaded by disease ; every disease which essentially depends upon a disturbance in the internal disposition of the tissues is always made up of the sum of the separate changes occurring in such territories. But at the same time the pictures which are here offered to us afford a really æsthetical enjoyment through the delicacy of this arrangement, and I cannot deny that, as often as I look at a section of tendon, it is with a peculiar feeling of satisfaction that I contemplate these reticular arrangements, which effect a union between the exterior and the interior, and, excepting in bone, can in no structure be demonstrated with greater distinctness and clearness than in tendons.

Considering the structure of the *cornea* and the disposition of its parts, it would be most convenient, gent'emen, to proceed at once to the consideration of its history, still I prefer reverting to it hereafter, inasmuch as it is at the same time the most suitable object for the demonstration of pathological changes. I will therefore only observe here, that in the same way that tendons have their peripheral system of vessels, and that their internal parts are nourished by a delicate juice-conveying system of tubes, so also in the cornea only the most minute vessels extend a few lines over its border, so that the central parts are completely destitute of vessels, as indeed they were obliged to be, in order to allow of the transparency of the tissue.

I should like, on the other hand, in connection with the foregoing tissues, to speak of one which has generally met with but little special preference in histology, but is perhaps more likely to have some interest in your eyes, I mean the *umbilical cord*. Its substance (the so-called jelly (gelatina) of Wharton*) is also formed by one of those tissues which certainly contain vessels, but yet really possess none. The vessels which are transmitted through the umbilical cord, do not immediately contribute to its nourishment, at least not in the sense in which we speak of nutrient vessels in other parts. For when we speak of nutrient vessels, we always mean vessels which have capillaries in the parts which are to be nourished. The thoracic aorta is not the nutrient vessel of the thorax, any more than the abdominal aorta, or the vena cava, is that of the abdominal viscera. We should expect, therefore, in the case of the umbilical cord to find umbilical capillaries in addition to the two

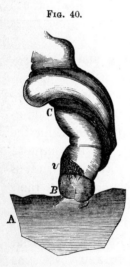

FIG. 40.

umbilical arteries and the umbilical vein. But these arteries and this vein run their course to the placenta, without giving off a single small vessel, and it is only when they have reached that body that they begin to ramify. The only capillary vessels which are found in the whole length of the umbilical cord of a somewhat developed fœtus do not extend more than about four or five lines (in rare instances a little farther), beyond the abdominal walls into that part of the cord which remains after birth. The

Fig. 40. The abdominal end of the umbilical cord of a nearly full-grown fœtus, injected. *A*. The abdominal wall. *B*. The permanent part of the cord with a congeries of injected vessels along its border. *C*. Its deciduous portion with the convolutions of the umbilical vessels. *v*. The limits of the capillaries.

* Lymphæductus, vel *gelatina, quæ eorum vices gerit*, alterum succum albumini ovorum similorem abducit (a placenta) ad funiculum umbilicalem. (Thom. Whart. Adenographia, Amstelædami, 1659, p. 233.)

farther up this vascular part extends, the greater the development of the navel. When the vascular layer is prolonged but a very short distance the navel is greatly depressed ; when it reaches a long way up, a prominent navel is the result. The capillaries mark the limits of the permanent tissue ; the deciduous portion of the cord has no vessels of its own.

This condition, which seems to be of great importance as regards the theory of nutrition, can be very easily seen with the naked eye in injected fœtuses of five months and upwards, and in new-born children. The vascular layer terminates by a nearly straight line.

Preparations of this sort do not, to be sure, furnish absolute proof, for there might happen to be a few minute vessels proceeding farther up, but invisible to the naked eye. But I formerly made this very point the subject of special investigation, and although I injected a number of umbilical cords, some from the arteries, and others from the veins, I never succeeded in discovering a single collateral vessel, however minute, that passed the limits of the persistent layer. The whole of the deciduous portion of the umbilical cord, that long portion which lies between its cutaneous end and its termination in the placenta, is entirely destitute of capillaries, and there really exist no other vessels in it than the three large trunks. Now these are all of them remarkable for the great thickness of their walls, which, as we have really only known since the investigations of Kölliker, are enormously rich in muscular fibres.

In a transverse section of the umbilical cord it may be observed, that the thick middle coat of the vessels is entirely composed of smooth muscular fibres, lying in immediate contact one with the other, and in such abundance as is scarcely to be seen in any completely developed vessel. This peculiarity explains the extraordinary great contractility of the umbilical vessels, which can be so readily seen in action on a large scale when mechanical stimuli are applied, when the vessels are divided with scissors or are pinched, or after the employment of electrical stimuli. Sometimes, upon the application of external stimuli, they even contract to such a degree that their canal is entirely closed, and thus after birth, even without the application of a ligature, as when, for example, the umbilical cord has been torn asunder, the bleeding may stop of itself. The thickness of the walls of these vessels is, therefore, easily comprehensible, for in addition to the muscular coat, which is of itself so thick, there is an internal, and, though it is certainly not very strongly developed, an external coat; and only after this do we come to the gelatinous, jelly-like tissue (*mucous tissue* (Schleimgewebe)) of the umbilical cord. Through these layers, therefore, nutrition would have to take place, if the umbilical vessels were the nutrient vessels of the cord. Now I certainly can-

Fig. 41.

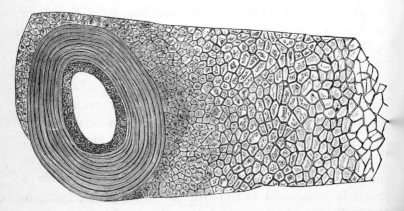

Fig. 41. Transverse section through a part of the umbilical cord. On the left is seen the section of an umbilical artery, with a very thick muscular coat, and to this, as one proceeds outwards, succeeds the gradually widening network of cells of the mucous tissue of the cord. 80 diameters.

not say with certainty whence the tissue of the umbilical cord derives its nourishment ; perhaps it receives nutritive matter from the liquor amnii, nor am I inclined to deny the possibility of nutriments passing through the walls of the vessels, or of the onward conveyance of nutritive materials from the small capillaries of the persistent portion.   In any case, however, a large extent of tissue lies at a distance from all vessels and from the surface, and is nourished and supported without the presence of any minute system of blood-vessels in it.   For a long space of time, indeed, no one troubled himself any further about this tissue, because it was designated by the name of jelly, and thereby summarily ejected from the number of the tissues and thrust into the ambiguous group of mere accumulations of organic materials.   I was the first to show that it is really a well-constructed tissue of a typical form, and that what constitutes the jelly in the more restricted sense of the term, is the expressible part of the intercellular substance, after the removal of which there remains a tissue containing a delicate network of anastomosing cellular elements, similar to that which we have seen to exist in tendons and other parts.   A section through the external layers of the umbilical cord exhibits a structure bearing great resemblance to the external layers of the cornea ; first, an epidermoidal stratum, beneath it a somewhat denser dermoid layer, and then the Whartonian jelly, which corresponds in texture to the subcutaneous cellular tissue, and is in some sort equivalent to it.   This has a peculiarly interesting bearing upon the tissues of a more advanced period, inasmuch as, by thus ranking the jelly with subcutaneous tissue, we at the same time establish its very close relationship to the *vitreous body*, which is the only remnant of tissue that, as far as I have until now been able to make out, persists in man in this condition of jelly. It is the last remnant of the embryonic subcutaneous tissue which in the development of the eye is inverted with the lens (which was originally epidermis, p. 38).

The proper substance of the umbilical cord consists of a reticulated tissue, the meshes of which contain mucus (mucin) and a few roundish cells, whilst its trabeculæ are composed of a striated fibrous substance. In this lie stellate corpuscles, and when a good preparation has been obtained by treatment with acetic acid, a symmetrical network of cells is brought to view, which splits up the mass into such regular divisions, that by means of the anastomoses which subsist between these cells throughout the whole of the umbilical cord, a uniform

FIG. 42.

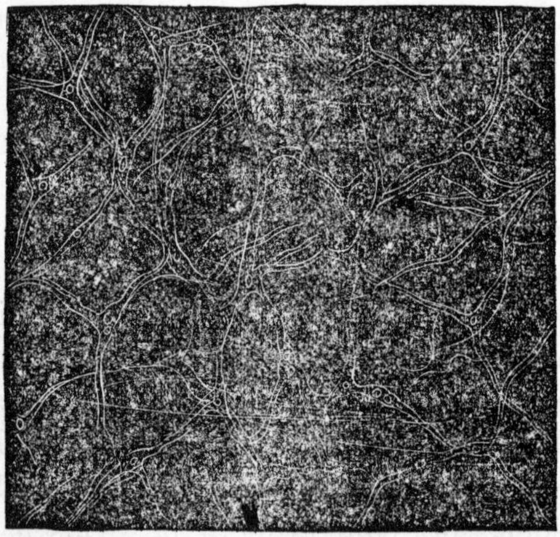

distribution of the nutritive juices throughout the whole of its substance is in this instance also rendered possible.

Fig. 42. Transverse section of the mucous tissue of the umbilical cord, exhibiting the network formed by the stellate corpuscles, after the application of acetic acid and glycerine. 300 diameters.

I have up to the present time, gentlemen, brought to your notice a series of tissues all of which agree in containing either very few capillary vessels, or none at all. In all these cases the conclusion to be drawn seems to be very simple—that, namely, the peculiar cellular, canalicular arrangement which they possess serves for the circulation of juices. It might, however, be supposed that this was an exceptional property, appertaining only to the non- or scantily-vascular and, generally speaking, hard, parts ; and I must therefore add a few words concerning the soft textures which possess a similar structure. All the tissues which we have hitherto considered, belong, in accordance with the classification which I have already given you, to the series of connective tissues ; fibro-cartilage, fibrous or tendinous tissue, mucous tissue, bone and the teeth, must one and all be considered as belonging to the same class. But to the same category belongs also the whole mass of what has usually been included under the name of *cellular tissue* (Zellgewebe), and for which the name proposed by Johannes Müller, *connective tissue* (Bindegewebe) is the most appropriate ; that substance, which fills up the interstices in the most different organs, sometimes in greater, sometimes in less, quantity—which renders the gliding of parts one upon the other possible, and formerly was imagined to enclose considerable spaces (cells in an inexact sense of the word), filled with a gaseous vapor or with moisture.

Of this kind is the peculiar interstitial, or connective, tissue, such as we meet with in the interior of the larger muscles between the several primitive fasciculi and in a still larger quantity between the several parcels, or bundles, of primitive fasciculi. Numerous arteries, veins, and capillaries lie in it ; and the arrangements for its nutrition are the most favorable that can be imagined. Notwithstanding this, however, there exists in it also, in addition to its blood-vessels, a more delicate system of nutrient channels, precisely similar to that with which we have just become acquainted ; only that, wherever it is specially required, in particular parts a peculiar change takes place in the cells, the place of the simple cell-networks and -fibres being gradually occupied by a more compact structure, which originates in a direct transformation of them, namely, the so-called *elastic tissue*.

A few months after I had made known my first observations concerning the systems of tubes existing in the connective tissues, Donders published his concerning the transformation of the cells of connective, into the elements of elastic, tissue—a discovery which has essentially contributed to the completion of the history of connective tissue. If this tissue, namely, be examined at points where it is liable to be much stretched, and where consequently it must be endowed with great power of resistance, the elastic fibres will be found arranged and distributed in it in the same way that the cells and

Fig. 43.

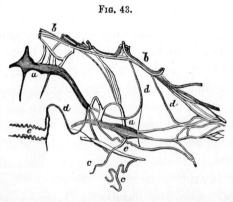

Fig. 43. Elastic networks and fibres from the subcutaneous tissue of the abdomen of a woman. *a, a.* Large elastic bodies (cell-bodies), with numerous anastomosing processes. *b, b.* Dense elastic bands of fibres, on the border of larger meshes. *c, c.* Moderately thick fibres, spirally coiled up at the end. *d, d.* Finer elastic fibres, at *e* with more minute spiral coils. 300 diameters.

cell-tubules of connective tissue usually are, and the transformation of these latter into the former can gradually be traced with such distinctness, that there remains no doubt, that even the coarser elastic fibres directly result from a chemical change and condensation of the walls of the cells themselves. Where originally there lay a cell, provided with a delicate membrane and elongated processes, there we see the membrane gradually increasing in thickness and refracting the light more strongly, whilst the proper cell-contents continually decrease and finally disappear. The whole structure becomes in this way more homogeneous, and to a certain extent sclerotic, and acquires an incredible power of resisting the influence of reagents, so that it is only after long-continued action that even the strongest caustic substances are able to destroy it, whilst it completely resists the caustic alkalies and acids in the degree of concentration usually employed in microscopical investigations. The farther this change advances, the more does the elasticity of the parts increase, and in sections we usually find these fibres not straight or elongated, but tortuous, curled up, spirally coiled, or forming little zigzags (Fig. 43, c, e). These are the elements which in virtue of their great elasticity cause retraction in those parts in which they are found in considerable quantity, as, for example, in the arteries. The fine elastic fibres, which are those that possess the greatest extensibility, are usually distinguished from the broader ones which certainly do not present themselves in tortuous forms. As far as regards their origin, however, there seems to be no difference between the two kinds ; both are derived from connective-tissue cells, and their subsequent arrangement is only a reproduction of the original plan. In the place of a tissue, consisting of a basis-substance and anastomosing, reticulated cells, there afterwards arises a tissue with its basis-substance mapped out by large elastic networks with extremely compact and tough fibres.

It has not up to the present time positively been determined, whether in the course of this transformation the condensation (sclerosis) of the walls of the cells proceeds to such a pitch as entirely to obliterate their cavity, and thus completely destroy their powers of conduction, or whether a small cavity remains in their interior. In transverse sections of fine elastic fibres, it looks as if the latter were the case, and there is therefore ground for the supposition, that in the transformation of the corpuscles of connective tissue into elastic fibres, nothing more than a condensation and thickening, and at the same time a chemical metamorphosis of the membrane, takes place, but that ultimately, however, a very small portion of the cell-cavity remains. What sort of a substance it is that constitutes the elastic parts, has not been determined, because it is not possible to accomplish their solution by any means; with a part of the products of the decomposition of this tissue we are, indeed, acquainted, but nothing further is known concerning its chemical constitution. But from this no decision can be arrived at with respect either to its composition, or position in a chemical point of view with regard to other tissues.

This kind of transformation prevails to an extraordinary extent in the skin, especially in the deeper layers of the corium proper, and to it is chiefly owing the extraordinary resistance of this tissue which we so gratefully acknowledge when daily testing it in the soles of our shoes. For the firmness of the individual layers of the skin depends essentially upon the greater or less quantity of elastic fibres contained in them. The most superficial part of the corium immediately beneath the rete mucosum is formed by the papillary portion (Papillarkörper), by which we are to understand not only the papillæ themselves, but also a continuous layer of coriaceous substance running along horizontally beneath them; it is under this that the coarse elastic networks begin, whilst only fine elastic fibres, and these in a fascicular form, ascend into the papillæ themselves, at the base of which they begin to form fine and close-meshed networks (Figs. 16, *P*, *P;* 83, *A, e; D, c*). These latter are connected inferiorly with the very thick and coarse elastic network which pervades the middle and toughest portion of the skin, the *corium* proper; below this comes a more coarsely meshed network within the less firm, but nevertheless very solid, undermost layer of the cutis, which passes inferiorly into the adipose or subcutaneous tissue.

In the places where such a transformation into elastic tissue has taken place, there are frequently scarcely any distinct cells to be found. This is the case not merely in the skin, but also especially in certain parts of the middle coat of arteries, and particularly in the aorta. Here the network of elastic fibres attains such a preponderance, that it is only with great care that minute cellular elements can here and there be detected. In the skin, on the other hand, in addition to the elastic fibres, a somewhat greater number of small corpuscles are found, which have retained their cellular nature, though they are certainly so extremely minute that they must be specially sought for. They generally lie in the interstices of the large-meshed networks, where they either form a system with perfect anastomoses and small meshes, or else appear in the shape of more isolated, roundish bodies, in consequence of the individual cells not being very distinctly connected with one another. This is especially the case in the papillary portion of the skin, which both in its continuous layer and in the papillæ contains nucleated cells, in direct contrast with the corium proper, which at the same time is less vascular. But a far greater number of vessels was certainly needed in the former part, inasmuch as they have at the same time to furnish nutritive material for the whole

Fig. 44.

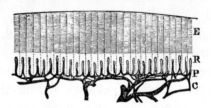

stratum of cuticle which lies above the papillæ ; nevertheless, however, there is left only a small quantity of juice at the disposition of the papillæ as such. Every papillæ, therefore corresponds to a certain (vascular) district of the superjacent cuticle, whilst on the other hand it is itself resolved into as many elementary (histological) districts as there are elements (cells) in it.

In the scrotum the subcutaneous tissue (the *dartos*) presents peculiar interest, from the fact of its being particularly rich in vessels and nerves, quite in accordance with the peculiar import of the part ; and besides from its possessing an enormous quantity of muscular tissue, consisting, in fact, of those little cutaneous muscles, which I lately described to you (p. 58). These are the really active elements of the contractile tunica dartos. In this very part in which formerly a contractile connective substance was considered to exist, the quantity of the little cutaneous muscles is extremely large, and the

Fig. 44. Vertical section from an injected preparation of the skin. *E.* **Epidermis.** *R.* Rete mucosum. *P.* Papillæ of the skin, with their ascending and descending vessels (loops). *C.* Cutis. 11 diameters.

rugæ of the scrotum are produced solely and exclusively by the contraction of these minute fasciculi, which, especially after they have been coloured with carmine, can very easily be distinguished from the connective tissue.

FIG. 45.

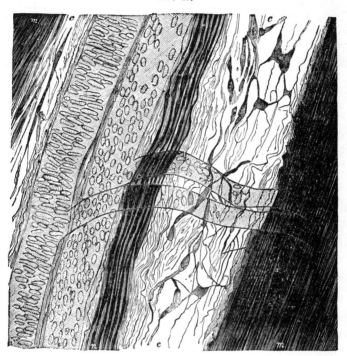

They are of pretty nearly the same breadth, broader for the most part than the bundles of connective tissue; and in them the individual elements are arranged in the shape of long, smooth fibre-cells. Every muscular fasciculus, after it has been treated with acetic acid, presents at regular intervals those peculiar, long, frequently

Fig. 45. Section from the tunica dartos of the scrotum. Side by side and parallel are seen, an artery (*a*), a vein (*v*), and a nerve (*n*); the first two with small branches. On the right and left of them organic muscular fasciculi (*m, m*), and in the interspaces soft connective tissue (*c, c*), with large anastomosing cells and fine elastic fibres. 300 diameters.

staff-shaped nuclei, and between them is seen a delicate division of the substance into separate cells, the contents of which have a slightly granular appearance. These are the wrinklers of the scrotum (*corrugatores scroti*). Besides, we also find in the extremely soft membrane a certain number of fine elastic elements, and in greater quantity the ordinary, soft, wavy connective tissue, with a great number of relatively voluminous, spindle-shaped and reticulated, granular, nucleated, cells.

These persistent cells of connective tissue had previously been totally overlooked, its fibrils having been regarded as its real elements. If, namely, the individual constituents of connective tissue be separated from one another, little bundles are obtained of a wavy form and streaky, fibrillar appearance. According to Reichert, indeed, this appearance is merely due to the formation of folds, an idea which ought not perhaps to be admitted to the extent in which it was advanced, but which has not been altogether refuted, inasmuch as a complete isolation of the fibrils can never be effected excepting by artificial means. At all events a homogeneous basis-substance, which holds the fasciculi together, must be assumed to exist in addition to the fibrils. This, however, is a question of subordinate importance. On the other hand, it is extremely important to know, that wherever this lax tissue is met with, whether beneath the cutis, in the interspaces of muscle, or in serous membranes, it is pervaded by cells which for the most part anastomose (so as in longitudinal sections to form parallel rows, in transverse ones networks), and separate the bundles of connective tissue from one another, in much the same way that the corpuscles of bone separate its different lamellæ. In addition, the most manifold vascular connections are everywhere met with; indeed, the vessels are so numerous, that a special nutrient canalicular system in the tissue might even appear altogether unnecessary. But this tissue also, however favourably its capillary channels may be disposed, stands in need of an arrangement of such a nature as to render *a special distribution of the nutritive juices to the separate cellular districts possible.* It is only when we conceive the absorption of nutritive matter to be a consequence of the activity (attraction) of the elements of the tissue themselves, that we are able to comprehend how it is that the individual districts are not exposed every moment to an inundation on the part of the blood, but the proffered material is, on the contrary, taken up into the parts only in accordance with the requirements of the moment, and is conveyed to the individual districts in such a quantity, that in general at least, as long as any possibility of its maintenance exists, one part cannot be essentially defrauded by the others.

LECTURE VI.

MARCH 3, 1858.

NUTRITION AND CIRCULATION.

Arteries—Capillaries—Continuity of their membrane—Its porosity—Hæmorrhage by transudation (per diapedesin)—Veins—Vessels during pregnancy.
Properties of the walls of vessels:
1. Contractility—Rhythmical movement—Active or irritative hyperæmia—Ischæmia—Counter irritants.
2. Elasticity and its importance as regards the rapidity and uniformity of the current of blood—Dilatation of the vessels.
3. Permeability—Diffusion—Specific affinities—Relations between the supply of blood and nutrition—Glandular secretion (liver)—Specific action of the elements of the tissues.
Dyscrasia—Its transitory character and local origin—Dyscrasia of drunkards—Hæmorrhagic diathesis—Syphilis.

I HAVE endeavoured, gentlemen, in the last two lectures, to present to you a somewhat detailed picture of the more delicate arrangements which prevail in the body for the conveyance of the different currents of nutritive juices, and particularly for the conveyance of those currents in which the juices themselves are more hidden from observation. Allow me to-day to pass on to the consideration of the larger channels and nobler juices, which, according to prevailing opinion, stand more in the foreground.

The distribution of the blood takes place, as is well known, within the vessels in the following manner: The arteries divide into finer and finer branches, and whilst they thus divide, the character of their walls gradually undergoes such alterations, that at last minute canals, the so-called capillary vessels, appear, provided with a membrane as simple as any that is ever met with in the body. The histological appearances which present themselves in these different vessels are as follows :

On isolating an *artery* we find that its walls are relatively very thick, and in those arteries which can be followed with the naked eye, not only the well-known three coats are distinguished with the help of the microscope, but in addition to these, a fine epithelial layer, which invests the internal surface and is not wont to be included in the class of structures usually termed coats The internal and external coats are essentially formations of connective tissue, which in the larger arteries display a continually increasing quantity of elastic fibres ; between them lies the relatively thick middle, or circular-fibre, coat, which, as being the seat of the muscular fibres, constitutes what may be almost termed the most important component of the arterial walls. These muscular fibres are found in the greatest abundance in the middle-sized and smaller arteries, whilst in the very large ones, and especially in the aorta, elastic layers form the predominant constituent even of the circular-fibre coat. In small arteries, on microscopical examination, there may be easily observed within this coat (Comp. Figs. 26, *b*, *b ;* 45, *a*) little transverse striations, corresponding to the individual fibre-cells, and encircling the vessel in such dense array that we find fibre-cell by the side of fibre-cell without any interruption. The thickness of this layer can be readily estimated in consequence of the well-marked limits set to it upon the in- and out-side by the longitudinal-fibre coats ; the only deceptive appearance is presented by certain round bodies, which are to be seen here and there in the substance of the circular-fibre coat, but only at the border of the vessel (Figs. 26, *b*, *b*; 46 ,*m*, *m*), and which look like round cells or nuclei scattered through the tissue. These are fibre-cells seen in apparent transverse section. The layer formed by the middle coat may be most distinctly seen, however, after the addition of acetic acid, which causes the appearance of a great number of oblong nuclei.

It is this layer which, generally speaking, confers upon the arteries their specific character, and distinguishes them most clearly from the veins. There are, indeed, numerous veins in the body which possess considerable layers of muscular tissue—for example, the superficial cutaneous veins; still, in the case of the smaller vessels, the occurrence of a distinctly marked circular-fibre coat

Fig. 46.

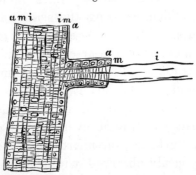

is so peculiarly characteristic of arterial vessels, that, wherever we meet with such a structure, we are at once inclined to assume the vessel to be arterial.

These vessels, which must be included among the

Fig. 46. A minute artery from the sheath of the tendon of one of the extensors of a hand just amputated. *a*, *a*. External coat. *m*, *m*. Middle coat, with well-developed muscular layer. *i*, *i*. Internal coat, partly with longitudinal folds, partly with longitudinal nuclei, in the side-branch brought well into view in consequence of the two external coats having been torn away. 300 diameters.

larger ones, although even when full of blood they only appear to the naked eye like red filaments, pass gradually into smaller ones, and with a power magnifying three hundred diameters, we see them breaking up into branches, into which, even when they are very small, the three coats are at first continued. It is only in the smallest branches that the muscular coat finally disappears, the intervals between the individual transverse fibres becoming wider and wider, and the internal coat (the nuclei of which lie in a longitudinal direction and cross those of the middle coat at right angles (Fig. 26, *D, E,*)), at the same time appearing more and more distinctly through it. The external coat also may be followed for a short distance farther (being in many places, as in the brain, rendered more evident by the interspersion of pigment or fat, Fig. 26, *D, E*), till at last it also becomes lost to view, and only a simple capillary remains (Fig. 3, *c*). The general supposition, therefore, is that the proper capillary membrane most nearly corresponds to the internal coat of the larger vessels, and it is usually considered that the more complete a vessel becomes, the greater is the number of the coats which develop themselves around it. The real developmental relations which these parts bear to one another have, however, been by no means accurately determined.

Within the true *capillary* region there is nothing further worthy of notice in the vessels than the nuclei I have previously mentioned, which correspond to the longitudinal axis of the vessel, and are so imbedded in its membrane, that it is impossible to discover any traces of a surrounding cell-wall. The capillary membrane is seen to be quite uniform, absolutely homogeneous and continuous (Fig. 3, *c*). Whilst even as lately as twenty years ago, it was a matter of discussion whether there did not exist vessels which were destitute of true walls, and were nothing more than channellings or excavations in the parenchyma of organs, as well as whether vessels could not be produced by the formation of new tracks in communication with the old channels by the forcing asunder of the neighboring parenchyma; there can, at the present time, be no longer any doubt as to the vascular system's being everywhere continuously closed by membranes. In these it is not possible to descry any porosity Even the minute pores, which have recently been observed in different parts, have not, up to the present time, met with their counterparts in the capillary membrane, and when the porosity of this membrane is spoken of, the expression can only be admitted in a physical sense, as applying to invisible, really molecular interstices. A film of collodion is not more homogeneous, nor more continuous, than the membrane of a capillary. A series of possibilities, which used to be admitted, as that, for example, the continuity of the capillary membrane did not exist at certain points, simply fall to the ground. A "transudation" or diapedesis of the blood through the walls of vessels without the occurrence of any rupture cannot for an instant be admitted; and although we cannot in every individual case point out the exact site of the rupture, it is, notwithstanding, quite inconceivable that the blood with its corpuscles should be able to pass through the walls in any other way than through a hole in them. This is such a very natural deduction from ascertained histological facts, that all discussion upon the point is impossible.

After the capillaries have pursued their course for a time, small veins begin gradually to form out of them, and generally run back in the neighbourhood of the arteries (Fig. 45, *v*). In them the characteristic circular-fibre coat of the arteries is in general wanting, or at least it is very much less developed. In its place we find in the middle coat of the larger veins toughish layers, which are not characterized so much by the absence of muscular elements as by the greater abundance of elastic elements which run in a longitudinal direction and are found in greater or less quantity in different localities.

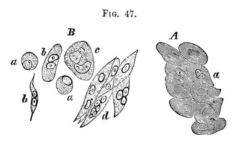

Fig. 47.

In an inward direction there follow next the softer and more delicate layers of connective tissue of the internal

Fig. 48.

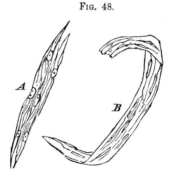

Fig. 47. *A*. Epithelium from the femoral artery ('Archiv f. path. Anat.,' vol. iii., figs. 9 and 12, p. 596). *a*. Division of nucleus.

B. Epithelium from veins of considerable size. *a, a*. Largish, granular, round, uni-nuclear cells (colourless blood-corpuscles?) *b, b*. Oblong and spindle-shaped cells, with divided nuclei and nucleoli. *c*. Large, flat cells, with two nuclei, of which each has three nucleoli, and is in process of division. *d*. Coherent epithelium, with the nuclei in a state of progressive division, one cell having six nuclei. 320 diameters.

Fig. 48. Epithelium from the vessels of the kidney. *A*. Flat, spindle-shaped cells with longitudinal folds and large nuclei from a new-born child. *B*. Ribbon-like, nearly homogeneous, plate of epithelium with longitudinal nuclei from an adult. 350 diameters.

coat, and lying on this is found, in the last place, a flat, extremely translucent layer of epithelium, which is very prone to protrude out of the cut end of the vessel, and gives the impression of spindle-shaped cells, so that it may easily be mistaken for spindle-shaped muscular cells. The smallest veins likewise possess this epithelium, but, with this exception, are, properly speaking, entirely composed of connective tissue provided with longitudinal nuclei (Fig. 45, *v*).

These relations undergo no essential change even when the individual constituents of the vascular system experience the most extreme enlargement. This is best seen in *pregnancy*, in which not merely in the uterus, but also in the vagina, the Fallopian tubes, the ovaries, and the ligaments of the uturus, both the large and small arteries and veins, as well as the capillaries, exhibit a very high degree of dilatation, so that the rest of the tissue, in spite of its having likewise in no inconsiderable degree become enlarged, is thereby virtually thrust into the background. Nevertheless, however, parts of this puerperal sexual apparatus are extremely well adapted for displaying the relation between the histological elements and the *vascular* (arterial) districts. In the fimbriæ of the Fallopian tubes, for example, every plexus or loop formed towards the borders by the greatly dilated capillaries encloses a certain number of large connective tissue cells, of which only a few lie in immediate contact with the vessels. In the alæ vespertilionum we find, moreover, very beautifully displayed, a condition which is of frequent occurrence in the appendages of the generative organs, and similar to what we lately considered in the scrotum ; the vessels, namely, are accompanied by flat bundles of smooth muscle in considerable quantity which do not belong to them, but only follow the course of the vessels, and in part receive the vessels into them. This is an extremely important feature, inasmuch as the contraction of these ligaments, in which muscular tissue is not generally considered to exist, is by no means solely to be ascribed to the blood-vessels, as James Traer only a short time ago endeavoured to establish ; on the contrary, we find thickish, flat bundles of muscle which run through the middle of the ligaments, and during menstrual excitement enable contractions to take place, similar to those which we can follow with such great distinctness in external portions of the genital passages.

If now the question be raised how far the individual elements of the vessels are of importance in the body, it is at once evident that the contractile elements play the most important part in the coarser processes of the circulation, whilst the elastic constituents come next, and the simply permeable, homogeneous membranes last. Let us first consider the import of the *muscular elements*, and more particularly in those vessels which are chiefly provided with them, namely the arteries.

When an artery is acted upon by any influence which causes a contraction of its muscular tissue, it must of course become narrower, inasmuch as the contractile cells lie in rings around the vessel ; this contraction may under certain circumstances proceed until the canal is almost entirely obliterated, and the natural consequence then is that less blood penetrates into the corresponding part of the body. When, therefore, an artery is in any way exposed to a pathological irritant, or when it is excited by some physiological stimulus, its proper action cannot be displayed in any other way than by its becoming narrower. Now, indeed, that the muscular elements of the walls of the vessels have become known, the old doctrine might again be taken up, that, namely, the vessels, like the heart, originated a kind of rhythmical pulsating movement, which was capable of directly furthering the onward movement of the blood, so that an arterial hyperæmia would be the result of an increased pulsation in the vessels.

We are indeed acquainted with one isolated fact which is a proof that a real rhythmical movement does take place in the arterial walls ; and this was first observed by Schiff in the ears of rabbits. Its rhythm, however, does not at all correspond with that of the well-known arterial pulsation ; the only counterpart to it exists in the movements which had previously been observed by Wharton Jones in the veins of the wings of bats, and proceed in an extremely slow and quiet manner. I have studied these phenomena in bats, and convinced myself that the rhythm coincindes neither with the cardiac nor the respiratory movements ; it is quite a peculiar, but comparatively not very forcible, movement, and takes place after tolerably long pauses, longer ones than are observed in the case of the circulation and shorter than those which occur in respiration. In the ears of rabbits, also, the contractions of the arteries are far slower than the cardiac and respiratory movements.

After excluding these phenomena, which manifestly ought not to be explained in such a way as to support the old view of the local occurrence of pulsation, the essential fact remains, that the muscular fibres of a vessel contract upon the application of every stimulus which sets them in action, but that this contraction is not propagated in a peristaltic manner, but is confined to the spot irritated, or, at most, extends a little beyond, and continues for a certain length of time at this spot. The more muscular the vessel is, the more lasting and forcible is the contraction and the greater is the obstruction experienced by the current of blood. The . smaller the vessels, the more rapidly, on the contrary, do we see the contraction succeeded by a dilatation, which, however, is not in its turn followed by a contraction, as it would have to be to constitute a pulsation, but persists for a longer or shorter time. This dilatation is not of an active, but of a passive nature, and results from the pressure of the blood upon the wall of the vessel which has become fatigued and opposes less resistance.

If we now proceed to examine the phenomena which

Fig. 49.

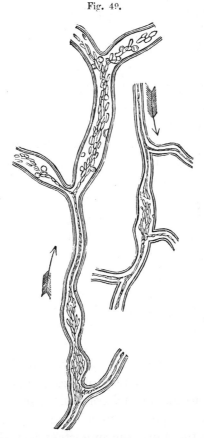

Fig. 49. Irregular contraction of small vessels from the web of a frog's foot after the application of stimuli. Copied from Wharton Jones.

are usually grouped together under the title of active hyperæmia, there can be no doubt but that the muscular tissue of the arteries is generally essentially concerned therein. We very commonly find we have to deal with processes in which the muscular fibres of the vessels have really been stimulated, and the contraction is succeeded by a state of relaxation, such as scarcely ever occurs in an equally marked manner in the rest of the muscles—a state which is manifestly the expression of a kind of fatigue and exhaustion, and is the longer persistent, the more energetic the stimulus which was applied. In small vessels with few muscular fibres, therefore, it often seems as if the stimuli really induced no contraction, in consequence of the extreme rapidity with which a state of relaxation is seen to set in, continuing for a considerable time, and allowing of an increased influx of blood.

This same condition of relaxation we can experimentally most easily produce by cutting the nerves supplying the vessels of a part, whilst the contraction can be effected to a very great extent by submitting these nerves to a very energetic stimulus. That our acquaintance with this kind of contraction is of so late a date, is explained by the fact that the stimuli applied to the nerves must be very powerful, and that, as Claude Bernard has shown, only strong electric currents are sufficient for the purpose. On the other hand, the conditions which ensue upon the section of the nerves are in most parts so complicated, that the dilatation escaped observation, until the lucky spot was discovered also by Bernard, and by the section of the sympathetic nerves in the neck a reliable and convenient field for observation was thrown open to experiment.

We obtain therefore the important fact that, whether the widening of the vessel, or, in other words, the relaxation of its muscular fibres, be produced directly by a paralysis of the nerve or an interruption of the nervous influence, or whether it be the indirect result of a previous stimulation, giving rise to exhaustion—that, I say, in every case we have to deal with a kind of paralysis of the walls of the vessel, and that the process is incorrectly designated active hyperæmia, inasmuch as the condition of the vessels in it is always a completely passive one. All that has been built up upon this assumed activity of the vessels, is, if not exactly built upon sand, still of an extremely ambiguous nature, and all the conclusions that have besides been drawn with regard to the important influence which the activity of the vessels was supposed to have upon the conditions of nutrition of the parts themselves, fall at the same time to the ground.

When an artery is really in action, it gives rise to no hyperæmia ; the more powerfully it acts, the more does it occasion anæmia, or, as I have designated it, *ischæmia*, and the less or greater degree of activity in the artery determines the greater or less quantity of blood which in a unit of time can stream into a given part. *The more active the vessel, the less the supply of blood.* If, then, we have to deal with an hyperæmia the result of irritation, the most important point, therapeutically, is just this : to place the vessels in such a state of activity as will enable them to offer resistance to the onward rush of blood. This we can accomplish by means of what is called counter-irritation, a higher degree of irritation in an already irritated part, stimulating the fatigued muscular fibres of the vessel to persistent contraction, and thereby diminishing the supply of blood and leading the way to a regulation of the disturbance. In the very cases in which reaction, that is, regulatory activity, is most called for, the chief point is to overcome that state of passiveness which maintains the (so-called active) hyperæmia.

If we now pass from the muscular to the *elastic* constituents of the vessels, we meet with a property which is of very great importance, on the one hand in the veins, the activity of which is in many cases to be wholly referred to their elastic elements, on the other hand, in the arteries, and particularly in the aorta and its larger branches. In these the elasticity of the walls has the effect of compensating for the loss which the pressure of the blood experiences from the systolic dilatation of the vessels, and of converting the uneven current produced by the jerking movements of the heart into an even one. If the walls of the vessels were not elastic, the stream of the blood would unquestionably be rendered very much slower, and at the same time, pulsation would take place throughout the whole extent of the vascular apparatus as far as the capillaries, for the same jerking movement which is communicated to the blood at the commencement of the aortic system would continue even into the smallest ramifications. But every observation we make in living animals teaches us that within the capillaries the stream is a continuous one. This equable onward movement is effected by the elasticity of the walls of the arteries, in virtue of which they return the impulse which they receive from the in-rushing blood with the same force, and by this means maintain a regular onflow of the blood during the time occupied by the following diastole of the heart.

If the elasticity of the vessel be considerably diminished, without its becoming stiff and immoveable (from calcareous incrustations) in the same degree, the dilatation, which it undergoes from the pressure of the blood, is not again compensated ; the vessel remains in a dilated condition, and thus are gradually produced the well-known forms of *ecstasis*, such as we are familiar with in the arteries under the name of aneurysms, and in the veins under that of varices. In these processes, we have not so much, as has been represented of late, to deal with primary disease of the inner coat, as with changes which are situated in the elastic and muscular middle coat.

If therefore it is the muscular elements of the arteries that have the most important influence upon the quantity of blood to be distributed, and the mode of its distribution, in the several organs, and the elastic elements that are chiefly concerned in the production of a rapid and equable stream, they nevertheless exercise only an indirect influence upon the nutrition of the parts which lie outside the vessels themselves, and in this matter, we are obliged to betake ourselves, as a last resource, to the *simple, homogeneous membrane of the capillaries*, without which indeed not even the constituents of the walls of the larger vessels provided with vasa vasorum would be able to maintain themselves for any lengthened period. The difficulty which here presents itself has, as you know, during the last ten years, been chiefly got over by the assumption of the existence of *diffusive currents* (endosmosis and exosmosis) between the contents of the vessels and the fluid in the tissues ; and by regarding the capillary wall as a more or less indifferent membrane, forming merely a partition between two fluids, which enter into a reciprocal relation with one another ; while the nature of this relation would be essentially determined by the state of concentration they are in and their chemical composition, so that, according as the internal or the external fluid was the more concentrated, the diffusive stream would run inwardly or outwardly, and, according to the chemical peculiarities of the individual juices, certain modifications would arise in these currents. Generally speaking, however, the chemical side of this question has been but little regarded.

It cannot be denied that there are certain facts which cannot well be explained in any other manner, especially in cases where essential alterations have taken place in the state of concentration of the juices, for example, in that form of cataract which Kunde has artificially produced in frogs by the introduction of salt into their intestinal canal or subcutaneous cellular tissue. But in proportion as, after a physical study of the phenomena of diffusion, the conviction has been acquired that the membrane which separates the fluids is not an indifferent substance, but that its nature exercises a directly controlling influence upon the permeating powers of the fluids, it becomes impossible that a like influence should be denied the capillary membrane. We must not, however, go so far, as to ascribe to this membrane all the peculiarities observable in the interchange of material, and so explain how it happens, that certain matters which enter into the composition of the blood are not distributed in equal proportion to every part, but leave the vessels at some points in greater, at others in less, quantity, and at others not at all. These peculiarities depend, manifestly, on the one hand, upon the different degrees of pressure to which the column of blood is subjected in certain parts, and, on the other, upon special preperties of the tissues ; and we are irresistibly compelled, both by the consideration of simply pathological, and particularly by that of pharmaco-dynamical, phenomena to admit that there are certain *affinities* existing between definite tissues and definite substances, which must be referred to peculiarities of chemical constitution, in virtue of which certain parts are enabled in a greater degree than others to attract certain substances from the neighbouring blood.

If we consider the possibility of such attraction with a little more attention, it is peculiarly interesting to observe the behaviour of parts, which are at a certain distance from the vessel. If we apply a definite stimulus, for example, a chemical substance, a small quantity of an alkali I will suppose, directly to any part, we see that this shortly afterwards takes up more nutritive matter, so that even in a few hours its size becomes considerably increased, and that, whilst before we were perhaps scarcely able to distinguish anything in its interior, we now find an abundant, relatively opaque material within it, in no wise composed of alkali which had made its way in, but essentially containing substances of an albuminous nature. Observation shows that the process in all vascular parts begins with hyperæmia, so that the idea readily presents itself that the hyperæmia is the essential and determining cause. But if we investigate the matter more minutely, we find it difficult to understand how the blood, which is in the hyperæmic vessels, can contrive only to act just upon the irritated part, whilst other parts lying in the immediate vicinity are not affected in the same manner. In all cases in which the vessels are the immediate originators of disturbances which take place in a tissue, these are most marked in the immediate neighbourhood of the vessels and in the district which they supply (vascular (or vessel-) territory). If we introduce an irritating, as, for example, a decomposing body into a blood-vessel, a fact that has been established by me upon a large scale when tracing out the history of embolia, we by no means see that the parts at a distance from the vessel are the principal seats of active change, but that this is in the first instance manifested in the wall of the vessel itself and then in the adjoining histological

elements.   But if we apply the stimulus directly to the
tissue, the central point of the disturbance will always
continue to be that at which the stimulus produced its
effect, just the same whether there are vessels in the
neighbourhood or not.

We shall hereafter have occasion to return to this subject, and my only object here was to lay this fact before
you in its general features, and thus repel the ordinary
conclusion, which is as convenient as it is fallacious, that
hyperæmia (in itself passive) exercises a directly regulating influence upon the nutrition of tissues.

If a special proof were still required in order to complete the refutation of this assumption, which in an anatomical point of view is utterly untenable, we find a
most apposite argument in the experiment above mentioned of the section of the sympathetic.   In an animal
the sympathetic may be divided in the neck ; thereupon
a state of hyperæmia ensues in the whole of that half of
the head, the ears become dark red, the vessels greatly
dilated, the conjunctiva and nasal mucous membrane
turgidly injected.   This may continue for days, weeks,
or months, without the least appreciable nutritive disturbance necessarily arising therefrom ; the parts,
although gorged with blood, are yet, as far at least as
we are at present able to judge of this, in the same state
of nutrition as before.   If we apply stimuli sufficient to
produce inflammation to these parts, the only thing that
we remark is, that the inflammation runs its course more
quickly, without exhibiting either in itself or in the nature of its products anything essentially unusual.

The greater or less quantity of blood, therefore, which
flows through a part is not to be regarded as the only
cause of the changes in its nutrition.   There is, I suppose, no doubt that, when a part, which is in a state of
irritation, receives more blood than usual, it is also able

to attract a larger quantity of material from the blood with greater readiness than it otherwise would have done, or than it would be able to do, if the vessels were in a state of contraction or less filled with blood. If, therefore, it were to be objected to my view that in such conditions the most favorable effects are often produced by local abstractions of blood, this would be no proof of its incorrectness. If we cut off or diminish the supply of nutritive matter, we must, of course, prevent the part from absorbing more than its wont, but, *vice versâ*, we cannot by offering it a larger quantity of nutritive material straightway compel it to take up more than it did ; these are two entirely independent cases. However apt one may be to conclude (and however much I may be disposed to allow, that at the first glance there is something very plausible in such a conclusion) that, from the favourable effect which the cutting off of the supply of blood has in putting a stop to a process which arose from an increase of it, the process depended upon this increased supply, yet I am of opinion that the practical fact cannot be interpreted in this way. It is not so much an increase of quantity, either in the blood as a whole or in that portion of it contained in an individual part, which is required in order that a like increase should forthwith take place in the nutrition of that part, or of the whole body, as that, in my opinion, particular conditions should obtain in the tissues (irritation) altering the nature of their attraction for the constituents of the blood, or that particular matters should be present in the blood (specific substances), upon which definite parts of the tissues are able to exercise a particular attraction.

If you apply this doctrine to the humoro-pathological conception of the processes, you will be able to deduce from it that I am far from contesting the correctness of the humoral explanations in general, and that I rather cherish the conviction that particular substances which find their way into the blood are able to induce particular changes in individual parts of the body by their being taken up into them in virtue of the specific attraction of individual parts for individual substances. We know, for example, that a number of substances are introduced into the body which possess special affinities for the nervous system, and that among this number again there are some which stand in a closer connection with certain very definite parts of the nervous system, as for instance with the brain, the spinal cord or sympathetic ganglia, and others again with particular parts of the brain, spinal cord, etc. On the other hand, we see that certain materials have some special relation to definite secreting organs ; that they penetrate and pervade them by a kind of elective affinity ; that they are excreted by them ; and that, when there is a too abundant supply of such materials, a state of irritation is produced in these organs. But an essential condition in all these cases is, that the parts which are believed to have a particular elective affinity for particular matters, should really exist, for a kidney which loses its epithelium is thereby deprived of its secreting power. Another condition is that the parts should possess a relation of affinity, for neither a diseased, nor a dead, kidney has any longer the affinity for particular substances which the gland, when living and healthy, possessed. The power of attracting and transforming definite substances can be maintained at most for a short time in an organ, which no longer continues in a really living condition. We are therefore, in the end, always compelled to regard the individual elements as the active agents in these attractions. An hepatic cell can attract certain substances from the blood which flows through the nearest capillary vessel, but it must in the first place exist, and in the next be in the ejoyment of its special properties, in order to exercise this attraction. If the living element become altered, if a disease set in which causes changes in its molecular, physical, or chemical peculiarities, then its power of exercising this special attraction will at the same time also be impaired.

Let us consider this example with still greater attention. The hepatic cells are almost in direct contact with the walls of the capillaries, from which they are only separated by a thin layer of delicate connective tissue. If now we were to imagine that the peculiar property possessed by the liver of secreting bile, merely consisted in a particular disposition of the vessels of the organ, we should indeed in no wise be justified in doing so. Similar networks of vessels, in a great measure of a venous nature, are found in several other places, for example, in the lungs. But the peculiarity of the secretion of bile manifestly depends upon the liver-cells, and only so long as the blood flows past in the immediate neighbourhood of the hepatic cells, does the particular attraction of matter continue which characterizes the action of the liver.

When the blood contains free fat, we see that after a time the hepatic cells take it up in minute particles, and that if the supply continues, the fat becomes more abundant and is gradually separated in the form of largish drops within the hepatic cells (Fig. 27, *B*, *b*). That which we see in the case of fat in a more palpable form, we must conceive to occur in the case of many other substances in a state of more minute division. Thus for the due performance of secretion it will always be essential that the cells exist in a certain, special condition; if they become diseased, if a condition be developed in them connected with some important chemical change in their contents, for example, an atrophy, ultimately causing the destruction of the parts, then the power pos-

sessed by the organ of forming bile will at the same time
continually become more limited. We cannot conceive
a liver without liver-cells ; they are, as far as we know,
the really active elements, since even in cases in which
the supply of blood has become limited owing to obstruction in the portal vein, the hepatic cells are able to produce bile, although perhaps not in the same quantity.

This fact derives peculiar value from its occurrence in
the liver, because the matters which constitute the bile
do not, as is well known, exist pre-formed in the blood,
and we must therefore suppose the constituents of the
bile to arise not by a process of simple secretion, but by
one of actual formation in the liver. This question has,
as you are aware, recently become invested with a still
greater degree of interest in consequence of the observation of Bernard that the property of producing sugar is
also inherent in these elements, whereby the blood is
supplied upon so gigantic a scale with a substance which
has the most decided influence upon the internal metamorphic processes and upon the production of heat. If,
therefore, we speak of the action of the liver, we can,
both in regard to the formation of sugar as well as that
of bile, mean nothing but the action of its individual elements (cells), an action which consists in their attracting
matters from the passing current of blood, in their effecting within their cavity a transmutation of these matters,
and returning them in this transmuted form either to
the blood, or yielding them up to the bile-ducts in the
shape of bile.

Now I demand for cellular pathology nothing more
than that this view, which must be admitted to be true
in the case of the large secreting organs, be extended also
to the smaller organs and smaller elements ; and that, for
example, an epidermis-cell, a lens-fibre or a cartilage-cell
be, to a certain extent, admitted to possess the power of

deriving from the vessels nearest to them (not always indeed directly, but often by transmission from a distance), in accordance with their several special requirements, certain quantities of material ; and again that, after they have taken this material up, they be held to be capable of subjecting it to further changes within themselves, and this in such a manner that they either derive therefrom new matter for their own development ; or that the substances accumulate in their interior, without their reaping any immediate benefit from it ; or finally that, after this imbibition of material, even decay may arise in their structure and their dissolution ensue. At all events it seems necessary to me that great prominence should be assigned to this *specific action of the elements of tissues*, in opposition to the specific action of the vessels, and that in studying local processes we should principally devote ourselves to the investigation of processes of this nature.

It will now, I think, be most suitable for us next to enter a little more in detail upon the consideration of the facts which form the basis of the humoro-pathological system—upon the study of the so-called *nobler juices*. If the blood be considered in its normal influence upon nutrition, the most important point is not its movement, nor the greater or less afflux of it, but its intimate composition. When the quantity of blood is great, but its composition does not correspond to the natural requirements of the parts, nutrition may suffer ; when the quantity is small, nutrition may proceed in a comparatively very favourable manner, if every single particle of the blood contain its ingredients mixed in the most favorable proportions.

If the blood be considered as a whole in contradistinction to other parts, the most dangerous thing we can do is to assume what has at all times created the greatest confusion, namely, that we have in it to deal with a fluid in itself independent, but upon which the great mass of tissues more or less depend. The greater number of the humoro-pathological doctrines are based upon the supposition, that certain changes which have taken place in the blood are more or less persistent ; and just in the very instance where these doctrines have practically exercised the greatest influence, in the theory, namely, of chronic dyscrasiæ, it is usually conceived that the change is continuous, and that by inheritance peculiar alterations in the blood may be transmitted from generation to generation, and be perpetuated.

This is, I think, the fundamental mistake of the humoralists, the real hinge upon which their errors turn. Not that I doubt at all that a change in the composition of the blood may pertinaciously continue, or that it may propagate itself from generation to generation, but I do not believe that it can be propagated *in the blood itself* and there persist, and that the blood is the real seat of the dyscrasia.

My cellulo-pathological views differ from the humoropathological ones essentially in this, that I do not regard the blood as a permanent tissue, in itself independent, regenerating and propagating itself out of itself, but as in a state of constant dependence upon other parts. We need only apply the same conclusions which are universally admitted to be true as regards the dependence of the blood upon the absorption of new nutritive matters from the stomach, to the tissues of the body themselves also. When the drunkard's dyscrasia is spoken of, nobody of course imagines that every one who has once been drunk labours under a permanent alcoholic dyscrasia, but the common opinion is, that, when continually fresh quantities of alcohol are ingested, continually fresh changes also declare themselves in the blood, so that its altered state must continue as long as the supply of fresh noxious matters takes place, or as, in consequence of a previous supply, individual organs remain in a diseased condition. If no more alcohol be ingested, if the organs which had been injured by the previous indulgence in it be restored to their normal condition, there is no doubt but that the dyscrasia will therewith terminate. This example, applied to the history of all the remaining dyscrasiæ, elucidates in a very simple manner the proposition, that *every dyscrasia is dependent upon a permanent supply of noxious ingredients from certain sources.* As a continual ingestion of injurious articles of food is capable of producing a permanently faulty composition of the blood, in like manner persistent disease in a definite organ is able to furnish the blood with a continual supply of morbid materials.

The essential point, therefore, is to search for the *local origins* of the different dyscrasiæ, to discover the definite tissues or organs from which this derangement in the constitution of the blood proceeds. Now I am quite willing to confess that it has not in many cases hitherto been possible to find out these tissues or organs. In many cases, however, success has been obtained, although it cannot be said in every instance in what way the blood has become changed. Thus we have that remarkable condition, which may very well be referred to a dyscrasia, the scorbutic condition, purpura, and the petechial dyscrasia. In vain will you look around for decisive information as to the nature of this dyscrasia, and as to the kind of change experienced by the blood when purpura or scurvy show themselves. What has been found by one has been contradicted by another, and it has even been shown that sometimes no change had taken place in the proportions of the grosser constituents of the blood. There remains in this case, therefore, a *quid ig-notum*, and you will, I am sure, deem it excusable, if we are unable to say whence a dyscrasia proceeds, of which we are altogether unacquainted with the nature. However, the knowledge of the nature of the change in the blood does not involve an insight into the requisite conditions for the dyscrasia, and just as little is the reverse the case. In the case of the hæmorrhagic diathesis, also, it must at all events be regarded as an important step in advance, that we are in a number of instances able to point to a definite organ as its source, as, for example, to the spleen or liver. The chief point now is to determine what influence the spleen or the liver exercises upon the special composition of the blood. If we were acquainted with the nature of the changes effected in the blood by the influence of these organs, it might not perhaps be difficult from our knowledge of the diseased organ also at once to infer what kind of change the blood would experience. But it is nevertheless an important fact that we have got beyond the mere study of the changes in the blood, and have been able to ascertain that there are definite organs in which the dyscrasia has its root.

In conformity herewith we must conclude that, if there is a syphilitic dyscrasia in which a virulent substance circulates in the blood, this cannot be permanently present there, but that its existence must be due to the persistence of local depots (Heerde), whence new quantities of noxious matter are continually being introduced into the blood. By following this track we arrive at the conclusion which we have already mentioned, and which is of extreme importance in a practical point of view, that, namely, every permanent change which takes place in the condition of the circulating juices, must be derived from definite points in the body, from individual organs or tissues ; and this fact, moreover, is educed, that certain organs and tissues exercise a more marked influence upon the composition of the blood than others ; that some bear a necessary relation to this fluid, others only an accidental one.

LECTURE VII.

MARCH 6, 1858.

THE BLOOD.

Fibrine—Its fibrillæ—Compared with mucus, and connective tissue—Homogeneous condition.

Red blood-corpuscles—Their nucleus and contents—Changes of form—Blood-crystals (Hæmatoidine, Hæmine, Hæmatocrystalline).

Colourless blood-corpuscles—Numerical proportion—Structure—Compared with pus-corpuscles—Their viscosity and agglutination—Specific gravity—Crusta granulosa—Diagnosis between pus-, and colourless blood-corpuscles.

I INTEND to lay before you to-day, gentlemen, some further particulars with regard to the history of the blood.

I concluded my last lecture by impressing upon you the necessity of localizing the different dyscrasiæ ; employing the term localize, not in its ordinary sense, as the dyscrasiæ have heretofore been considered as localized, but rather in a genetical meaning, in accordance with which we constantly refer the dyscrasiæ to a pre-existing local affection, and regard some one tissue as the source of the persistent changes in the blood.

If now we consider the different dyscrasiæ with regard to their importance and their source, two great categories of dyscrasic conditions may at the very outset be distinguished, according namely as the morphological elements of the blood become changed, or the deviation is more of a chemical one, and seated in the fluid constituents.

Among these latter, it is the *fibrine*, which, in conse-

166

quence of its coagulability, first, and that very soon after the blood has been removed from the living body, assumes a visible form, and which for this reason has frequently passed for a morphological constituent of the blood. This notion concerning it has of late been maintained in many quarters, and has indeed always had a traditional existence in medicine, inasmuch as from ancient times fibrine was constantly brought forward in addition to the red constituents of the blood as a special element, and it was the custom to estimate the quality of the blood, not only from the number of the blood-corpuscles, but frequently in a much more positive manner from the amount of fibrine.

This dissociation of fibrine from the other fluid constituents of the blood is, to a certain extent, of real value, because fibrine, like the blood-corpuscles, is quite a peculiar substance, and so exclusively confined to the blood and the most closely allied juices, that it really may be viewed as connected rather with the blood-corpuscles than with the mere fluids which circulate as serum. If we consider the blood in its really specific constituents, in those, by means of which it becomes blood, and is distinguished from other fluids, it cannot be denied that, on the one hand, the corpuscles with their hæmatine, and, on the other, the fibrine of the liquor sanguinis are the elements in which the specific differences must be sought for.

If now we next proceed to consider these constituents a little more closely, the morphological description of fibrine is comparatively rapidly made. On examining it, as it appears in blood-coagula, it is nearly always found in the form described by Malpighi, the fibrillar. Its fibres generally form extremely fine interlacements, delicate networks, in which they usually cross and join one another in a somewhat tortuous form. The greatest

variations exhibited by these fibres when forming out of
the blood have reference to their size and breadth ;

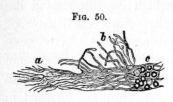

these are peculiarities concerning which it has not
hitherto been possible to form
any certain judgment. I meet
with these variations pretty
frequently, but without being
in a position to assign the causes which determine them.
The extremely fine and delicate fibres are those usually
met with ; but sometimes we find far broader, and
almost ribbon-like fibres, which are much smoother, but
in other respects, cross and interlace in pretty nearly
the same manner. Essentially, therefore, there is always
present in a clot a network composed of fibres, in the
meshes of which the blood-corpuscles are enclosed. If
a drop of blood be allowed to coagulate, fine filaments
of fibrine can be seen everywhere shooting up between
the blood-corpuscles.

With regard to the nature of these fibres, we may
observe that there are only two other kinds which, his-
tologically speaking, bear at all a near resemblance to
them. The one kind occurs in a substance which,
singularly enough, effects an approximation between the
most ancient, perfectly antique, craseological ideas and
the modern ones, namely in mucus. In the old Hippo-
cratical system of medicine the whole mass of fibrine is,
as is well known, included under the terms *phlegma*,
mucus, and when we compare mucus with fibrine, we
are obliged to confess that there does indeed exist a
great similarity between them in the form they assume
upon coagulation. In a similar manner to fibrine,

Fig. 50. Coagulated fibrine from human blood. *a*, Fine, *b*, coarser and broader
fibrils. *c*, Red and colourless blood-corpuscles enclosed in the coagulum. 280
diameters.

mucus also forms into fibres, which frequently become
isolated and then coalesce, so as to give rise to certain
figures.   The other substance which belongs here is the
intercellular, or, if you will, the gelatine-yielding substance of connective tissue, the collagen (gluten of earlier
writers).   The fibrils of connective tissue only differ in
that they are not usually reticulated, but run a parallel
course, whilst in other respects they resemble those of
fibrine in a high degree.   The intercellular substance of
connective tissue presents another point of resemblance
with fibrine in the great analogy of its behaviour with
reagents.   When we expose it to the action of diluted
acids, especially the ordinary vegetable acids, or also
weak mineral acids, the fibres swell up and disappear
before our eyes, so that we are no longer able to say
where they are.   The mass swells up, every interspace
disappears, and it looks as if the whole were composed
of a perfectly homogeneous substance.   If we slowly
wash it and again remove the acid, a fibrous tissue may,
if the action have not been too violent, once more be
obtained, after which the previous condition can be produced afresh, and changed again at pleasure.   This
behaviour has hitherto remained unexplained, and for
this very reason Reichert's view, which I have already
mentioned, that the substance of connective tissue, is
really homogeneous and the fibres are only an artificial
product, or an optical delusion, has something alluring
in it.   In fibrine, however, the individual fibres can,
much more distinctly than is the case with connective
tissue, be so completely isolated, that I cannot help
saying that I regard the separation into single fibres as
really taking place, and not merely as an artificial one,
or as a delusion on the part of the observer.

But it is very interesting to observe that this fibrillar
stage of fibrine is invariably preceded by a homogeneous

one, just as connective tissue originally wears the form
of a homogeneous intercellular substance (mucus) from
which fibres are only by degrees, if I may so express
myself, excreted, or, to employ the usual term, differentiated. So fibrine, too, which is first of all gelatinous,
becomes differentiated into a fibrillar mass. And indeed
in the case of inorganic substances also we find certain
analogous appearances. From deposits of calcareous
salts or silicic acid, which were originally perfectly gelatinous and amorphous, solid granules and crystals are
gradually separated.

The name fibrils may therefore still be retained to
designate the usual form in which fibrine presents itself,
but at the same time it must be borne in mind, that this
substance originally existed in a homogeneous, amorphous, gelatinous condition, and can again be reduced
to it. This reduction can not only be effected artificially,
but takes place also naturally in the body itself, so that
where we have previously found fibrils, we may afterwards meet with the fibrine in a homogeneous condition, as, for example, in the vessels, where aneurysmal
coagula, and others, are gradually converted into a
homogeneous mass of cartilaginous density.

Now, with reference to the second portion of the
blood, the *blood-corpuscles*, I may express myself briefly,
as they are well-known elements. I have already
remarked that nearly all the histologists of the present

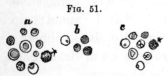

Fig. 51.

time are agreed that the coloured corpuscles of the blood
of man and the higher mammalia contain no nuclei, but
that they are simple vesicles,

Fig. 51. Nucleated blood-corpuscles from a human fœtus, six weeks old.
a. Homogeneous cells varying in size, with simple, relatively large nuclei, of which

concerning the cellular nature of which doubts might be permitted, if we did not happen to know that, at certain periods of the development of the embryo, they do contain nuclei. An ordinary red blood-corpuscle must therefore be considered as composed of a closed membrane, containing a tolerably tough mass, which is the seat of the colour. Now, in man the blood-corpuscles are, as is well known, flat, disc- or plate-shaped bodies, with a central depression on each surface, and, when regular in form, constitute, as it were, a ring, in the centre of which the colour is fainter from the diminished thickness.

Fig. 52.

The contents are generally somewhat summarily regarded as consisting of hæmatine, or the colouring matter of the blood. They are, however, unquestionably very complex, and what is called hæmatine forms merely a part of them; how great a part it has not been hitherto possible to determine. Whatever other matters are contained within the blood-corpuscle belong entirely to its chemistry. Certain changes produced by the action of external media constitute all that can be seen of them. We observe that the blood-corpuscles, according as they imbibe oxygen, or contain carbonic acid, appear light or dark, whilst they alter their form a little. We know, further, that

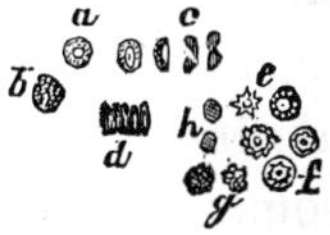

a few are slightly granular, but the greater number more homogeneous; at * a colourless corpuscle. *b.* Cells with extremely small, but well defined nuclei, and distinctly red contents. *c.* After the addition of acetic acid the nuclei are seen in some instances shrivelled and jagged, in several, double; at * a granular corpuscle. 280 diameters.

Fig. 52. Human blood-corpuscles from an adult. *a.* An ordinary disc-shaped, red blood-corpuscle; *b*, a colourless one; *c*, red corpuscles seen in profile, and standing upon their rims. *d.* Red corpuscles arranged in the form of rouleaux of money. *e.* Red corpuscles which have become irregular in outline, and shrivelled through loss of water (exosmosis). *f.* Shrivelled red corpuscles, with tuberculated margins, and a projection, like that produced by a nucleus, upon the flat surface of the disc. *g.* A still more shrivelled state. *h.* The highest degree of shrivelling (melanic corpuscles). Magnified 280 diameters.

by the action of chemical fluids, certain quantities of
water are abstracted from the corpuscles, and that they
then shrivel up and experience peculiar changes in form,
which might very easily give rise to errors. These are
not unimportant conditions, and I will therefore now add
a few words concerning them.

When a blood-corpuscle is exposed to a loss of water
by the action of a strongly concentrated liquid upon it,
the first thing we observe is that, as fast as fluid exudes,
little prominences arise on the surface of the corpuscle,
at first very much scattered, sometimes at the border,
sometimes more towards the middle, and in the latter
case, occasionally bearing a deceptive resemblance to a
nucleus (Fig. 52, *e*, *f*). This has been the source of the
erroneous assumption of nuclei, which have been so
much described. If a blood-corpuscle be watched for a
considerable time whilst under the action of concentrated
media, more and more protuberances are seen to arise,
and the surface of the corpuscle becomes less in diameter.
At the same time, little folds and knobs form with continually increasing distinctness on the surface, and the
cell becomes jagged, stellate, and angular (Fig. 52, *g*).
Jagged bodies of this sort are to be seen every moment
on examining blood which has been for some time exposed to the air. Even mere evaporation will produce
this change. We can effect it with great rapidity by
altering the composition of the serum by the addition of
salt or sugar. If the abstraction of water continue, the
corpuscle grows smaller still, and ultimately becomes
smooth again, and at the same time globular (Fig. 52, *h*),
or even perfectly spherical, whilst its colour appears
much more intense, and the contained mass assumes
quite a deep blackish-red hue. Hence we are able to
draw the not uninteresting conclusion, that this exosmosis consists essentially in a withdrawal of water, dur-

ing which perhaps one or more other matters pass out. as, for example, salt, but the essential constituents remain behind. The hæmatine does not follow the water ; the membrane of the blood-corpuscles keeps it back, so that when a large quantity of fluid is lost, the hæmatine in the interior must of course become proportionately increased in density.

The reverse is the case when we employ diluted fluids. The more diluted the fluid, the more does the blood-corpuscles enlarge ; it swells up and becomes paler. On treating blood-corpuscles, which have become smaller from the action of concentrated fluids, with water, we see them pass back from the globular into the angular form, and from this into the discoidal one ; after which they continually become more and more globular, often assume very peculiar shapes, and again grow paler. This process may, if the dilution of the blood be effected with great precaution, be continued until the blood-corpuscles scarcely seem to retain a trace of colour, though they still remain visible. In ordinary cases, when much liquid is added at once, such a violent revolution is produced in the economy of the blood-corpuscle, that an escape of the hæmatine immediately ensues. We then obtain a red solution, in which the colouring matter is free and dissolved in the fluid. I call your attention to this peculiarity, because it is continually occurring in the course of investigations, and because it explains one of the most important phenomena in the formation of pathological deposits of pigment, in which we meet with a precisely similar escape of hæmatine from the blood-corpuscles (Fig. 54, *a*). The expression generally made use of under such circumstances is, that the blood-corpuscles are dissolved, but it has long been a well-known fact that, as was first shown by Carl Heinrich Schultz, although there apparently no longer exist any cells, yet their membranes may, by means of an aqueous solution of iodine, again be rendered visible, whence it is evident that it was only the high degree of distension and the extraordinary thinness of the membranes which prevented the corpuscles from being seen. Indeed, very violent action on the part of substances chemically different is required, in order to effect a real destruction of the blood-corpuscles. If, immediately after they have been treated with a very concentrated solution of salt, water be added in large quantity, we may succeed in bringing things to such a pass that the contents of the corpuscles are abstracted without their swelling up, and their membranes remain behind visible. This was the reason why Denis and Lecanu asserted that the blood-corpuscles contained fibrine ; for they believed that, by treating them first with salt and then with water, they were able to demonstrate its presence in them. This so-called fibrine is, however, as I have shown, nothing more than the membranes of the blood-corpuscles ; real fibrine is not contained in them, although their walls are certainly composed of a substance which has more or less affinity to albuminous matters, and may, when obtained in large masses, present appearances reminding one of fibrine.

Now with regard to the substances contained in the blood-corpuscles, they happen quite recently to have become invested with great interest in consequence of the more morphological products which have been observed to arise out of them, and which have produced a kind of revolution in the whole theory of the nature of organic matters. I refer here to the peculiar forms of coloured crystals. which can, under certain circumstances, be obtained from the colouring matter of the blood, and which have acquired not only on their own account great chemical, but also very considerable practical, interest.

We have already become acquainted with three different kinds of *crystals*, of which hæmatine seems to be the common origin.

To the first form, with which I at one time busied myself much, I have given the name of *Hæmatoidine.* This is one of the most frequent of metamorphic products, and is spontaneously formed in the body out of hæmatine, and that indeed often in such large quantities that its excretion can be perceived with the naked eye. This substance in its perfect form presents itself in the shape of oblique rhombic columns, and is of a beatiful yellowish-red, or frequently, when in thicker pieces, deep rubyred, colour, and forms one of the most beautiful crystals we are acquainted with. In little plates too it is not uncommonly met with, and frequently bears a considerable resemblance to the crystalline forms of uric acid. In the majority of cases the crystals are very small,

Fig. 53.

not merely microscopical, but even somewhat difficult of observation with the microscope. A man must either be a very keen observer, or provided with special preparatory knowledge, else he will frequently discover in the spots where the hæmatoidine is lying nothing more than little streaks, or an apparently shapeless mass. But, upon more accurate inspection, the streaks resolve themselves into minute rhombic columns, the mass into an aggregation of crystals. This substance may be considered as the regular, typical, ultimate form into which hæmatine is converted in any part of the body where large masses of blood continue to lie for any length of time. An apoplectic effusion in the brain, for example, cannot be repaired by any other process than by a large portion of the blood undergoing this form of crystalliza-

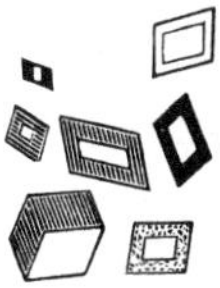

Fig. 53. Crystals of Hæmatoidine in different forms (Comp. 'Archiv. f. path. Anat.,' vol. i, p. 391, plate iii, fig. 11). Magnified 300 diameters.

tion, and if we afterwards find a coloured cicatrix at the spot, we may feel perfectly assured that the colour is dependent upon the presence of hæmatoidine. When a young woman menstruates, and the cavity of the Graafian vesicle, from which the ovum has been extruded, becomes filled with coagulated blood, the hæmatine is gradually converted into hæmatoidine, and we afterwards find at the spot where the ovum had lain, the beautiful deep-red colour of the hæmatoidine crystals, which remain as the last memorials of this episode. In this manner we can count the number of apoplectic attacks, or calculate how often a young girl has menstruated. Every extravasation may leave behind its little contingent of hæmatoidine crystals, and these, once formed,

Fig. 54.

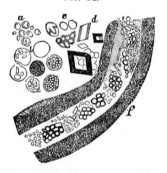

remain in the interior of the organ, in the shape of compact bodies endowed with the greatest powers of resistance.

With respect to the peculiarities of hæmatoidine, it has, in a theoretical point of view, another special claim to

Fig. 54. Pigment from an apoplectic cicatrix in the brain ('Archiv,' vol. i, pp. 401, 454, plate iii, fig. 7). *a*. Blood-corpuscles which have become granular and are in process of decolorization. *b*. Cells from the neuroglia, some of them provided with granular and crystalline pigment. *c*. Pigment-granules. *d*. Crystals of Hæmatoidine. *f*. Obliterated vessel with its former channel filled with granular and crystalline red pigment. 300 diameters.

our interest, from its presenting to us a series of properties, which render it conspicuous as the only substance in
the body, at least, that we are as yet acquainted with,
which is allied to the colouring matter of the bile (Cholepyrrhine). By the direct action of mineral acids, or after
previous treatment and preparation by means of alkalies,
the same, or precisely similar, colour-tests are obtained,
which are yielded by the colouring matter of the bile
when treated with mineral acids, and it seems also from
other facts, that we have here a body before us, which is
very intimately connected with the colouring matter of
the bile. This circumstance derives its especial interest
from its being supposed, for other reasons also, that the
coloured constituents of the bile are products of the decomposition of the red colouring matter of the blood.
In the interior of extravasations there really does arise a
yellowish red substance which may be designated as a
newly formed kind of biliary colouring matter.

The second kind of crystals which arise out of hema-
tine was discovered later; they are very similar to the
preceding ones, but differ from them in that they do not
occur as a spontaneous product in the body, but must be
artificially produced. They are more of a dark brownish

Fig. 55.

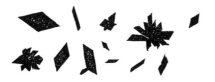

colour and usually form flat rhombic plates with more
acute angles; they are in an extraordinary degree capable of resisting tests, and also do not, when acted upon

Fig. 55. Crystals of Hæmine, artificially procured from human blood.   300 diameters.

by the mineral acids, exhibit the peculiar play of colours afforded by hæmatoidine. This second kind of crystals has received the name of *Hæmine* from their discoverer Teichmann. Quite recently Teichmann has himself begun to entertain doubts as to whether it is not really a sort of hæmatine. These forms do not present as yet the slightest pathological interest, but, on the other hand, they have proved of very great importance in forensic medicine on account of their having been recently employed as one of the surest tests for the examination of blood-stains. I myself have been in a position to make experiments of this sort in forensic cases. For this purpose the best mode of proceeding is to mix dried blood in as compact a form as possible with dry, crystallized, powdered common salt, and then to add to this mixture glacial acetic acid, and evaporate at a boiling heat. When this has been done, crystals of hæmine are found where the blood-corpuscles or the substance previously lay, in which the presence of hæmatine was doubtful. This is a reaction which must be ranked among the most certain and reliable ones with which we are acquainted. There is no other substance in which we know such a transformation to take place, but hæmatine. This test is extremely important, because it is applicable in the case of extremely minute quantities, only they must not be spread over too large a surface. It would therefore not be easy of application in a case where we had to deal with a cloth which had been dipped into a thin, watery, fluid coloured with blood. Yet I was able, in the case of a murdered man, on the sleeve of whose coat blood had spurted, and where some of the drops were only a line in diameter, from these minute specks to produce innumerable crystals of hæmine, though of course microscopical ones. In cases in which the ordinary chemical tests would necessarily absolutely fail on account of the smallness of the quantity, we are still able to obtain hæmine. When the mass of blood is so very small, the size of the crystals is certainly also extremely minute, and we then find, as in the case of hæmatoidine, small needles of an intensely brown colour and provided with acute angles.

The third substance which belongs to this series, is the so-called *Hæmato-crystalline*, a substance about the discovery of which the learned still dispute, for the simple reason that it was found out piecemeal. The first observation concerning it was made by Reichert in extravasations in the uterus of the guinea-pig, in a preparation which, I think, had already lain for some little time in spirits. This observation of his acquired especial significance because he showed that these crystals in certain respects behaved like organic substances, inasmuch as they became larger through the action of certain agencies, and smaller through that of others, without any change of form, a phenomenon which, up to that time, had not been known to take place in crystals. Afterwards these crystals were again discovered by Kölliker, but Funke, Kunde, and especially Lehmann, have examined them more closely. The result has been that they are very different in different classes of animals, but hitherto it has not been possible to discover any definite reason for their existence, or to obtain any insight into the nature of the substance itself. In man the crystals are tolerably large. At first it was believed that they only occurred in the blood of certain organs, but it has since turned out that they occur everywhere, though they are obtained with greater readiness in certain morbid conditions. In a few very rare cases it happens that they are found already formed in the blood of the dead bodies of animals. These crystals are very easily destructible ; both when they dry up and when they become moist, or are brought into contact with any fluid medium, they perish, and they are therefore only observed in certain transitional stages, which must be exactly hit upon, in the destruction of blood-corpuscles. The well-developed forms in man are perfectly rectangular bodies ; but very frequently they are extremely small, and nothing is seen but simple spicules which shoot up into the object at certain spots in large masses. There is besides this peculiarity about them, that they retain the property which hæmatine itself has of becoming bright red with oxygen and dark red with carbonic acid. It is still, however, a frequent subject of discussion whether their whole substance is composed of colouring matter, or whether in this case also the crystals are really colourless and merely impregnated with pigment ; this much, however, may be regarded as certain, that the colour has something very characteristic about it, and that the existence of a close connection between it and the ordinary colouring matter of the blood cannot be doubted.

If we now revert to the natural morphological elements of the blood, we meet with the *colourless corpuscles* as its third constituent. They are present in comparatively small quantity in the blood of a healthy man. To three hundred red corpuscles we reckon about one colourless one. As they generally present themselves in the blood, they are spherical corpuscles, which are sometimes a little larger, sometimes a little smaller than, or

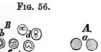

FIG. 56.

of the same size as, ordinary red blood-corpuscles, from which they are, however, strikingly distinguished by the want of all colour and by their perfectly spherical form.

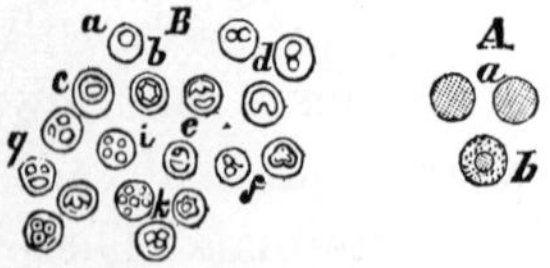

In a drop of blood which has become quiet, the red cor-

Fig. 56. Colourless blood-corpuscles from a vein of the pia-mater of a lunatic. *A.* Examined when fresh ; *a* in their natural fluid, *b* in water. *B.* After the addi-

puscles are usually found aggregated in rows, presenting the familiar form of rouleaux of money, with their flat discs one against the other (Fig. 52, *d*) ; in the interspaces may be observed here and there one of these pale, spherical bodies, in which in the first instance, when the blood is quite fresh, nothing more can be distinguished than an occasionally slightly granular-looking surface. If water be added, the colourless corpuscles are seen to swell up, and in proportion as they absorb the water, a membrane first becomes distinct ; then granular contents gradually come into view with more and more clearness, and at last some indication is perceived of the presence of one or several nuclei. The apparently homogeneous globule is gradually transformed into a structure with delicate walls, and often so fragile, that when water is incautiously added, the external parts begin to fall to pieces, and in the interior a somewhat granular mass displays itself, which becomes looser and looser, and discloses within it a nucleus generally in process of division, or several nuclei. These may be made to display themselves with much greater rapidity, by treating the object with acetic acid, which renders the membrane translucent, dissolves the nebulous contents, and causes the nucleus to coagulate and shrivel up. The nuclei then are seen to be dark bodies with sharply defined outlines, and one or more in number according to circumstances. In short, we obtain in this way in the majority of cases the view of an object which presents the peculiar appearance that one of our *confrères* now present, Dr. Güterbock, first proclaimed to be the special characteristic of pus-corpuscles. The question concerning the resemblance or want of re-

tion of acetic acid : *a—c*, cells with a single, granular nucleus, which becomes progressively larger, and is finally provided with a nucleolus. *d.* Simple division of the nuclei. *e.* A more advanced stage of the division. *f—h.* Gradual division of the nuclei into three parts. *i—k.* Four and more nuclei. 280 diameters.

semblance between the colourless cells of the blood and
pus-corpuscles still continues to occupy the attention of
observers, and it will probably still require a number of
years before the views entertained with regard to the
connection between the colourless corpuscles and pyæmia
have been rendered so clear that relapses on one side
or the other will not now and then recur. There is
namely this source of error, that upon examining a number of persons, in the blood of several among them corpuscles will be found which have only a single nucleus,
and that a very large one and not unfrequently provided
with a nucleolus, whilst in the blood of others no corpuscles will be seen which do not contain several nuclei.
Now, since these latter bear a great resemblance to pus-
corpuscles, those observers, who had previously chanced
to meet with nothing but uni-nuclear corpuscles in normal blood, cannot be blamed for believing, in another
case in which they see multi-nuclear ones, that they have
something essentially different before them, namely, pus-
corpuscles in the blood, and that the case is one of pyæmia. But, strange to say, the corpuscles with one nucleus form the exception, and you may look for a long
time without finding blood in which all the cells have
only one nucleus. Oddly enough to-day, while occupied in preparing the microscopical objects, I stumbled
upon a specimen of blood, in which scarcely
anything but cells with one nucleus are to be
met with, and these in extremely large number ; it was taken from a man who died of
smallpox, and in whom a very highly remarkable acute hyperplasia of the bronchial glands existed.

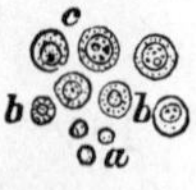

Now, one might be inclined to believe that these are

FIG. 57.

Fig. 57. Colourless blood-corpuscles in variolous leucocytosis. *a.* Free or naked
nuclei. *b, b.* Colourless cells with small, simple nuclei. *c.* Larger, colourless cells,
with large nuclei and nucleoli. 300 diameters.

different qualities of blood. But in opposition to such an idea it must be remarked, that, although in the cases in which the one or the other kind of corpuscles exist in large quantities, we have to deal with a pathological phenomenon, yet that, when we do not find such large quantities, we have before us only an earlier or a later stage of the development of the elements. For one and the same blood-corpuscle may, in the course of its life, have one or several nuclei, the one belonging to an earlier, the several to a later, stage of its existence. You must always bear in mind, that the change is seen to take place in the same individual in a short time, indeed often in the course of a few hours, so that in blood which had previously only contained one sort, afterwards quite a different one may be found—a proof of the rapidity of the change to which these bodies are subjected.

Allow me, gentlemen, to add a few words with regard to the more palpable relations which the individual constituents of the blood present towards one another. It is, as you well know, generally assumed that of the morphological constituents only two are accessible to the grosser perception of the naked eye, namely, the red corpuscles in the clot, and the masses of fibrine, which under certain circumstances form a buffy coat, but that, on the other hand, the colourless cells are not to be perceived by the unaided sight. This is a notion which I consider myself bound to correct. The colourless corpuscles, whenever they are present in considerable numbers, become very distinctly manifest to the more practised eye during the separation of the constituents of the blood, and especially when the coagulation is accompanied by movement; and they then exhibit a peculiarity, with which it is as well that one should be acquainted when one is required to pass judgment upon specimens derived from post-mortem examinations, and the ignorance of which has led to great errors. The colourless corpuscles possess namely, as was brought to light in the discussion which Herr Ascherson, now here present, had some time ago with E. H. Weber, the peculiar property

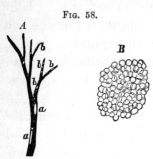

FIG. 58.

of being sticky, so that they readily adhere to one another, and under certain circumstances also cling fast to other parts, when the red corpuscles do not present this phenomenon. This tendency to adhere to other parts is particularly evident when several of the corpuscles are at the same time placed in a position which enables them to stick together. Thus, in blood in which there is an actual increase in the number of colourless cells, it is extremely common for agglutinations to take place among them, as soon as the pressure, under which the blood flows, is diminished ; in every vessel, in which the stream becomes slower, and the pressure weaker, an agglutination of the corpuscles may take place.

The adhesiveness (viscosity) of the colourless blood-corpuscles produces besides this effect, that, as has been shown by Herr Ascherson, when the blood is flowing as usual through the capillary vessels, the colourless corpuscles generally float rather more slowly than the red, and that, whilst these move along more in the centre of the vessel in a continuous stream, a comparatively large vacuity is left at the circumference, within which the

Fig. 58. *A.* Fibrine clot from the pulmonary artery, and corresponding to its terminal branches ; at *a, a* beset with largish patches, composed of heaps of white cells ; at *b, b, b* with specks of an analogous nature. Natural size.

B. A portion of one of these specks or heaps, composed of thickly crowded, colourless blood-corpuscles. Magnified 280 diameters.

colourless corpuscles move, and that indeed often with such constancy, that Weber came to the conclusion that every capillary lay within a lymphatic vessel, in the inside of which the colourless blood- or lymph-corpuscles floated.   But there cannot be the least doubt but that the canals in question are single ones, in which the colourless corpuscles float along closer to the walls than the red ones ; and it is in this peripheral space that, whilst the corpuscles move on, we see one here and there stick fast for a moment, then tear itself away and again move on slowly, so that the name of the *slug-gish layer* (träge Schicht), applied to this part of the stream, has been universally adopted.

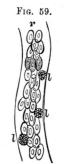

FIG. 59.

These two peculiarities, first, that, when the current becomes weaker, the corpuscles here and there cling to the walls of the vessel, and in some measure adhere to them, and, secondly, that they gather together and become conglomerated into largish masses, combine to produce this effect, that, when there exists a large number of colourless corpuscles in the blood, and death occurs, as it does in ordinary cases, after a gradual weakening of the propelling force, the colourless corpuscles collect in vessels of every description, into small heaps, and generally lie upon the outside of the later formed blood-clot.

If, for example, we pull out of the pulmonary artery the generally very tough clot of blood which fills it, minute granules will perchance be found upon its surface (Fig. 58, *A*), little beads of a white colour, which look like specks of pus, or are connected several of them toge-ther in the form of a string of pearls.   This appearance

Fig. 59. Capillary vessel from the web of a frog's foot.   *r*. The central stream of red corpuscles.   *l, l, l*. The sluggish, peripheral layer of the stream with the colourless corpuscles.   Magnified 280 diameters.

most frequently presents itself at those points where the number of the bodies is normally the largest, namely in the interval between the orifice of the thoracic duct, and the capillaries of the lungs. The naked eye can with tolerable ease detect in these clots the greater or less quantity of colourless corpuscles. Under circumstances inducing the presence of a very large number of them, whole heaps of them may be seen, investing different parts of the coagulum like a sheath, and if one of these heaps be placed under the microscope, many thousands of colourless corpuscles are seen crowded together.

If the coagulation of the blood takes place, when it is more at rest, another appearance is presented with great distinctness, as may be seen in the vessels used to receive the blood after venæsection. When the fibrine does not coagulate very quickly, as is the case in inflammatory blood, the blood-corpuscles begin, in consequence of their greater specific gravity, to sink through the fluid. This subsidence proceeds, as is well known, to such a pitch, that, after the fibrine has been removed by stirring, the serum becomes perfectly clear, in consequence of the corpuscles' falling to the bottom. On defibrinating blood rich in colourless corpuscles, and allowing it to stand, a double sediment forms, a red and a white one. The red one constitutes the deeper, the white one the more superficial stratum, and the latter looks exactly as if a layer of pus were lying upon the blood. When the blood has not been deprived of its fibrine, yet coagulates slowly, the subsidence of the corpuscles does not take place so completely, but only the highest part of the liquor sanguinis becomes free from corpuscles ; and when after this the fibrine coagulates, we obtain the well-known *crusta phlogistica*, the *buffy coat*, and on looking for the colourless corpuscles, we find them forming a separate layer at the lower border of the buffy coat. This peculiarity is simply explained by the different specific gravity of the two kinds of blood-corpuscles. The colourless ones are always light, poor in solid matter and very delicate in structure, whilst the red ones are as heavy as lead in comparison, owing to their richness in hæmatine. They therefore reach the bottom with comparatively great rapidity, whilst the colourless ones are still engaged in falling. If two bodies of different specific gravities be allowed to fall from a sufficient height in the open air, the lighter one will, you know, in a similar manner, reach the ground after the other, owing to the resistance of the air.

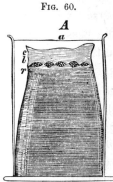

Fig. 60.

In the coagulation which takes place in blood derived from venæsection, this white clot does not usually form a continuous, but an interrupted, layer, composed of little heaps or nodules adhering to the under side of the buffy coat. Hence Piorry, who was the first to observe this appearance, but completely misinterpreted it, seeing that he referred it to an inflammation of the blood itself (Hæmitis) and established the doctrine of Pyæmia, upon it, termed this form of buffy coat *crusta granulosa*. It really consists of nothing more than large accumulations of colourless corpuscles.

Under all circumstances this layer resembles pus in appearance, and since, as we have already seen, the colourless blood-cells individually are constituted like pus-corpuscles, you see that we are liable not only in the case of a healthy person to take colourless blood-cells for

Fig. 60. Diagram of a bleeding-glass with coagulated hyperinotic blood. *a.* The level of the liquor sanguinis. *c.* The cup-shaped buffy coat. *l.* The layer of lymph (Cruor lymphaticus, Crusta granulosa), with the granular and mulberry-like accumulations of colourless corpuscles. *r.* The red clot.

pus-corpuscles, but still more so in pathological conditions when the blood or other parts are full of these elements. You can imagine how apt the question is to
present itself, which has already been seriously raised by
Addison and Zimmermann, whether pus-corpuscles are
not merely extravasated colourless blood-cells, or *vice
versâ*, whether the colourless blood-cells found within
the vessels are not pus-corpuscles which have been admitted into them from the exterior. We are here called
upon for the first time to make the practical application
of the principles which I laid down with regard to the
specific nature and heterology of elements (p. 92.) A
pus-corpuscle can be distinguished from a colourless
blood-cell by nothing else than its mode of origin. If
you do not know whence it has come, you cannot say
what it is ; you may conceive the greatest doubt as to
whether you are to regard a body of the kind as a pus-
or a colourless blood-corpuscle. In every case of the
sort the points to be considered are, where the body
belongs to, and where its home is. If this prove to be
external to the blood, you may safely conclude that it is
pus ; but if this is not the case, you have to do with
blood-cells.

LECTURE VIII.

MARCH 10, 1858.

BLOOD AND LYMPH.

Change and replacement of the constituents of the blood—*Fibrine*—Lymph and its
coagulation—Lymphatic exudation—Fibrinogenous substance—Formation of
the buffy coat—Lymphatic blood, hyperinosis, phlogistic crasis—Local formation of fibrine—Transudation of fibrine—Formation of fibrine in the blood.
Colourless blood-corpuscles (lymph-corpuscles)—Their increase in hyperinosis and
hypinosis (Erysipelas, pseudo-erysipelas, typhoid fever)—Leucocytosis and
leukæmia—Splenic and lymphatic leukæmia.
The spleen and lymphatic glands as blood-making organs—Structure of lymphatic
glands.

THE last time, gentlemen, I introduced to your notice
the individual morphological elements of the blood, and
endeavored to portray their special peculiarities. Allow
me to begin to-day with a few words concerning their
origin.

From the facts which have been ascertained with
regard to the first development of the elements of the
blood, important conclusions may be drawn respecting
the nature of the changes which take place in the mass
of the blood in deceased conditions. Formerly the blood
was regarded more as a juice shut up by itself, which
was indeed to a certain extent connected with the parts
external to it, but yet was in itself endowed with real
durability, and it was assumed that it could retain pecu-

liar properties for lengthened periods, nay, that these might cling to it for many years. Of course it was impossible at the same time to entertain the opinion, that the constituents of the blood were of a perishable nature, and that new elements were added to it, to replace the old ones. For the durability of a part as such presupposes either that all its individual particles are durable, or that these individual particles are continually producing fresh ones within the part which bear impressed upon them all the peculiarities of the old ones. In the case of the blood, therefore, one would have to assume that its constituents really did subsist for years, and could for years present the same changes, or one would have to imagine that the blood transmitted something from one particle to another, and that from a parent blood-cell to its progeny something hereditary was handed down. Of these possibilities the former has, I believe, at the present time been pretty generally discarded. No one, I think, now imagines that the individual constituents of the blood last on for years. On the other hand, the possibility that the corpuscles of the blood are renewed by propagation, and that certain peculiarities which are introduced into the blood at a certain time, are transmitted from corpuscle to corpuscle, cannot straightway be rejected. But the only phenomena pointing to such a propagation of the blood, concerning which we possess any positive information, belong to an early period of embryonic life. There it appears from observations which were only the other day again confirmed by Remak, the existing blood-corpuscles undergo direct division, the process being that, in a corpuscle which during the early stages of its development had displayed itself as a nucleated cell, first of all a partition of the nucleus takes place (Fig. 51, c) ; and that then the whole cell becomes constricted in the middle, and gradually is really seen to pass into a state of complete division. At this early period it is therefore certainly allowable to regard a blood-corpuscle as endowed with qualities which are propagated from the first series of cells to the second, and from this to the third, and so on.

In the blood of a fully developed human being, nay even in that of a fœtus in the later months of pregnancy, these phenomena of partition are no longer known, and not a single one of the facts which can be adduced from the history of development speaks in favour of an increase of the cellular elements taking place in fully developed blood by means of direct division, or any other formative process taking its rise in the blood itself. As long as the possibility was regarded as demonstrated, that cells might arise out of simple cytoblastema by means of the direct precipitation of different substances, so long was it possible to conceive new precipitates as forming in the liquor sanguinis from which cells were produced. But this view also has been abandoned. All the morphological elements of the blood, whatever may be their nature, are at present considered to be derived from sources external to the blood. On all hands recourse is had to organs which do not communicate with the blood directly, but rather by the means of intermediate channels. The principal organs which here come into play are the lymphatic glands. *Lymph* is the fluid which, whilst it conveys certain substances to the blood which come from the tissues, at the same time brings along with it the corpuscular elements out of which the blood-cells continually recruit their numbers.

With regard to two of the constituents of the blood, there can, I think, be scarcely any doubt but that this is the view which is perfectly warranted, I mean with regard to the fibrine and the colourless corpuscles. As for the fibrine, the properties of which I brought to your notice last time, it is a very essential and important fact that the fibrine which circulates in lymph differs in certain respects from that contained in the blood, which we see on examining different extravasations, or blood drawn from a vein. The fibrine of lymph has this special peculiarity, that under ordinary circumstances it coagulates within the lymphatic vessel neither during life nor after death, whilst blood in many instances coagulates even during life, and regularly does so after death, so that coagulative power is attributed to blood as being one of its regular properties. In the lymphatics of a dead animal or human corpse, no coagulated lymph is met with, yet the coagulation takes place directly the lymph is brought into contact with the air, or has changes imparted to it by some diseased organ.

The explanation of this peculiarity has been attempted in very different ways. For my own part I must still adhere to the view that there is, properly speaking, no perfectly developed fibrine contained in lymph, but that it becomes perfect either by contact with the atmospheric air, or in abnormal conditions by the introduction into it of altered matters. Normal lymph contains a substance which is very readily converted into fibrine, and is, when it has once coagulated, scarcely to be distinguished from fibrine, but which, as long as it continues to circulate with the ordinary stream of lymph, cannot be regarded as really perfect fibrine. This is a substance, of which I had demonstrated the presence in various exudations, especially in pleuritic fluids, long before my attention had been drawn to its occurrence in lymph.

In many forms of pleurisy the exudation long remains fluid, and a number of years ago a peculiar case came under my notice, in which on puncturiug the thorax a liquid was evacuated which was perfectly clear and fluid, but in a short time after its evacuation had its whole mass pervaded by a coagulum, as is often enough the case with fluids from the abdominal cavity. After I had removed this coagulum from the liquid by stirring it, in order to convince myself of its identity with ordinary fibrine, the next day a fresh coagulum displayed itself, and this took place also on the following days. This coagulative power lasted fourteen days, although the operation had been performed in the midst of the heat of summer. This therefore was a phenomenon essentially differing from the ordinary coagulation of the blood, and somewhat difficult to explain upon the supposition that real fibrine existed completely developed in the fluid, but it seemed to indicate that it was only under the influence of the atmospheric air that the fibrine was produced from a substance which must indeed have been nearly related to fibrine, but yet could not be real fibrine. I therefore propose to give it the distinctive name of *fibrinogenous* substance, and when I afterwards had come to the conclusion that it was the same substance which we find in lymph, I was enabled to extend my view so as to include the proposition, that in lymph also fibrine is not contained in a perfect form.

This same substance, which is distinguished from ordinary fibrine by its requiring to be a longer or shorter time in contact with atmospheric air before it can become coagulable, is also found under certain circumstances in the blood of the peripheral veins, so that even by an ordinary venæsection performed on the arm blood may be obtained, distinguished from ordinary blood by the slowness of its coagulation. Polli named this coagulative substance *brady-fibrine*. Such cases occur especially in inflammatory diseases of the respiratory organs, and most frequently give rise to the formation of a *buffy coat* (crusta pleuritica, crusta phlogistica). You all know that the ordinary crusta phlogistica forms in the blood of

pneumonia or pleurisy the more readily the greater the
wateriness of the liquor sanguinis, and the poorer the blood
is in solid constituents, but it is an essential requisite that
the fibrine should coagulate slowly. If the duration of
the process be noted watch in hand, the conviction will
soon be acquired that a very much longer time passes
than is requisite for ordinary coagulation. From this
frequent phenomenon, as it is met with in the ordinary
formation of a crust upon the surface of inflamed blood,
gradual transitions are observed to a greatly increased
prolongation of the period during which fluidity is retained.

The most extreme instance of this kind as yet known
occurred in a case observed by Polli. In a vigorous man,
suffering from pneumonia, who came under treatment in
the summer, at a time which does not offer the external
conditions most favourable to slowness of coagulation, the
blood, which flowed from the opened vein, took a week
before it began to coagulate, and not until the end of a
fortnight was the coagulation complete. In this case,
too, occurred the other phenomenon which I had observed in the pleuritic exudations, namely, that decomposition (putrefaction) took place in the blood at an
unusally late period in proportion to this lateness of
coagulation.

Now since phenomena of this kind are observed to
occur with especial frequency in chest affections, a frequency so especial indeed that the buffy coat was long
since designated *Crusta pleuritica*, there would seem to
be some grounds for inferring from this, that the function
of respiration has a definite influence upon the occurrence or non-occurrence of the fibrinogenous substance
in the blood. At all events, the peculiarity possessed by
the lymph is under certain circumstances transmitted to
the blood, so that either the whole of the blood partakes

of it, and that in a higher degree, the greater the disturbance under which the respiration labours; or, in addition to the ordinary, quickly coagulating matter, a second which coagulates more slowly is found. It frequently happens, namely, that two sorts of coagulation subsist side by side in the same blood, one early and the other late, especially in the cases in which direct analysis shows an increase of fibrine, a *hyperinosis*. These hyperinotic conditions appear therefore to indicate that in them an increased supply of lymphatic fluid is introduced into the blood, and that the matters which are afterwards found in the blood are not the products of an internal transformation of its constituents, and that therefore the original source of the fibrine must not be sought for in the blood itself, but in those parts from which the lymphatic vessels convey the increased supply of fibrine.

In explanation of these phenomena, I have ventured to advance the hypothesis, somewhat bold perhaps, though I consider it perfectly able to sustain discussion, namely, that *fibrine generally, wherever it occurs in the body external to the blood, is not to be regarded as an excretion from the blood, but as a local production;* and I have endeavored to introduce an important change in the views entertained with regard to the so-called phlogistic crasis in relation to its localization. Whilst it had previously been the custom to regard the altered composition of the blood in inflammation as a condition existing from the very outset, and especially denoted by a primary increase in the fibrine, I on the contrary have shown the crasis to be an occurrence dependent upon the local inflammation. Certain organs and tissues have inherent in them in a higher degree the power of producing fibrine and of favouring the occurrence of large quantities of fibrine in the blood, whilst other organs are by far less adapted for its production.

I have, moreover, pointed out the fact, that those organs which with especial frequency exhibit this peculiar
combination of a so-called phlogistic state of the blood
with a local inflammation are generally abundantly provided with lymphatic vessels and connected with large
masses of lymphatic glands, whilst all those organs which
either contain very few lymphatics, or in which these
vessels are scarcely known to exist, do not exercise any
influence worth naming upon the amount of fibrine in
the blood.   Former observers had already remarked
that there were inflammations occurring in very important organs, as for example, in the brain, in which the
phlogistic crasis was, properly speaking, not at all met
with.   Now it is precisely in the brain that we have
scarcely any evidence of the existence of lymphatics. In
those cases, on the contrary, in which the composition of
the blood is earliest altered, namely, in diseases of the
respiratory organs, we find an unusually abundant network of lymphatics.   Not merely the lungs are pervaded
by, and covered with, them, but the pleura also has extremely numerous connections with the lymphatic system, and the bronchial glands constitute almost the greatest accumulations of lymphatic-gland substance possessed
by an organ in the whole body.

On the other hand, we are acquainted with no fact
which shows it to be possible that, in consequence of a
simple increase of the pressure of the blood, or of a
simple change in the conditions which influence its circulation, an exudation of fibrinous fluids could in any
organ take place into its parenchyma, or upon its surface, from the blood.   It is certainly generally imagined
that, when the current of the blood attains a certain
strength, fibrine begins to appear in the exudation, but
this has never been proved by experiment.   Nobody has
ever been able, by the production of a mere change in

the force of the current of the blood, to induce the fibrine to transude directly as it is wont to do in certain inflammatory processes; for this some irritation is always required. The greatest obstructions may be induced in the circulation, exudations of serous fluids may be experimentally produced upon the largest scale, but that peculiar fibrinous exudation which the irritation of certain tissues provokes with so much ease, never ensues upon these occasions.

That the fibrine in the blood itself is produced by a transformation of the albumen, is a chemical theory, which has no other evidence in its favour than the fact that albumen and fibrine have a strong chemical resemblance, and that, on comparing the questionable formula for fibrine with the equally questionable one for albumen, it is very easy to imagine how, by the abstraction of a couple of atoms, the transition from albumen to fibrine might be effected. But our being able in this manner to deduce one of the formulæ from the other does not afford the slightest proof that an analogous transformation occurs in the blood. It may possibly take place in the body, but even then it would at any rate be more probable that it was accomplished in the tissues, and that from them the fibrine was conveyed away into the blood by means of the lymph. This is, however, the more doubtful, because rational formulæ for the chemical composition of albumen and fibrine have not yet been determined, and the incredibly high atomic numbers in the empirical formulæ point to a very complex grouping of the atoms.

Let us therefore hold fast the well-ascertained fact that fibrine can only be made to exude upon any surface by the occurrence of some irritation, that is, local change, in addition to the disturbance in the circulation. This local change, however, is, as results from experiment, alone sufficient to cause the exudation of fibrine, even when no obstruction arises in the circulation. Such obstruction is not therefore in any way needed in order that the production of fibrine may commence at any given point. On the contrary, we see that the cause of the greatest differences in the nature of exudations is to be found in the special constitution of the irritated parts. On the simple application of an irritating substance to the surface of the skin, there arises, when the irritation, whether chemical or mechanical in its nature, is only slight in degree, a vesicle, a serous exudation. If the irritation is more violent, a liquid exudes, which in the vesicle appears quite fluid, but coagulates after its evacuation. If the fluid from a blister raised by a cantharides-plaster be received into a watch-glass and exposed to the air, a coagulum forms, showing that there is fibrinogenous substance in the fluid. But we sometimes meet with conditions of the body, in which an external stimulus is sufficient for the production of blisters containing a fluid which directly coagulates. I had, last winter, a patient in my wards, whose feet had remained in a state of anæsthesia ever since they had been frozen, and I employed as a remedy, amongst other things, local baths containing aqua regia. After a certain number of these baths, blisters, which varied in diameter up to two inches, and were found, when opened, to be filled with large, jelly-like masses of coagulum, formed upon every occasion on the anæsthetic part of the soles of the feet. In other persons probably ordinary blisters would have formed, containing a fluid, which would not have coagulated until after its evacuation. Such a difference manifestly depends upon a difference, not in the composition of the blood, but in the disposition of the part affected. The difference between that form of pleurisy, which from its very commencement furnishes coagulable and coagulating fluids, and that in which the exudation is coagulable, but not coagulating, certainly points to peculiarities in the local irritation.

I do not think therefore that we are entitled to conclude that in a person who has an excess of fibrine in his blood, there is on that account also a greater tendency to fibrinous transudation ; on the contrary, I should rather expect that in a patient who produces at a certain point a large quantity of fibrine-forming substance, much of it would pass from that point into the lymph and finally into the blood. The exudation may therefore in such cases be regarded as the surplus of the fibrine formed *in loco*, for the removal of which the lymphatic circulation did not suffice. As long as the current of lymph does suffice, all the foreign matters which are formed in the irritated part are conveyed into the blood ; but, as soon as the local production becomes excessive, the products accumulate, and in addition to the hyperinosis, a local accumulation of fibrinous exudation will also take place. On account of the shortness of the time which is allotted to us, we cannot follow up this subject in its whole extent, but still I hope that you will at least completely grasp the fundamental idea which has guided me. Here, too, we have another example of that dependence of a dyscrasia upon a local disease to which I but a short time ago called your attention as being the most important result of all our investigations concerning the blood.

Now it is a very remarkable fact, and one which adds weight to this very view of mine, that it is *very rarely that a considerable increase of fibrine takes place without a simultaneous increase in the colourless blood-corpuscles*, and that therefore the two essential constituents which we find in the lymph we again meet with in the blood. In every case of hyperinosis we may rely upon discovering an increase in the colourless corpuscles, or, in other words, every irritation of a part, which is abundantly provided with lymphatics, and freely connected with lymphatic glands, occasions also the introduction of large numbers of colourless cells (lymph-corpuscles) into the blood.

This fact is especially interesting, inasmuch as you will perceive from it, that not only organs richly provided with lymphatic vessels can occasion this increase, but that certain processes also are more calculated than others to lead to the introduction of considerable quantities of these elements into the blood, namely all those which are early conjoined with serious disease in the lymphatic system. If you compare an erysipelatous, or a diffuse phlegmonous (according to Rust pseudo-erysipelatous), inflammation in its effects upon the blood with a simple superficial inflammation of the skin, such as occurs in the course of the ordinary acute exanthemata, or after traumatic or chemical irritation, you will at once see how great the difference is. Every erysipelatous or diffuse phlegmonous inflammation has the peculiarity of early affecting the lymphatic vessels and producing swellings in the lymphatic glands. In such a case we may feel assured that an increase in the number of the colourless corpuscles is taking place. Further, we find the significant fact, that there are certain processes which simultaneously cause an increase of fibrine and colourless corpuscles, and others again which only occasion an increased production of the latter. To this latter category belong the whole series of simple diffuse inflammations of the skin, in which also no considerable formation of fibrine takes place in the diseased parts. On the other hand, a number of conditions belong to it, which with regard to the quantity of fibrine may be designated as *hypinotical*, all the processes namely which belong to the typhoid class, and agree in producing considerable swelling now of one, and now of another, kind in the lymphatic glands, but do not produce any local exudation of fibrine. Thus typhoid fever causes these changes not only in the spleen, but also in the mesenteric glands.

The condition in which the increased proportion of colourless corpuscles in the blood appears to be dependent upon an affection of the lymphatic glands, I have designated by the name of *Leucocytosis*. Now you know that another matter has long been the subject of my studies, the affection named by me *Leukæmia*, and our next business must be to determine how far genuine leukæmia differs from these leucocytotical conditions. In the very first cases of leukæmia which came before me, a very essential property was discovered to exist, namely, that there was no essential variation in the proportion of fibrine in the blood. Afterwards it was found out that the proportion of fibrine might, according to the particular circumstances of the case, be greater or less than, or the same as, usual, but that a continually augmenting increase of the colourless blood-corpuscles invariably took place ; and that the coincidence of this increase with a diminution in the number of the coloured (red) corpuscles became more and more marked, so that as a final result a condition was attained, in which the number of the colourless corpuscles was almost equal to that of the red ones, and striking phenomena were displayed, even when the coarser modes of observation were employed. Whilst in ordinary blood we can seldom count more than one colourless corpuscle to about three hundred coloured ones, there are cases of leukæmia in which the increase of the colourless ones reaches such a height, that to every three red corpuscles there is one colourless one, or even two ; or in which indeed the greater numbers are in favour of the colourless corpuscles.

In dead bodies the increase in the colourless corpuscles generally appears more considerable than it really is, from reasons which I but a short time ago pointed out to you (p. 184) ; for these corpuscles possess extraordinary adhesiveness and accumulate in considerable masses wherever there is a retardation in the stream of blood, so that in the dead body the greatest number is always found in the right heart.   Once, before I left Berlin, this singular case occurred to me, that, when I punctured the right auricle, the physician who had treated the case cried out, astonished, " Why, there's an abscess there !" So like pus did the blood appear.   This puriform condition of the blood does not indeed pervade the entire circulating stream ; the whole of the blood never looks like pus, because a comparatively large number of red corpuscles always continues to exist ; still it sometimes happens that blood flowing from a vein even during life exhibits whitish streaks, and that, when the fibrine has been removed by stirring, and the defibrinated blood is allowed to stand, a voluntary separation at once takes place, the whole of the blood-corpuscles, red and colourless, gradually sinking to the bottom of the vessel, and there forming a double sediment, a lower red stratum, covered by an upper, white and puriform one.   This is explained by the difference in the specific gravity of the two kinds of corpuscles and the time they take to sink (p. 186).   In this way too we are enabled very readily to distinguish leukæmic from chylous (lipæmic) blood in which a milky appearance of the liquor sanguinis is produced by the admixture of fat, for, if the fibrine be removed, after some time there forms not a white sediment, but a cream-like layer on the surface.

In the histories of all the known cases of leukæmia we only find it once as yet recorded that the patient, after he had been for some time the subject of medical treatment, left the hospital considerably improved in health.

In all the other cases the result was death. I do not wish by any means to infer from this that the disease in question is absolutely incurable ; I hope on the contrary that for it too remedies will at length be discovered ; but it is certainly a very important fact that we have in it, much, as in the progressive atrophy of muscles, to deal with conditions, which, when abandoned to themselves, or subjected to any one of the hitherto known methods of treatment, continually grow worse and ultimately lead to death. These cases possess, in addition, the remarkable peculiarity that, usually towards the close of life, a genuine *hæmorrhagic diathesis* is developed and hæmorrhages ensue, which occur with especial frequency in the nasal cavity (under the form of exhausting epistaxis) but may also, under certain circumstances, take place in other parts of the body, as for example on a very large scale in the form of apoplectic clots in the brain, or of melæna in the intestinal canal.

Now, upon investigating whence this curious change in the blood takes its origin, we find in the great majority of cases that it is a certain, definite organ which presents itself over and over again with convincing constancy as the one essentially diseased, an organ which frequently, even at the outset of the malady, forms the chief object of the complaints and distress of the patients, namely, the *spleen*. In addition, a number of lymphatic glands are very frequently diseased, but the affection of the spleen stands in the foreground. Only in a few cases have I found the change in the spleen the less and that in the lymphatic glands the more prominent, and in these, matters had proceeded to such a pitch, that lymphatic glands, at other times scarcely observable, had developed themselves into lumps the size of walnuts, and that indeed in some few places there appeared to be scarcely anything else than glandular substance. Of the

glands which lie between the inguinal and lumbar glands
we are wont to hear but little, nor have they indeed even
a suitable name.   Some of them lie in the course of the
iliac vessels, and some in the real pelvis.   But in two of
these cases of leukæmia I found them so enlarged that
the whole cavity of the pelvis proper was, as at were,
stuffed full of glandular substance, between which the
rectum and the bladder only just dipped in.

I have therefore distingushed two forms of leukæmia,
namely, the *ordinary splenic*, and the *lymphatic, form*,
which are certainly not unfrequently combined.   The
distinction rests not only upon the circumstance, that in
the one case the spleen, in the other the lymphatic glands,
constitute the starting point of the disease, but also upon
the fact that the characteristic morphological elements
which are found in the blood are not precisely similar.
Whilst namely in the splenic forms these elements are
generally comparatively large and perfectly developed
cells with one or more nuclei, and in many cases bear a
particularly great resemblance to the cells of the spleen,
we notice in the well-marked lymphatic forms that the
cells are small, the nuclei large in proportion and single,
usually sharply defined, with dark outlines and somewhat
granular, whilst the cell-wall is frequently in such close
apposition to them that an interval can scarcely be demonstrated.   In many instances it looks as if perfectly
free nuclei were contained in the blood.   In these (the
lymphatic) cases, therefore, it seems that the enlargement of the glands alone, which is accompanied in its
progress by a real increase in the number of their elements (hyperplasia), also conveys a larger number of cellular elements into the lymph and through this into the
blood, and that, just in proportion to the predominance
of these elements, the formation of the red cells suffers
obstruction.   This is in a few words the history of these

processes. Leukæmia is thus a sort of permanent, progressive leucocytosis, whilst this on the other hand in its simple forms constitutes a transitory process, connected with fluctuating conditions in certain organs.

You see therefore that there are at least three different conditions here, bordering one upon the other : hyperinosis, leucocytosis and leukæmia, between which and the lymphatic fluids there exists an intimate connection. The one series, that namely which is distinguished by an increase in the quantity of fibrine, is rather to be referred to the accidental condition of the organs from which the lymphatic fluids are derived, whilst those states which are induced by an increase in the number of cellular elements are rather regulated by the condition of the glands through which these fluids have flowed. These facts can hardly, I think, be interpreted in any other manner than by supposing that the spleen and lymphatic glands are really intimately concerned in the development of the blood. This has become still more probable since we have succeeded in obtaining chemical evidence also in support of it. Herr Scherer upon two occasions examined leukæmic blood which I had submitted to him, in order to compare it with the matters he had discovered in the spleen, and the result was that hypoxanthine, leucine, uric, lactic, and formic, acid, were found there. In one case of leukæmia a liver which I had kept for several days became entirely covered with granules of tyrosine ; in another, leucine and tyrosine crystallized in large masses out of the contents of the intestines. In short, everything points to an increased action in the spleen, which normally contains these substances in considerable quantity.

A good many years elapsed (after 1845) during which I found myself pretty nearly alone in my views. It has only been by degrees and indeed, as I am sorry to be obliged to confess, in consequence rather of physiological than pathological considerations, that people have come round to these ideas of mine, and only gradually have their minds proved accessible to the notion, that in the ordinary course of things the lymphatic glands and the spleen are really immediately concerned in the production of the formed elements of the blood ; and that in particular the corpuscular constituents of this fluid are really descendants of the cellular bodies of the lymphatic glands and the spleen which have been set free in their interior and conveyed into the current of the blood. And let this serve as an introduction to the consideration of the question of the origin of the blood-corpuscles themselves.

You will probably recollect, gentlemen, from the time of your studies, that the lymphatic glands used to be regarded as coils of lymphatic vessels. The afferent lymphatics may, as is well known, even with the naked eye be seen breaking up into smaller branches, disappearing within the glands, and finally again emerging from them. From the results of the mercurial injections which even in the last century were made with such great care, the only inference to be drawn appeared to be, that the afferent lymphatic vessel formed a number of convolutions, which interlaced in various ways and were finally continued into the efferent vessel, so that the gland was composed of nothing else than the thickly crowded coils of the afferent vessels. The whole attention of modern histologists has been directed to the task of confirming this tortuous transit of the lymphatic vessels through the gland, but after many years of labour spent in vain, the attempt was at length abandoned.

At the present moment there is, I should suppose, scarcely an histologist who believes in the perfect continuity of the lymphatic vessels throughout the gland, but

Kölliker's view is generally adopted, that the lymphatic glands interrupt the current of the lymph, the afferent vessel resolving itself into the parenchyma of the gland and reconstituting itself out of it. This condition we cannot well compare with anything else than a kind of filtering apparatus, something like our ordinary sand or charcoal filters.

When a gland is cut across, a structure is frequently brought to view resembling that of a kidney. At those points where the afferent vessels break up, a firmer substance is seen to lie, half surrounded by which a kind of hilus marks the spot at which the lymphatic vessels again forsake the gland. Here there is found a reticular tissue with an often distinctly areolar or cavernous structure, into which, besides the efferent lymphatic vessels, blood-vessels also enter on their way into the proper substance of the gland. Kölliker has accordingly distinguished a cortical and a medullary substance ; but the so-called medullary substance scarcely retains the character of glandular tissue. This is found chiefly in the cortical substance, which is of greater or less thickness, and it is therefore best to call the medullary substance simply the hilus, since afferent and efferent vessels lie there in close contact, just as in the hilus of the kidneys the ureters and veins emerge, whilst the arteries enter. The essential part of the gland is therefore the periphery, the often kidney-like cortical substance.

In this can be distinguished, whenever the gland is at all well developed (and in some cases of pathological en-largement it is extremely distinct) even with the naked eye, little, roundish, white or grey granules lying side by side. When the part is moderately well filled with blood, around each granule may be pretty nearly always discerned a red circle of vessels. These granules have long been called *follicles*, but it was doubtful whether they were distinct formations or mere convolutions of the lymphatic vessel protruding on the surface.

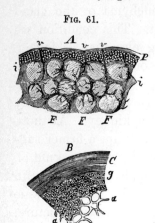

FIG. 61.

Upon more delicate microscopical examination, the proper (glandular) substance of the follicles can easily be distinguished from the fibrous meshwork (stroma) which bounds them on all sides, and is externally continuous with the connective tissue of the capsule. The internal substance is chiefly composed of little cellular elements, which lie pretty loosely, being merely enclosed in a fine network of star-shaped, often nucleated trabeculæ. If we attempt to search for the lymphatic vessels in the cortical substance, but very little can be discovered of them in the stroma, and if a gland be injected, the injection penetrates right into the middle of the follicles. If a mesenteric gland be examined during chylification, that is perhaps three or four hours after a meal at which fat has been taken in abundance, its whole substance appears white and perfectly milky, and on examining individual parts of it microscopically, the minute fat-drops of the chyle may be detected every where lying between the cellular elements of the follicles. It seems, therefore, that the current of lymph forces its way between these elements, and

Fig. 61. Sections through the cortical substance of human mesenteric glands. *A*. View of the whole cortical substance slightly magnified: *P*, investing adipose tissue and capsule, through which blood-vessels *v, v, v* enter. *F, F, F*. Follicles of the gland, into which the blood-vessels in part plunge, at *i, i* the interstitial tissue separating the follicles (stroma).

B. More highly magnified (280 times). *C*. The tissue of the capsule with parallel fibrils. *a, a*. The reticulum, partly empty, partly filled with the nucleated contents. The whole corresponds to the outer part of a follicle.

that no really free channel for it exists, seeing that the
elements lie crowded together like the particles in a
charcoal filter, so that the lymph trickles out again on
the other side in a more or less purified state. The follicles should accordingly be regarded as spaces filled with
cellular elements but variously intersected by a trabecular network, and thus they can no longer be held to be
convolutions or dilatations of the lymphatics, but must
be viewed as interposing themselves in the course of
these vessels after they have broken up into a series of
ramifications continually increasing in minuteness.

Of the minute elements contained in the follicles, the
cells of the parenchyma, some appear to become separated

FIG. 62.

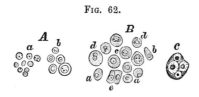

and afterwards to mingle with the blood as colourless
blood- or lymph-corpuscles. The more the glands become enlarged, the more numerous are the cellular elements which pass into the blood, and the larger and more
perfectly developed are the individual colourless cells of
the blood wont to be.

The same condition seems to prevail in the spleen.
Originally we all imagined that the veins were the chan-

Fig. 62. Lymph-corpuscles from the interior of the follicles of a lymphatic gland.
A. As usually seen; *a*, free nuclei, with and without nucleoli, simple and divided.
b. Cells with smaller and larger nuclei, which are closely invested by the cell-wall.
B. Enlarged cells from a hyperplastic bronchial gland in a case of variolous pneumonia (comp. in Fig. 57 the colourless blood-corpuscles from the same source). *a*.
Largish cells with granules, and single nuclei. *b*. Club-shaped cells. *c*. Larger
cells with larger nuclei and nucleoli. *d*. Division of nuclei. *e*. Club-shaped cells
in close apposition (cell-division ?). *C*. Cells with an endogenous brood. 300
diameters.

nels by which the colourless corpuscles were conveyed away from the spleen ; but in this instance also I have come to the conclusion that their removal is in all probability effected by means of the lymphatic vessels.

LECTURE IX.

MARCH 13, 1858.

PYÆMIA AND LEUCOCYTOSIS.

Comparison between colourless blood- and pus-corpuscles—Physiological re-absorption of pus; incomplete (inspissation, cheesy transformation), and complete (fatty metamorphosis, or milky transformation). Intravasation of pus.

Pus in the lymphatic vessels—Retention of matters in the lymphatic glands—Mechanical separation (filtration)—Coloration by tattooing—Chemical separation (attraction): Cancer, Syphilis—Irritation of lymphatic glands, and its relation to leucocytosis.

Digestive and puerperal (physiological) leucocytosis—Pathological leucocytosis (Scrofulosis, typhoid fever, cancer, erysipelas).

Lymphoid apparatuses: solitary and Peyerian follicles in the intestines—Tonsils and follicles of the tongue—Thymus—Spleen.

Complete rejection of pyæmia as a dyscrasia susceptible of demonstration morphologically.

In a practical point of view the question of *pyæmia* forcibly intrudes itself upon us in connection with the changes which we have last considered, and as this must still be reckoned among the most controvertible of subjects, you will, I hope, allow me to enter a little more particularly into its details.

What is to be understood by pyæmia? It has generally been conceived to be a condition, in which the blood contains pus, and as pus is essentially characterized by its morphological constituents, what is meant of course is, that pus-corpuscles are to be seen in the blood. Now that we have found out, however, that the colour-

less corpuscles of the blood as they usually appear and
are to be observed in people in the best state of health,
resemble pus-corpuscles in every respect (p. 180), one
essential point in the question is thus at the very outset
got rid of. In order, however, to render the subject to
some extent perspicuous, it is necessary to enter into the
consideration of the different points of view which are
here involved a little more in detail.

Colourless blood-cells are so like pus-corpuscles as easily
to be mistaken for them, so that if in any specimen we
meet with such elements, we can never say with certainty
off-hand whether we have to deal with colourless blood-,
or pus-corpuscles. Formerly, and to some extent even
up to our own times, the view was very generally entertained that the constituents of pus pre-existed in the
blood; that pus was only a kind of secretion from the
blood, in somewhat the same way that urine is; and that
it could also like a simple fluid return into the blood.
This view explains, you see, the conception which has
been so long preserved in the doctrine of the so called
physiological reabsorption of pus.

It was imagined that the pus might be again taken up
into the blood from the different points at which it had
been deposited, and that a favourable turn was thereby
effected in the disease, inasmuch as the reabsorbed pus
was thus at last removed from the body. The tale went
that in the case of a patient with pus in the cavity of the
pleura the disease might terminate in the evacuation of
purulent urine or purulent fæces, without the pus having
previously made its way directly from the pleura into the
urinary passages or the intestinal canal. It is therefore
admitted to be possible that pus may be reabsorbed and
conveyed away in substance. Afterwards, when the doctrine of pyæmia had more and more gained ground, these
cases were distinguished by the name of physiological re-

absorption of pus, from that which was considered to be pathological, and the only question that remained was, in what way the first process with its favourable and the second with its malignant issue could be accounted for. This matter finds its simple solution in the fact that *pus as pus is never reabsorbed.* There is no form, by which pus in substance can disappear by the way of reabsorption ; it is always the fluid part of the pus which is taken up, and therefore what is called the reabsorption of pus may be referred to the two following possibilities.

In the first case, the pus with its corpuscles is at the time of the reabsorption still more or less intact. Then the pus becomes of course thicker in proportion as the fluid disappears. This constitutes the long known *thickening (inspissation)* of pus, whereby is produced what the French term " pus concret," which consists of a thick mass, containing the pus-corpuscles in a shrivelled condition, when not only the fluid between the pus-corpuscles (pus-serum) but a part also of that present in them has disappeared.

Fig. 63.

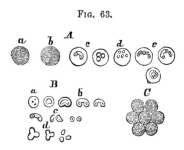

Fig. 63. *A*. Pus-corpuscles, *a* fresh, *b* after the addition of a little water, *c—e* after treatment with acetic acid, the contents cleared up, the nuclei which were in process of division, or already divided, visible, at *e* with a slight depression on their surface. *B*. Nuclei of pus-corpuscles in gonorrhœa; *a* simple nucleus with nucleoli, *b* incipient division, with depressions* on the surface of the nuclei, *c* progressive bi-partition, *d* tri-partition. *C*. Pus-corpuscles in their natural position with regard to one another. 500 diameters.

* By many held to be nucleoli.

Pus consists essentially of cells, which in their ordinary condition lie close to one another (Fig. 63, *C*, and between which a small quantity of intercellular fluid (*pus-serum*) exists. Within the pus-corpuscles themselves lies a substance which is likewise provided with a great quantity of water ; for nearly every specimen of pus, although it may look very thick when fresh, contains such a large amount of water that it loses a great deal more by evaporation than a corresponding quantity of blood. The latter only gives the impression of being more watery because it contains a great deal of free (intercellular), but relatively little intracellular, fluid, whilst in pus on the contrary there is a greater quantity of water in the cells, and less without them. When then reabsorption takes place, the greatest part of the intercellular fluid first disappears, and the pus-corpuscles draw nearer to one another ; soon, however, a part of the fluid from the cells

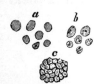

Fig. 64.

themselves also vanishes, and in proportion as this is the case, they become smaller, more irregular, angular, and uneven, they assume the most singular forms, lie closely pressed together, refract the light more strongly on account of their containing a greater quantity of solid matter, and present a more homogeneous appearance.

This kind of inspissation is by no means so rare a process as it is often assumed to be, but on the contrary of extremely frequent occurrence, and almost even more important than frequent. This is namely one of the processes which lead to the formation of the much discussed

Fig. 64. Inspissated, cheesy pus. *a*. Shrivelled pus-corpuscles, diminished in size, somewhat distorted, and looking more homogeneous and solid than usual. *b*. Similar corpuscles with fat granules. *c*. Their natural position with regard to one another. 300 diameters.

cheesy products which have recently been all included under the term tubercle, and concerning which it has been shown, especially by Reinhardt, that they must to a very considerable extent really be referred to pus as their origin, and therefore be regarded as inflammatory products. Hereafter, we shall see that these observations have been employed for the deduction of false conclusions concerning tubercle itself; but that by inspissation inflammatory products can be converted into things which are called tubercles, is indubitable. It is precisely in the history of pulmonary tuberculosis that this operation plays a very prominent part. You have only to imagine shrivelled-up cells like these inclosed within the alveoli of the lungs and undergoing inspissation of their contents in one alveolus after another, and you will at length obtain a cheesy hepatization such as is usually described under the name of *tubercular infiltration..*

This imperfect reabsorption, in which only the fluid constituents are reabsorbed, leaves the mass of solid constituents lying in the part as a *caput mortuum*, as a mass deprived of vitality and no longer capable of life. This is the kind of inspissation which we see occur on a large scale in the case of imperfect reabsorption of pleuritic exudations, when very large layers of a crumbling substance remain behind in the sac of the pleura; and also round about the vertebral column in caries of the verte-

FIG. 65.

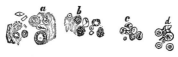

Fig. 65. Inspissated hæmorrhagic pus from a case of empyema, some of it in process of disintegration. *a.* The natural mass, containing granular débris, shrivelled pus- and blood-corpuscles. *b.* The same mass treated with water; a few granular, decolorized blood-corpuscles have become evident. *c* and *d.* After the addition of acetic acid. 300 diameters, and at *d* 520.

bræ (Spondylarthocace), cold abscesses, etc. In all
these cases the reabsorption is at an end as soon as the
fluid has disappeared. Herein consists the evil import
of these processes. For the solid parts which are not
reabsorbed, either remain lying in the part as such, or
they may afterwards soften, in which case, however, they
do not usually undergo reabsorption, but for the most
part give rise to ulceration. At all events what is reabsorbed is not pus, but a simple fluid composed in great
part of water, a few salts, and a very small quantity of
albuminous matter, and there can be no question but
that we have here presented to us one of the most incomplete forms of reabsorption.

The second form of purulent reabsorption is that which
constitutes the most favourable case, when the pus really
disappears and no essential part of it need remain behind. But here too the pus is not reabsorbed as pus,
but first undergoes a fatty metamorphosis ; every single
cell sets fatty particles free within it,
breaks up and at last nothing further
remains than fatty granules and intervening fluid. Then therefore there exist
no longer either cells or pus ; and their
place is occupied by an emulsive mass, a
kind of milk, composed of water, some albuminous matter and fat, and in which even sugar has on various occasions been demonstrated, whereby a still greater analogy
with real milk is brought about. It is this *pathological
milk* which afterwards comes to be reabsorbed—once
more therefore not pus, but fat, water, and salts. These
are the processes which may be denominated " physiolo-

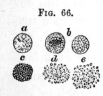
Fig. 66.

Fig. 66. Pus engaged in retrograde fatty metamorphosis (fatty degeneration). *a.*
Commencement of the change. *b.* Fat-granule cells with nuclei still distinct.
c. Granule-globule (inflammatory globule). *d.* Disintegration of the globule. *e.*
Emulsion, milky débris. 350 diameters.

gical reabsorption of pus ;" a reabsorption, in which pus is not reabsorbed as such, but either only its fluid constituents, or its solid ones after they have been considerably altered by an internal transformation.

There is however certainly one case in which pus in substance may become the object, not exactly of a reabsorption, but at any rate of an *intravasation*, and where this intravasated pus may circulate within the vessels ; I mean the case in which a vessel receives a wound or is perforated and pus passes through the opening into its interior. An abscess may lie close to a vein, burst through the walls, and evacuate its contents into the vessel. Still more easily can such a transit be effected in lymphatic vessels which run into open abscesses. The only question therefore is how far we are entitled to consider this case as a frequent one. As far as the veins are concerned, the possibility of such an occurrence has been for the last twenty years confined within somewhat narrow limits, and the notion of the reabsorption of pus in substance through the medium of the veins has been more and more abandoned ; but about its taking place by means of the lymphatics people still pretty frequently talk, and indeed they have frequently occasion to do so.

But it is almost a matter of indifference whether the pus really finds its way into lymphatic vessels from the outside, or, whether, as others assume to be the case, it owes its origin to inflammation in the lymphatic vessels ; u¹timately, the question is always this, how far a lymphatic vessel filled with pus is capable of effecting an evacuation of its contents into the circulating stream of blood, and producing a genuine pyæmia. The possibility of such an occurrence must as a rule be denied, and indeed for a very simple reason. All the lymphatic vessels which are in a condition to take up pus in this way are peripheral ones, whether they arise from external or internal parts, and only after a somewhat lengthened course do they gradually reach the blood-vessels. In all, interruptions are formed by the lymphatic glands, and since we know that the lymphatic vessels do not pass through the glands as wide, tortuous, and interlacing canals (p. 208), but that, after they have broken up into fine branches, they enter into spaces which are filled with cellular elements, it is manifest, that no pus-corpuscle can pass a gland.

This is a very important point of view which curiously enough is generally overlooked, although it meets with the best possible confirmation in the daily experience of the practical physician. In proof of the inevitable obstruction to the passage of solid particles through the lymphatic glands, a very pretty experiment is afforded by a custom prevalent amongst the lower classes of our population, the well-known practice of tattooing the arms and occasionally other parts. When a workman or a soldier has a number of punctures made upon his arm, and arranged so as to represent letters, signs, or figures, nearly always, in consequence of the great number of punctures, some of the superficial lymphatic vessels are injured. It could not indeed well happen otherwise than that, when whole regions of skin are circumscribed by the pricks of a needle, at least some few lymphatic vessels should be hit upon. Afterwards a substance is rubbed in which is insoluble in the fluids of the body, such as cinnabar, gunpowder, or the like, and which, remaining in the parts, causes a permanent coloration of them. But in the rubbing in a certain number of the particles find their way into lymphatic vessels, are carried along in spite of their heaviness by the current of lymph, and reach the nearest lymphatic glands, where they are separated by filtration. We never find that any particles are conveyed beyond the lymphatic glands and make their way to more distant points, or that they deposit themselves in any way in the parenchyma of internal organs. No, the mass always settles in the nearest group of glands. On examining the infiltrated glands it is easy to convince oneself that the size of the deposited particles is less than that even of the smallest pus-corpuscle.

Fig. 67.

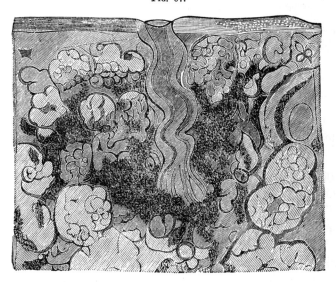

In the object which I place before you (Fig. 67) the spot has accidentally been hit upon, at which the lymphatic vessel enters into the gland, and whence, enclosed within the trabeculæ of connective tissue which are prolonged from the capsules between the follicles, it proceeds in a spiral form, and finally breaks up into its branches. Where these pass into the neighbouring follicles, which are here

Fig. 67. Section through the cortical substance of an axillary gland from an arm, the skin of which had been tattooed. A large lymphatic vessel is seen entering from the cortical substance, gently winding and breaking up into fine branches. Round about are follicles, for the most part filled with connective tissue. The dark, finely granular mass represents the deposit of cinnabar. 80 diameters.

indeed in great part filled with connective tissue, they have poured out the whole mass of cinnabar, so that in part it still lies within the intervening trabeculæ, but yet in part has penetrated into the follicles themselves. The preparation comes from the arm of a soldier who had the

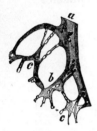

FIG. 68.

figures rubbed in in 1809, so that the mass has remained nearly fifty years in the same place. None of it has penetrated farther than this spot; even the next layer of follicles does not contain any. The particles are however so small, and the majority of them so minute in comparison with the cells of the gland, that they cannot at all be compared to pus-corpuscles. Now when such molecules as these are unable to pass, when such extremely minute particles cause an obstruction, it would be somewhat bold to imagine that pus-corpuscles, which are relatively large, could effect a passage.

This arrangement, gentlemen, by means of which the free current of fluid is interrupted in the lymphatic glands, and the coarser particles are retained there in quite a mechanical manner, admits, as may readily be conceived, of no other kind of reabsorption from the periphery through the medium of the lymphatic vessels than that of simple fluids. We should indeed be mistaken, if we were to consider the whole action of the lymphatic glands to consist merely in their being interposed like filters between the different portions of the lymphatic vessels. They have manifestly another part to play, inasmuch as the substance of the glands indubitably takes up

Fig. 68. Reticulum of an axillary gland filled with cinnabar, from an arm which had been tattooed (Fig. 67). *a.* Part of an inter-follicular trabecula with a lymphatic vessel; *b* one of its larger branches entering into a follicle; *c, c* the anastomosing, nucleated networks of the reticulum; the dark granules are particles of cinnabar. 300 diameters.

into itself certain ingredients from the fluid mass of the lymph, retains them, and thereby also alters the chemical constitution of the fluid, so that it quits the gland all the more altered because it must at the same time be assumed that the gland yields up certain constituents to the lymph, which did not previously exist in it.

I will not here enter into minute details, since the history of every *malignant tumour* affords the best examples in support of this position. When an axillary gland becomes cancerous, after previous cancerous disease of the mamma, and when during a long period only the axillary gland remains diseased without the group of glands next in succession or any other organs becoming affected with cancer, we can account for this upon no other supposition than that the gland collects the hurtful ingredients absorbed from the breast, and thereby for a time affords protection to the body, but at length proves insufficient, nay, perhaps at a later period itself becomes a new source of independent infection to the body, inasmuch as a further propagation of the poisonous matter may take place from the diseased parts of the gland. Equally instructive examples are afforded by the history of *syphilis*, in which a bubo may for a time become the depository of the poison, so that the rest of the economy is affected in a comparatively trifling degree. As Ricord has shown, it is precisely in the interior of the real substance of the gland that the virulent matter is found, whilst the pus at the circumference of the bubo is free from it; only so far as the parts come into contact with the lymph conveyed from the diseased part, do they absorb the virulent matter.

If we apply these facts to the reabsorption of pus, we are not, even in the case when it has really made its way into lymphatic vessels, at all entitled to conclude that as an immediate consequence of this irruption the blood be-

comes infected with the constituents of pus ; on the contrary a retention of the pus-corpuscles will probably take
place within the glands, and even the fluids which succeed in passing them, will during that passage lose a
great part of their noxious properties.   Secondary glandular swellings show themselves in various forms after
peripheral infection.   How can they be explained otherwise than upon the supposition, that every contaminat-
ing (miasmatic) substance, which is to be regarded as
essentially foreign or, if I may so express myself, hostile,
to the body, by penetrating into the substance of the
gland, produces in it a state of more or less marked irritation which very frequently increases to a real inflammation of the gland ?   I shall hereafter revert to the subject of irritation and enter a little more fully into the consideration of the meaning which should be attached to it,
and I will therefore here only make this remark, that
according to my investigations the irritation of a gland
consists in its falling into a state in which there is an
increased formation of cells in it—its follicles becoming
enlarged, and after a time exhibiting a much greater
number of cells than before.   In proportion to the extent
of these processes we then see the colourless elements of
the blood also increase.   Every considerable irritation of
a gland is followed by an increase in the proportion of
lymph-corpuscles in the blood, and every process therefore which is accompanied by glandular irritation, will
also have the effect of supplying the blood with larger
quantities of colourless blood-corpuscles, or, in other
words, of producing a leucocytotic condition.   If then the
opinion be entertained that pus has been absorbed, and
that pus is the cause of the disturbances which have declared themselves, nothing is easier than to demonstrate
the presence of cells in the blood which have the appearance of pus-corpuscles and are often present in such large

quantities as to form accumulations (Fig. 58) which may be seen, in the dead body, with the naked eye, looking like minute spots of pus ; or as to constitute large, continuous or granular layers on the inferior surface of the buffy coat of blood taken from a vein (Fig. 60). Apparently the proof is as plausible as possible. The observer starts with the supposition that pus has found its way into the blood ; he examines the blood and really discovers elements, having all the appearance of pus-corpuscles, and in very great numbers. Even if it be admitted that colourless blood-cells may look like pus-corpuscles, still the conclusion which has been repeatedly arrived at in cases of pyæmia, is very seductive, namely, that on account of the great multitude, they cannot possibly be colourless blood-, but must be pus-corpuscles. This was the conclusion arrived at years ago by Bouchut on the occasion of an epidemic of puerperal fever which he then took to be pyæmia, but has very recently, founding his opinion upon the same observations, declared to have been acute leukæmia. It is moreover the same conclusion which Bennett came to in the much-discussed matter of priority between us, when he observed a case of indubitable leukæmia some months before I saw my first case, and inferred from the presence of colourless corpuscles in larger numbers than in any instance upon record, that it was a case of "suppuration of the blood." This conclusion of his indeed was not original, but was based upon the hæmitis of Piorry of which I lately spoke (p. 187), this physician having conceived the blood itself to become inflamed and engender pus, a state which was afterwards denominated spontaneous pyæmia by the Vienna school.

Now all these errors proceeded from the circumstance that such an enormously great number of colourless corpuscles were found in the blood. Now-a-days their

occurrence can be just as simply explained according to
our theory of hæmatopoiesis, as it previously seemed
explicable only according to that of pyæmia. Irritation
of the lymphatic glands explains without any difficulty
the increase in the colourless, pus-like cells in the blood,
and that too in all cases—not only in those where
pyæmia was expected to be found, but also in those
where it was not expected, but where the blood, notwithstanding, exhibited the same quantity of colourless
corpuscles as in genuine pyæmia answering to our
clinical notions of the disease.

Thus it has been shown that every meal produces a
certain state of irritation in the mesenteric glands, inasmuch as the constituents of the chyle which are conveyed
to these bodies, act as a physiological stimulus to them.
The milk which we drink, the fatty matters in our soups,
the various kinds of fat distributed in a state of minute
division throughout the more solid articles of our food,
find their way in the form of extremely minute globules
into the lacteals and diffuse themselves there just like the
cinnabar in the glands ; but the smallest of the fatty
molecules after a time force their way through the gland.
For such minute bodies therefore there still exists a real
permeability in the channels of the gland, but even they
are for a time retained, and it always takes a long time
before the mesenteric glands after a meal again become
entirely free from fat, and the propulsion of this substance through them is manifestly effected by a proportionately strong pressure. At the same time we observe
an enlargement of the gland, and likewise after every
meal an increase in the number of colourless corpuscles
in the blood—a *physiological leucocytosis*, but no pyæmia.

In proportion as *pregnancy* advances, as the lymphatic
vessels in the uterus dilate, and the interchange of material in the organ increases with the development of the

fœtus, the lymphatic glands in the inguinal and lumbar regions become considerably enlarged, and that sometimes to such an extent, that, if we were to find them in a similar state at any other time, we should regard them as inflamed. This enlargement conveys into the blood an increased quantity of fresh particles of a cellular nature, and thus from month to month the number of colourless corpuscles augments. At the time of birth we may see in the defibrinated blood of nearly every puerperal woman, whether suffering from pyæmia or not, the colourless corpuscles forming a pus-like sediment. This too is a physiological form which is far from being a pyæmic one. But if care be taken to select a puerperal woman, offering symptoms of disease which correspond with those usually presented by pyæmia, nothing is easier than to find these numerous colourless multi-nuclear cells, which are precisely such as are supposed to corroborate the presence of pyæmia. These are fallacious conclusions which result from imperfect knowledge of the normal conditions of life and development. As long as we are exclusively bent upon proving the presence of pyæmia, all this may have the appearance of being a great and new occurrence, and we may, when we examine the blood of a woman in child-bed, consider ourselves justified in concluding that she has pyæmia even before its symptoms declare themselves. But we may examine when we will, we shall always find some traces of leucocytosis, just as it has already long been known that it is very common for a buffy coat to form in the case of pregnant women, because their blood generally has conveyed into it a larger quantity than usual of a more slowly contracting fibrine (hyperinosis). This is accounted for by the increased nutrition of the uterus, and by the changes, so nearly allied to inflammatory processes, which are going on in the uterine system, and are associated with a certain amount of irritation in the lymphatic glands immediately in connection with it.

If we proceed a step farther and consider pathological cases, we meet with these leucocytotic conditions in the whole of that series of diseases which are complicated with glandular irritation, and in which the irritation does not lead to a destruction of the glandular substance. During the progress of an attack of scrofula, in which, if the disease run a somewhat unfavourable course, the glands are destroyed, either by ulceration, or cheesy thickening, calcification, etc., an increased introduction of corpuscles into the blood can only take place as long as the irritated gland is still in some degree capable of performing its functions, or still continues to exist ; as soon however as the gland is withered or destroyed, the formation of lymph-cells likewise ceases and with it the leucocytosis. In all cases, on the other hand, in which a more acute form of disturbance prevails, connected with inflammatory tumefaction of the glands, an increase in the colourless corpuscles always takes place in the blood. So it is in typhoid fever, in which we observe such extensive medullary (markige) swellings of the abdominal glands ; so it is in cancer patients, when irritation of the lymphatic glands manifests itself ; so, lastly is it in the course of the processes which come under the denomination of malignant erysipelas and are so early wont to be accompanied by glandular swellings. Such is the meaning of this increase in the colourless elements which ultimately always refers us to an increased development of lymph-corpuscles within the irritated glands.

It is now of importance that I should point out to you, that at present our conceptions concerning lymphatic glands are much more comprehensive than they were a short time ago. The most recent histological investigations have shown that, in addition to the ordinary well-known lymphatic glands, which are of a certain size, a great number of smaller apparatuses exist in the body which possess precisely the same structure, but do not exhibit such a complex arrangement as we find in a lymphatic gland. To this class belong above all the *follicles of the intestines*, both the solitary and the Peyerian. A Peyer's patch is nothing more than a lymphatic gland spread out as it were upon the surface ; the individual follicles of the patch, just as the solitary follicles of the digestive tract, correspond to the individual follicles of a lymphatic gland, only that the former, in man at least, are disposed in a single layer, the latter in several. The solitary and Peyerian glands have therefore nothing at all in common with the ordinary glands which pour their secretions into the intestinal canal ; on the contrary, they rather hold the position, and manifestly also fulfil the functions, of lymphatic glands.

To the same category belong in all probability also the analogous apparatuses which we find grouped together in such large masses in the upper part of the digestive tract, where they form the *tonsils* and the *follicles of the root of the tongue*. Whilst in the intestine the follicles lie spread out on an even surface, in these parts the surface is inverted and the individual follicles lie around the involuted membrane.

To the same category belongs moreover the *thymus gland*, which in its interior exhibits no other differences of structure excepting that the aggregation of the follicles reaches a still higher degree than in the lymphatic glands. Whilst in most of the lymphatic glands we have a hilus, where there are no follicles, this ceases to be the case in the thymus gland which has no hilus.

Finally, to the same class belongs also a very essential constituent of the *spleen*, namely, the *Malpighian or white bodies*, which in different persons are distributed in just as different numbers throughout the parenchyma of the spleen, as the solitary and Peyerian follicles in the intestine. In a section through the spleen we see the trabeculæ radiating from the hilus towards the capsule and enclosing certain districts of glandular substance, within which the red spleen pulp lies, interrupted here and there by a sometimes greater, sometimes less, number of white bodies (follicles) of larger or smaller size, single or in groups, and sometimes almost clustered. The structure of these follicles agrees exactly with that of the follicles of lymphatic glands.

We may therefore regard this whole series of apparatuses as nearly equivalent to the lymphatic glands properly so called, and a swelling of the spleen will, under certain circumstances, furnish just as abundant a supply of colourless blood-corpuscles, as is the case when a lymphatic gland enlarges. This possibility explains how it is that, for example, in cholera, where the change in the solitary glands and Peyer's patches forms the chief part of the disease, and where the swelling of the other lymphatic glands is much less marked, we meet at an extremely early period with a considerable increase in the colourless corpuscles. Hereby is explained moreover why, in such cases of pneumonia as are connected with great swelling of the bronchial glands, an increase in the number of colourless blood-corpuscles likewise takes place, which is generally wanting in those forms of pneumonia which are not connected with such swelling. The more the irritation extends from the lung to the lymphatic glands, the more abundantly noxious fluids are conveyed from the lung to the glands—the more manifestly does the blood undergo this change.

Upon examining these different pathological processes in this manner one by one, it is really impossible to discover anything at all, which in a morphological point of view, could even in a remote degree justify the assumption of a condition such as might be called pyæmia. In the extremely rare cases, in which pus breaks through into veins, purulent ingredients may, without doubt, be conveyed into the blood, but in such instances the introduction of pus occurs for the most part but once. The abscess empties itself, and if it be large, an extravasation of blood is more apt to ensue than the establishment of a persistent pyæmia. Perhaps we shall at some future time succeed, in the course of such a process, in discovering pus-corpuscles with well-defined characters in the blood ; at present, however, the matter stands thus, that it can most positively be maintained that nobody has hitherto succeeded in demonstrating, by arguments capable of supporting even gentle criticism, the existence of a morphological pyæmia. This name therefore must, as designating a definite change in the blood, be entirely abandoned.

LECTURE X.

MARCH 17, 1858.

METASTATICAL DYSCRASIÆ.

Pyæmia and phlebitis—Thrombosis—Puriform softening of thrombi—True and false
  phlebitis—Purulent cysts of the heart.
Embolia—Import of prolonged thrombi—Pulmonary metastases—Crumbling away
  of the emboli—Varying character of the metastases—Endocarditis and capillary
  embolia—Latent pyæmia.
Infectant fluids—Diseases of the lymphatic apparatuses and secreting organs—
  Chemical substances in the blood; salts of silver—Arthritis—Calcareous metastases—Diffuse metastatic processes—Ichorrhæmia—Pyæmia as a collective name.
Chemical dyscrasiæ—Malignant tumours, especially cancer—Diffusion by means of
  contagious parenchymatous juices.

GENTLEMEN,—I was interrupted the last time in my
description of pyæmia by the termination of the lecture,
just as I was about to discuss the nature of the connection
between this disease and certain affections of the vessels.
As soon as it was found necessary to abandon the original view, in accordance with which the mass of pus
which was believed to be seen in a vein, was considered
to have made its way in (been absorbed) through an
opening in its walls, or through its yawning extremity,
recourse was had to the doctrine of phlebitis, which is
still the one most current. It was imagined that the pus
which was regarded as the really noxious matter, was
furnished as a product of secretion by the wall of the

vessel (John Hunter). This doctrine, however, presented some difficulty, because it was soon pretty generally allowed that a primary purulent inflammation of the veins did not occur, but that, as was first distinctly shown by Cruveilhier, at the commencement a clot of blood is always present. Cruveilhier himself was so greatly surprised at this observation of his, that he connected a theory with it which was beyond all medical comprehension. He concluded namely from the impossibility of explaining why inflammations of the veins began with coagulation of the blood, that inflammation in every case whatever consisted in a coagulation of the blood. The impossibility of explaining phlebitis seemed to him to be got over by raising coagulation into a general law, and by referring every inflammation to a phlebitis on a small scale (capillary phlebitis). Cruveilhier was the more induced to assert this in consequence of his entertaining similar views with regard to other morbid processes, and believing that cysts, tubercles, cancer, and in short all important processes, accompanied by changes susceptible of anatomical demonstration, really ran their course within special, minute veins imagined by him. This manner of thinking, however, continued so entirely alien to that of the great majority of learned and unlearned physicians, that the separate conclusions propounded by Cruveilhier, which were adopted in medical science in part as drawn up by him, were altogether misunderstood.

Cruveilhier was right in this point, as indeed has since been more and more acknowledged, namely, that the so-called pus in the veins in the first instance never lies against the wall of the vein, but always first appears in the centre of the previously existing clot of blood which marks the outset of the process. He imagined that the pus was secreted from the wall of the vessel, but that it did not remain there, but by means of " capillary attraction" made its way to the centre of the clot. This was a very singular theory, which can only be approximatively comprehended by assuming, as it was still the custom to do in Cruveilhier's time, pus to be a simple fluid. But apart from these extremely obscure interpretations, the fact remains constant, against which even now no argument can be advanced, that before a trace of inflammation is visible, we find a clot, and that shortly afterwards in the middle of this clot a mass displays itself, which differs in appearance from the clot, whilst on the other hand it exhibits a greater or less resemblance to pus.

FIG. 69.

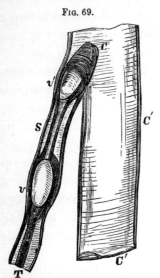

With this observation as my starting point, I have endeavoured to clear up the doctrine of phlebitis, as far as lies in my power, by substituting for the mysticism which pervaded Cruveilhier's interpretation, merely a statement of the real facts. We do not know that inflammation as such has any necessary connection with coagula ; on the contrary, it has turned out that the doctrine of stasis rests upon manifold misinterpretations. Inflammation may unquestionably exist when the current of blood within the vessels of the affected part is perfectly free and unobstructed. If we therefore leave inflammation on one side and confine our attention simply to the coagulation

Fig. 69. Thrombosis of the saphenous vein. *S.* Saphenous vein. *T.* Thrombus : *v, v'* thrombi seated on the valves (valvular) in process of softening, and connected by more recent and thinner portions of coagulum. *C.* Prolongation of the plug, projecting beyond the mouth of the vessel into the femoral vein *C'.*

of the blood, to the formation of the clot (thrombus), it seems most convenient to comprehend the whole of this process under the term *Thrombosis.* I have proposed to substitute this term for the different names, phlebitis, arteritis, etc., inasmuch as the affection essentially consists in a real coagulation of the blood *at a certain fixed spot.*

Upon investigating the history of these thrombi, we find that the puriform mass which is met with in their interior does not originate in the wall, but is produced by a direct transformation of the central layers of the clots themselves, a transformation indeed which is of a chemical nature, and during which, with a result similar to that which can be artificially obtained by the slow digestion of coagulated fibrine, the fibrine breaks up into a finely granular substance and the whole mass becomes converted into *débris.* This is a kind of softening and retrograde metamorphosis of the organic substance, in the course of which from the very commencement a number of extremely minute particles become visible ; the large threads of fibrine crumble into pieces, these again into smaller ones, and so on until after a certain time has elapsed the chief part of the mass is found to be composed of small, fine, pale granules (Fig. 70, *A*). In cases in which the fibrine is comparatively very pure, we frequently see scarcely anything else than these granules.

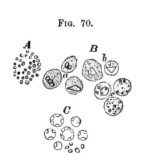

FIG. 70.

Fig. 70. Puriform mass of débris from softened thrombi. *A*. The granules seen in disintegrating fibrine, varying in size, and pale. *B*. The colourless blood-corpuscles set free by the softening, some of them in process of retrograde metamorphosis; *a*, with multiple nuclei, *b*, with simple, angular nuclei and a few fat-granules, *c*, non-nucleated (pyoid) corpuscles, in a state of fatty metamorphosis. *C*. Red blood-corpuscles undergoing decolorization and disorganization. 350 diameters.

You see, gentlemen, the microscope solves the difficulties in a very simple manner, by demonstrating that this mass, which looks like pus, is not pus. For we understand by pus a fluid essentially provided with cellular elements. Just as little as we can imagine blood without blood-corpuscles, just as little can pus exist without pus corpuscles. But when, as in the present instance, we find a fluid which is nothing more than a mass pervaded by granules, this may indeed, as far as external appearance goes, look like pus, but never ought to be regarded as real pus. *It is a puriform, but not a purulent substance.*

But now we frequently see that in addition to these granules a certain proportion of other structures show themselves, for example, really cellular elements (Fig. 70, *B*), which are round (spherical), or angular, present one, two, or more nuclei, frequently lie tolerably close to one another, and in reality exhibit a great similarity to pus-corpuscles, the distinction at most being that very often fat-granules occur in them, indicating that a process of disintegration is going on. Whilst therefore in individual cases there can, on account of the often very greatly preponderating mass of débris, exist no doubt as to what the observer has before him, in others considerable doubts may exist as to whether real pus is not present. These doubts cannot be removed in any other way than by an examination into the history of the development of the puriform mass. Now that we have already seen that colourless blood- and pus-corpuscles perfectly agree with one another in form, so that it is impossible to draw a real distinction between them, the question which suggests itself in cases where we find round, colourless cells in a clot of blood, whether these cells are colourless blood- or pus-corpuscles, can only be decided by determining whether the corpuscles were present in the thrombus from its very commencement, or only sprang up in it afterwards, or found their way into it in some other manner. Now upon accurately following up the different stages of the process, the very positive result is obtained that the corpuscles pre-exist, and that they do not arise within the clot, and are not forced into it. Even when quite recent thrombi are examined, the corpuscles are found in many places heaped up in great masses, so that, when the fibrine breaks up, they are set free in such numbers, that the débris are nearly as rich in cells as pus. It is with this process just as when water which is thoroughly impregnated with solid particles is frozen and then exposed to a higher temperature ; when the ice melts the enclosed particles must of course again come to light.

To this view of the matter one objection may be raised, to wit, that we do not see the red blood-corpuscles set free in a similar manner. The red corpuscles, however, perish very early ; they are soon seen to grow pale ; they lose a portion of their colouring matter and become smaller, whilst numerous dark granules appear at their circumference (Figs. 54, *a ;* 70, *C*), and in the majority of cases they entirely disappear, nothing but these granules at last remaining. Still there are also cases in which the red corpuscles retain their integrity within the softening mass. As a rule they certainly perish, and it is precisely upon this that depends the peculiarity of the transformation, by means of which a yellowish white fluid arises bearing the external appearance of pus. And for it too an explanation may be found without any particular difficulty, if it be borne in mind how very trifling is the power possessed by the red blood-corpuscles of resisting the most various reagents. If to a drop of blood you add a drop of water, you see the red corpuscles disappear before your eyes while the colourless ones remain behind.

That therefore, which according to the ordinary nomenclature is called suppurative phlebitis, is neither suppurative, nor yet phlebitis, but a process which begins with a coagulation, with the formation of a thrombus in the blood, and afterwards presents a stage in which the thrombi soften, so that the whole history of the process is contained in the history of the thrombus. But here I must impress upon you that I do not, as has been said of me in different quarters, deny the possibility of a real phlebitis, and that I have not in any way discovered that there is no such thing as phlebitis. *No! phlebitis certainly does exist.* But it is an inflammation which really affects the walls, and not the contents of a vessel. In the larger vessels the most different layers of their walls may become inflamed and enter upon every possible phase of inflammation, and yet all the while their channel remain entirely unaltered. In accordance with the views generally entertained the internal coat of the vessels was thought to be like a serous membrane, and as this readily furnishes fibrinous exudations or purulent masses, the same was supposed to be the case with the internal coat. Concerning this point a series of investigations was years ago set on foot, and I too have occupied myself at various times with it, but hitherto no experimenter, who carefully prevented the blood from streaming into the vessels, has succeeded in producing an exudation, which was deposited in their cavity. On the contrary, when the wall is inflamed, the "exuded matter" (Exsudatmasse) passes into the wall, which becomes thicker, cloudy, and subsequently begins to suppurate. Nay, even abscesses may form, which cause the wall to bulge on both sides like a variolous pustule, without any coagulation of the blood ensuing in the cavity of the vessel. At other times, certainly, phlebitis, properly so called (and in like manner arteritis and endocarditis), is the cause of thrombosis, in consequence of the formation of inequalities, elevations, depressions, and even ulcerations upon the inner wall which favour the production of the thrombus. Still, wherever phlebitis, in the usual sense of the word, takes place, the alteration in the coat of the vessel is almost always a secondary one, and indeed occurs at a comparatively late period.

The process runs its course in such a way that the most recent parts of the thrombus always consist of the blood which has most lately coagulated. The softening, the partial liquefaction, generally commences in the centre, in the oldest layers, so that, when the thrombus has attained a certain size, there exists in the midst of it a cavity of larger or smaller dimensions, which gradually enlarges and keeps approaching more and more closely to the wall of the vessel. But in general this cavity is shut off in an upward and downward direction by means of a more recent and tougher portion of the clot which, after the manner of a cap, takes care that, as Cruveilhier expresses himself, the "pus" remains sequestered, and all contact between the *débris* and the circulating blood is prevented. Only sideways does the softening extend until it at last reaches the wall of the vessel itself ; this becomes altered, it begins to grow thicker and at the same time cloudy, and ultimately even suppuration takes place within the walls.

The same thing which we have hitherto considered in the veins occurs also in the heart. In the right ventricle especially we not unfrequently see what are called purulent cysts between the trabeculæ of its wall. They project into the cavity like small rounded knobs, and form little pouches which, when cut open, contain a soft pulp that may present a completely pus-like appearance.

People have plagued themselves to an indefinite extent about these purulent cysts and invented all possible theories to account for them, until at length the simple fact came out, that their contents are frequently nothing more than a finely granular pulp of an albuminous substance, which does not offer even the slightest resemblance in its more intimate structure to pus. This was so far tranquillizing, as there is no observation as yet on record of the death of any patient from pyæmia who had sacs of this description even in pretty considerable number, but it ought to have struck those who are so much inclined to establish a connection between peripheral thromboses, which are however just the same thing, and pyæmia.

For the question naturally arises how far particular disturbances that can be designated by the name of pyæmia may, in consequence of the softening of the thrombi, be evoked in the body. To this in the first place we may answer that secondary disturbances certainly are very frequently occasioned, but not so much by the immediate introduction of the softened masses as fast as they become liquid into the blood, as by the detachment of larger or smaller fragments from the end of the softening thrombus which are carried along by the current of blood and driven into remote vessels. This gives rise to the very frequent process upon which I have bestowed the name of *Embolia*.

This is an occurrence which we can here only briefly touch upon. In the peripheral veins the danger proceeds chiefly from the small branches. By no means rarely do these become quite filled with masses of coagulum. As long however as the thrombus is confined to the branch itself, so long the body is not exposed to any particular danger ; the worst that can happen is that, in consequence of a peri- or meso-phlebitis,* an abscess

* See the Author's "Gesammelte Abhandl.," p. 484.

may form and open externally. Only the greater number of the thrombi in the small branches do not content themselves with advancing up to the level of the main trunk, but pretty constantly new masses of coagulum deposit themselves from the blood upon the end of the thrombus layer after layer, the thrombus is prolonged beyond the mouth of the branch into the trunk in the direction of the current of the blood, shoots out in the form of a thick cylinder farther and farther, and becomes continually larger and larger. Soon this *prolonged* thrombus (Fig. 71, *t*) no longer bears any proportion to the original (*autochthonous*) thrombus (Fig. 71, *c*), from which it proceeded. The prolonged thrombus may have the thickness of a thumb, the original one that of a knitting-needle. From a lumbar vein, for example, a plug may extend into the vena cava as thick as the last phalanx of the thumb.

FIG. 71.

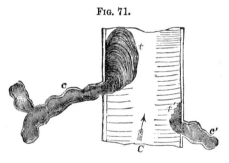

It is these prolonged plugs that constitute the source of real danger ; it is in them that ensues the crumbling away which leads to secondary occlusions in remote vessels. They are the parts from which larger or smaller

Fig. 71. Autochthonous and prolonged thrombi. *c, c'.* Smallish, varicose, lateral branches (circumflex veins of the thigh), filled with autochthonous thrombi which project beyond the orifices into the trunk of the femoral vein. *t.* Prolonged thrombus produced by concentrically apposed deposits from the blood. *t'.* Prolonged thrombus, as it appears after fragments (emboli) have become detached from it.

particles are torn away by the blood as it streams by (Fig. 71, t').

Through the vessel originally occluded no blood at all flows ; in it the circulation is entirely interrupted : but in the larger trunk through which the blood still continues its course, and into which only at intervals the thrombus-plugs project, the stream of blood may detach minute particles, hurry them away with it, and wedge them tightly into the nearest system of arteries or capillaries.

Thus we see, that as a rule all the thrombi at the periphery of the body produce secondary obstructions and metastatic deposits in the lungs. I long entertained doubts whether I ought to consider the metastatic inflammations of the lungs one and all as embolical, because it is very difficult to examine the vessels in the small metastatic deposits, but I am continually becoming more and more convinced of the necessity of regarding this mode of origin as the rule. When a considerable number of cases are compared statistically, the result obtained is that every time metastatic deposits occur, thrombosis is also present in certain vessels. Quite recently, for example, we have had a tolerably severe epidemic of puerperal fever, and in this it was found that, however manifold the forms the disease assumed, yet all those cases which were accompanied by metastases in the lungs, were also attended with thrombosis in the region of the pelvis or in the lower extremities, whilst in the inflammations of lymphatic vessels the pulmonary metastases were wanting. Such statistical results carry with them a certain amount of compulsory conviction, even where strict anatomical proof is wanting.

Into the pulmonary artery the introduced fragments of thrombus of course penetrate to different depths according to their size. Usually a fragment of the kind sticks fast where a division of the vessel takes place (Fig. 72, *E*), because the diverging vessels are too small to admit it. In the case of very large fragments even the principal trunks of the pulmonary artery are blocked up, and instantaneous asphyxia ensues ; other fragments again penetrate into the most minute arteries and there give rise to very minute, and sometimes miliary inflammations of the parenchyma. In explanation of these small and often very numerous deposits, I must mention a conjecture which only occurred to me whilst engaged in my more recent observations, but which I do not scruple to declare to be a necessary inference. I believe namely that, when a considerable fragment of a thrombus becomes wedged at a certain point in an artery, it may in its turn crumble away through the onward pressure of the blood, and thus the minute particles to which this crumbling of the larger plug gives rise be conveyed into the small branches into which the vessel breaks up. Thus alone does it seem to me that the fact can be explained, that in the district supplied by an artery of considerable size a number of little deposits of the same sort are often found.

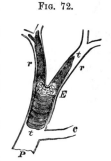

Fɪɢ. 72.

This whole series of cases has nothing whatever to do with the question, whether there is pus in the blood or not. We have in them to deal with bodies of quite a different nature, with fragments of coagula in a more or less altered condition, and according as this alteration has assumed this or that character, the nature of the pro-

Fig. 72. Embolia of the pulmonary artery. *P.* Moderately large branch of the pulmonary artery. *E.* The embolus, astride upon the angle (spur—Sporn), formed by the division of the artery. *t, t'.* The capsulating (secondary) thrombus: *t*, the portion in front of the embolus reaching to the next highest collateral vessel *c ;* *t'*, the portion behind the embolus, in a great measure filling up the diverging branches *r, r'*, and ultimately terminating in the form of a cone.

cesses which arise in consequence of the obstruction may
also be very different. If, for example, a gangrenous
softening has taken place at the original site of the coagulum, the metastatic deposit will also assume a gangrenous character, just as this would be the case if gangrenous matter were inoculated. So, *vice versâ*, it also
happens that the secondary disturbances, like those at
the spot whence the fragments were detached, run a very
favourable course, the embolus like the thrombus becoming converted into pigment and connective tissue, and at
the same time growing smaller.

This group of processes must be separated from those
ordinarily occurring in pyæmia all the more, because the
same processes are also met with on the other side of the

FIG. 73.

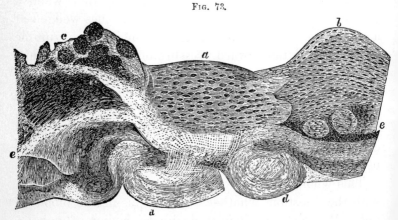

lungs in the regions belonging to the left side of the circulation, where they often run the same course and pre-

Fig. 73. Ulcerative endocarditis affecting the mitral valve. *a.* The free, smooth
surface of the mitral valve, beneath which the connective-tissue-corpuscles are enlarged and clouded, whilst the intervening tissue is denser than usual. *b.* A considerable hilly swelling caused by increasing enlargement and cloudiness of the tissue. *c.* A swollen part which has already begun to soften and break up. *d, d.* The
tissue at the lower part of the valves which is stil but little altered, with numerous
corpuscles, the results of proliferation. *e, e.* The commencement of the enlargement, cloudiness, and proliferation of the corpuscles. 80 diameters.

sent the same results, but are still less dependent upon an original phlebitis. Thus, for example, *endocarditis* by no means seldom forms the starting point of such metastases. Ulceration takes place in one of the valves of the heart, not by means of the formation of pus, but in consequence of an acute or chronic softening ; crumbling fragments of the surface of the valve are borne away by the stream of blood and reach with it far distant points. The kind of obstruction which these masses produce is altogether similar to that which the thrombi in the veins give rise to, but they present a different chemical constitution. Their minuteness also and their friability favour their penetration into the smallest vessels in a high degree. Therefore we do not so very unfrequently find the obstructing mass in minute microscopical vessels

FIG. 74.   FIG. 75.

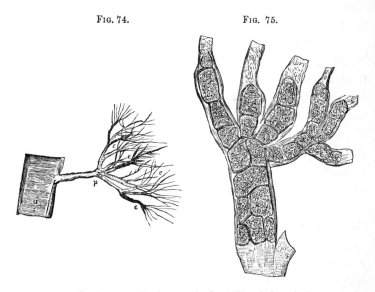

Fig. 74—75. Capillary embolia in the tufts (penicilli) of the splenic artery after endocarditis (Cf. Gesammelte Abhandlungen zur wiss. Medicin. 1856, p. 716). 74. Vessels of a tuft magnified 10 times, in order to show the position of the occluding emboli in the arterial district. 75. An artery filled a little before its division, and in the branches into which it next divides, with fragments of the finely granular embolic mass (Cf. Fig. 73, *c*). 300 diameters.

which are no longer to be followed with the naked eye,
and in them it usually extends as far down as a point of
division and somewhat beyond. This mass constantly
presents a finely granular appearance, and does not consist of the coarse débris that we find in the veins, but of
a very fine, yet at the same time dense, granular matter ;
chemically, it possesses the extremely convenient quality
for examination of being remarkably resistant to the ordinary tests, and thus readily distinguished from other matters. This is *capillary embolia* properly so called, one of
the most important forms of metastasis, which frequently
gives rise to minute deposits in the kidney, the spleen,
and the substance of the heart itself ; in certain cases
occasions sudden occlusions in the vessels of the eye or
brain, and according to circumstancs produces metastatic
deposits or sudden functional disturbances (amaurosis,
apoplexy). Here too one can clearly convince oneself
that in recent cases the wall of the vessel is quite unaltered at the seat of the affection ; nay here indeed the
doctrine of phlebitis would no longer suffice, since these
are not vessels which possess vasa vasorum, and concerning which it might be assumed that a secretion proceeded
from the wall inwards. In these cases it is impossible to
regard the occluding mass in any other light than as one
primarily existing in the vessel, and in no wise dependent upon the condition of its wall.

Perhaps this description has convinced you, gentlemen,
that two essential errors have existed in the doctrine of
pyæmia ; the one, that people thought they had found
pus-corpuscles in the blood, when only colourless blood-
corpuscles were really present ; the second, that they
thought they had found pus in vessels in which nothing
more than the products of the softening of fibrine existed.
Yet we have ascertained that this last class of cases certainly furnishes the most important source of genuine

metastatic deposits.   But in my opinion, the history of
the processes which have been called pyæmia is not confined to these conditions.   When the process runs its
course free from all complication, so that from the original seat of the disease (thrombosis in a vein, endocarditis,
etc.), only *solid* masses in an undecomposed state are detached and cause obstructions, the real process is in
many cases brought to notice only in consequence of the
metastasis.   There are cases which run their course so
latently that all the earlier stages of the affection are entirely overlooked, and that the first rigors which declare
themselves announce that the development of the metastatic processes has already set in.   Usually, however,
another condition must be taken into consideration,
which is not directly accessible either to the coarser or
more delicate modes of anatomical investigation ; I mean
certain *fluids*, which in themselves bear no immediate and
necessary relation to pus as such, but manifestly differ
very much from one another in their nature and origin.

Whilst I was engaged in the consideration of the
changes which lymph undergoes, I pointed out to you
(p. 220), that fluids which were taken up by lymphatic
vessels were not only freed in the filters of the lymphatic
glands from corpuscular elements, but were also in part
attracted and retained by the substance of the glands, so
as to display some activity within them.   Similar effects
appear to take place also elsewhere than in the glands.
Where the reabsorption was primarily effected by the
veins, this must, of course, always be the case.   There is
namely a series of peculiar phenomena which pervade all
infectious processes as a constant element.   These are
on the one hand the changes which the lymphatic and
lymphoid glands may undergo not so much at the
seat of the primary affection as rather in the body generally, and on the other hand the changes which the

secreting organs offer, through which the matters have to be excreted.

It was for some time believed that *tumefaction of the spleen* was characteristic of typhoid fever, inasmuch as it formed a parallel to the swellings of the mesenteric glands occurring in that disease. But more accurate observation has shown that a great number of feverish conditions which follow a more or less typhoid course, and affect the nervous system in such a manner that a state of depression is brought about in its most important central organs, set in with swelling of the spleen. The spleen is a remarkably sensitive organ, which swells not only in intermittent and typhoid fever, but also in most other processes in which noxious, infectant matters have been freely taken up into the blood. No doubt the spleen must always be considered in its near relationship to the lymphatic system, but its diseases in addition usually bear a very direct relation to analogous diseases of the important glands in its vicinity, especially the liver and the kidneys. In most cases of infection do these three organs exhibit corresponding enlargement connected with real changes in their interior ; but since these changes do not, even on microscopical examination, apparently present anything remarkable, the attention of the observer is chiefly attracted by the result which is obvious to the naked eye, namely, the great swelling. On careful comparison, however, a good deal is discovered, so that we can affirm with certainty that the gland-cells quickly become changed, and that disturbances early show themselves in the elements by means of which the secretion is to be accomplished. I shall revert to this subject hereafter. Allow me now, in elucidation of these conditions, in the first place to advert to one or two more obvious examples which are accessible to direct observation.

We know that when any one takes *salts of silver*, they penetrate into the different tissues of his body ; and if we do not employ them in a really corrosive and destructive manner, the silver penetrates into the elements of the tissues in a state of combination, the nature of which has not yet been satisfactorily made out, and, when it has been made use of long enough, produces a change of colour at the point of application. A patient who had in Dr. Von Graefe's out-patient room on the 10th November received a solution of nitrate of silver as a lotion, very conscientiously employed the remedy up to the present time (17th March) ; the result of which was that his conjunctiva assumed an intensely brown, nearly black appearance. The examination of a piece cut out of it showed that silver had been taken up into the parenchyma, and indeed in such a manner that the whole of the connective tissue had a slightly yellowish brown hue upon the surface, whilst in the deeper parts the deposition had only taken place in the fine elastic fibres of the connective tissue, the intervening parts, the proper basis-substance, being perfectly free. But deposits of an entirely similar nature take place also in more remote organs. Our collection contains a very rare preparation from the kidneys of a person who on account of epilepsy had long taken nitrate of silver internally. In it may be seen the Malpighian bodies, in which the real secretion takes place, a blackish blue colouring of the whole of the membrane of the coils of the vessels, limited to this part in the cortex, and appearing again, in a similar, though less marked form, only in the intertubular stroma of the medullary substance. In the whole kidney, therefore, besides the parts which constitute the real seat of their secretion, those only are altered which correspond to the ultimate system of capillaries in the medullary substance.

Of the well-known discoloration of the skin by silver I need not speak here.

Another instance is afforded us by *gout*. If we examine the concretions (tophi) in the joints of a gouty person, we find they are composed of very delicate, needle-shaped, crystalline deposits of all possible sizes, and consisting of urate of soda, with at most here and there a pus- or blood-corpuscle lying between them. We have here therefore also, as when silver has been employed, to deal with a material substance which is usually excreted by the kidneys, and that indeed not rarely in such large quantities, that deposits form even within the kidney itself and large crystals of urate of soda accumulate, especially in the uriniferous tubules of the medullary portion, so as sometimes to lead even to an occlusion of the tubules. If, however, this secretion does not proceed in a regular manner, the immediate result is an accumulation of urates in the blood, as has been shown in a very able manner by Garrod. Then at last deposits begin to form at other points, not throughout the whole body, nor uniformly in all parts, but at certain definite points and in accordance with certain rules.

Here we have to do with very different forms of metastasis from those with which we became acquainted whilst considering the nature of embolia. That the changes which ensue in the substance of the kidney, in consequence of the absorption of silver from the stomach. accord with what has in pathology since times of old been termed metastasis is unquestionable. This consists in a transferrence of matter from one spot to another, so that the same substance which had previously been present in the first comes and lodges in the second, and the secreting organ takes up minute particles of the matter into its own tissue. This is what we find constantly recurring in the history of all metastatic deposits of this kind, in which only matters in solution and not particles of a visible and mechanical nature are present in the blood. The urate of soda cannot be directly seen in the blood of the gouty person, unless it have previously been collected by the help of chemical processes ; and just as little the salts of silver.

I have moreover described a new form of metastasis which is certainly more rare but yet belongs to the same category. When calcareous salts are reabsorbed from the bones in large quantity, the bone-earth is generally excreted by the kidneys, likewise in large quantity, so that sediments form in the urine, the knowledge of which has straggled down to us in the history of osteomalacia [mollities ossium], from the notorious Mme. Supiot in the last century. But this regular excretion of the calcareous salts is not unfrequently impaired by disturbances in the functions of the kidneys, in the same way as in arthritis the excretion of urate of soda ; then there also arise metastatic deposits of bone-earth, but at other points, namely the lungs and the stomach. Considerable portions of the lungs sometimes become calcified without any injury to the permeability of the respiratory passages ; the diseased parts look like fine bathing sponge. The mucous membrane of the stomach becomes filled in like manner with calcareous salts, so that it feels like a rasp and grates under the knife without the glands of the stomach becoming directly implicated ; they are merely imbedded in a stiffened mass, and possibly even thus secretion might take place from them.

To these kinds of metastasis in which definite substances, though not in a palpable form, but in solution, find their way into the mass of the blood, careful attention must at all events be paid when we endeavour to unravel the complex mass of conditions which are com-

prehended under the term pyæmia. I see at least no other
possible way of explaining certain more diffuse processes,
which do not present themselves in the form of the ordinary circumscribed metastatic deposits. To this class belongs that metastatic pleurisy which develops itself without any metastatic abscesses in the lungs—that seemingly
rheumatic articular affection, in which no distinct deposit
is found in the joints—that diffuse gangrenous inflammation of the subcutaneous connective tissue which cannot
well be accounted for unless we suppose a more chemical
mode of infection. Here we have, as may be seen in
cases of variolous and cadaveric infection, to deal with a
transferrence of *corrupted, ichorous juices* into the body ;
and we must admit the existence of a dyscrasia (*ichorous
infection*) in which this ichorous substance which has
made its way into the body, displays its effects in an
acute form in the organs which have a special predi-
lection for such matters.

Now it may possibly happen that in the course of the
same case of illness the three different changes which we
have considered may coexist. An increase in the number of the colourless corpuscles (leucocytosis) may take
place to such an extent as to tempt one to believe in the
presence of a morphological pyæmia. This will at all
events always be the case when the process has been connected with extensive irritation of the lymphatic glands.
The formation of thrombi, moreover, and embolia with
metastatic deposits may occur. And finally there may
at the same time be taking place an absorption of ichorous or putrid juices (ichorrhæmia, septhæmia). These
three different conditions may present themselves as complications one of the other, but do not necessarily coincide. If it be wished therefore to retain the term pyæmia, let it be reserved for such complications as these,
only we must not *seek for a common central point in a*

purulent infection of the blood, but the term must be regarded as a collective name for several processes dissimilar in their nature.

I hope, gentlemen, that what I have now imparted to you will be sufficient to put you in possession of the chief bearings of the subject. Of course no real demonstration can be afforded without reference to distinct cases. You will, however, yourselves have sufficient opportunity for testing the exactitude of this description of mine, and I shall be glad if you find that important data have thereby also been furnished, by which clearer conceptions with regard to the really practical, and especially the therapeutical, questions arising out of the subject, may be obtained.

Now that we have become acquainted not only with corporeal particles, but also with certain chemical substances as the originators of dyscrasia, lasting for a longer or shorter time according as the supply of these particles and substances continues for a longer or shorter period, we may briefly revert to the question, whether, in addition to these forms, a kind of dyscrasia can be shown to exist in which the blood is the permanent seat of definite changes. We must answer this question in the negative. The more marked a really demonstrable contamination of the blood with certain matters is, the more manifest is the relatively acute course of the process. Just the very forms* in which medical men are most apt to console themselves—especially for the shortcomings of the therapeutical results, with the reflection that they have to do with the deeply rooted and incurable chronic dyscrasia—just these forms depend, I imagine, least of all upon an original change in the blood ; for these are pre-

---

* Tubercle, cancer, purpura, syphilis, etc.

cisely the cases, in the majority of which extensive alterations are discovered in certain organs or in individual
parts. I cannot assert that investigation has in this matter in any way been pushed to its utmost limits, I can
only say that every resource afforded by microscopical
or chemical analysis has hitherto been fruitlessly employed in investigating the part played by the blood in
these processes ; and that, on the other hand, we are in
most of them able to demonstrate important changes in
larger or smaller groups of the ultimate constituents of
organs ; and that on the whole the probability that the
dyscrasia should in these instances also be regarded as
secondary, and as derived from definite points in organs,
becomes stronger every day. I shall have to examine
this question a little more closely when I come to consider the theory of the propagation of malignant tumours,
in the case of which recourse is, you know, so often had
to the supposition that the malignancy has its root in the
blood which gives rise to the local affections. And yet
it is precisely in the course of these processes that it is
comparatively most easy to show the mode of propagation, both in the immediate neighbourhood of the diseased part, and in remote organs ; and it is in them we
find, that there is one circumstance which especially
favours the extension of such processes, namely the
abundance of parenchymatous juices in the pathological
formation. The drier a new formation is, the less in
general are its powers of infecting, both nearer and more
distant parts. The mode of propagation itself commonly
entirely agrees with what we have already said ; first of
all, a conveyance of the morbid matter though the
lymphatic channels, and then an affection of the lymphatic glands, takes place, and it is only by degrees that
processes of a similar nature declare themselves in more
remote organs. Or the process may here too in the first

instance encroach upon the walls of the veins, so that they become really cancerous, and after a certain time the cancer either grows directly through the walls into the vessel and there continues its course, or a thrombus forms at the point, which invests the cancerous plug in a greater or less degree and into which the mass of cancer grows.   Here, therefore, we see a diffusion of the disease may possibly take place in two different manners, but the diffusion of corpuscular elements only in one, when, namely, an irruption ensues into the veins.   An absorption of cancer-cells by means of the lymphatics cannot indeed in itself be ranked amongst impossibilities, but at all events this much is certain, that no propagation of the disease can take place until the lymphatic glands have in their turn undergone a complete cancerous transformation, and similar masses of cancer push on their growth from them into their efferent vessels.   In no case can a peripheral lymphatic vessel sweep along into the blood the cells of the cancer so simply as it does the fluid parts ; this is only conceivable and possible in the case of the veins.   But even in that case there is not the slightest probability that noxious matters are frequently diffused by their means, and for the simple reason that the metastases of cancer very frequently do not correspond with those with which we have become acquainted as occurring in embolia.   The usual form of metastatic diffusion in cancer follows rather the direction of the secreting organs. The lungs, as is well known, are much more rarely invaded by cancerous disease than the liver, not only after gastric and uterine, but also after mammary cancer which would necessarily rather produce cancer in the lungs, if it were anything corpuscular which was conveyed away, became stagnant and gave rise to a new eruption of the disease.   The manner in which the metastatic diffusion takes place seems, on the contrary, to render it probable that the transferrence takes place by means of certain fluids, and that these possess the power of producing an infection which disposes different parts to a reproduction of a mass of the same nature as the one which originally existed. We need only imagine a process similar to that which we see upon a large scale in small pox. The pus of small pox when directly inoculated does indeed induce the disease, but the contagium * is also volatile, and a person may have pustules over his skin after merely breathing air of a certain character. A similar state of things seems to prevail in cases, in which, in the course of heteroplastic processes, dyscrasiæ occur which do not burst out afresh at points which, according to the direction of the current of blood or lymph, would be most directly exposed to them, but at remote spots. As the salts of silver do not deposit themselves in the lungs, but pass through them to be precipitated only when they reach the kidneys or the skin, so an ichorous juice may pass from a cancerous tumour through the lungs without producing any change in them, and yet at a more remote point, as for example in the bones of a far distant part, excite changes of a malignant nature.

* *i. e.* Contagious matter.—*Transl.*

LECTURE XI.

MARCH 27, 1858.

PIGMENTARY ELEMENTS IN THE BLOOD. NERVES.

Melanæmia—Its relation to melanotic tumours and colorations of the spleen.
Red blood-corpuscles—Origin—Melanic forms—Chlorosis—Paralysis of the respiratory substance—Toxicæmia.
The nervous system—Its pretended unity.
Nerve-fibres—Peripheral nerves: their fasciculi, primitive fibres, and perineurium—Axis-cylinder (electrical substance)—Medullary substance (Myeline)—Non-medullated and medullated fibres—Transition from the one kind to the other: hypertrophy of the optic nerve—Different breadth of the fibres—Their terminations—Pacinian and tactile bodies.

GENTLEMEN,—I have still some observations to make to you in reference to the changes of the blood, more for the sake of completeness than because I am able to offer to you in doing so any decisive points of view.

In the first place I wish to mention one other condition which has recently been a great deal talked about, and might, when occasion offered, present increased interest to you, the so-called *melanæmia*. This is a condition most nearly connected with leukæmia, inasmuch we have in it to deal with elements, which, like the colourless corpuscles in leukæmia, make their way from definite organs into the blood and circulate with it. The number of recorded observations concerning this matter is already tolerably large, indeed I might almost say,

larger than perhaps is necessary, for it seems indeed that
here and there mistakes have slipped in, which should, I
think, be again removed from the history of the affection.
But unquestionably there is a state in which coloured
elements are met with in the blood that do not belong to
it. Isolated observations in support of this fact have
already for a considerable length of time * been upon
record, and indeed first occur in the history of melanotic
tumours, concerning which it has frequently been declared that in their neighbourhood minute black particles
are met with in the vessels, and the opinion put forward
that from this source the melanotic dyscrasia arose. But
this is not quite the condition which is meant when melanæmia is now-a-days spoken of. In the last ten years
not a single observation has been made known which in
any way adds to our knowledge concerning the passage
of the particles of melanotic tumours into the blood.

The first observation concerning that class of diseases
which in a narrower sense of the word is designated melanæmia, was made by Heinrich Meckel in the case of a
lunatic a short time after I had published my description
of leukæmia. Meckel found that here too the spleen was
enlarged in a very considerable degree and pervaded by
black pigment, and he therefore ascribed the change in
the blood to an absorption of coloured particles from the
spleen. The next observation I made myself (and that
too in a class of cases which afterwards proved very fruitful) in the case of an ague-patient, who had long been
afflicted with a considerable enlargement of the spleen ;
for I found in the blood of his heart cells containing pigment. Meckel had only observed free granules and

---

* Dr. Stiebel, sen., of Frankfort-on-the-Maine, calls my attention to the fact that
he had already in a review of Schönlein's Clinical Lectures (in Häser's ' Archiv '),
mentioned the occurr nce of pigment-cells in the blood.

            Note to the Second Edition.

flakes (Schollen) containing pigment. The cells which I discovered in many respects bore a resemblance to colourless blood-corpuscles ; they were spherical, but frequently also rather oblong, nucleated cells, within which a greater or less number of large black granules were to be seen. In this case also the occurrence of a large black spleen was again verified. Since that time attention has been continually more and more drawn to

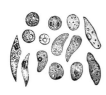

Fig. 76.

these conditions by Meckel himself and by a number of other observers in Germany, and last of all by Frerichs, and in Italy by Tigri. Tigri has not scrupled to designate the disease *milza nera*, from the blackness of the spleen in it, whilst according to the view of Meckel which has been expanded by Frerichs, it is rather one of the more severe forms of intermittent fever which is to be explained in this way.

It has been attempted to explain the serious import of these affections by supposing that the elements, which find their way into the blood, accumulate at certain points in the more minute capillary districts, and there produce stagnation and destruction. This was especially held to be the case in the capillaries of the brain, in which they were said to attach themselves after the manner of emboli to the points of division, and so occasion sometimes capillary apoplexies, sometimes the comatose and apoplectic forms of severe intermittent fever. Frerichs has added a new and important kind of obstruction, namely, that of the minute hepatic vessels, which is said ultimately to give rise to atrophy of the parenchyma of the liver.

Fig. 76. Melanæmia. Blood from the right heart (Cf. 'Archiv f. pathol. Anatomie und Physiologie,' vol. ii., fig. 8, p. 594). Colourless cells of various shapes filled with black, and in part angular, pigment-granules. 300 diameters.

If all this be the case, there would seem to exist an extremely important series of conditions directly dependent upon the dyscrasia. Unfortunately I can myself say but little concerning the matter, inasmuch as I have not since my first case again been in a position to observe anything similar. I cannot therefore form a decided opinion with regard to the value of the relations which have been laid down with respect to the connection of the secondary changes with the contamination of the blood. I only wish to remark that all the facts with which we are acquainted concerning these conditions, indicate that the contamination of the blood has its rise in a definite organ, and that this organ, as in the case of the colourless blood-corpuscles, is generally the spleen.

In the course of my description of the blood I have hitherto scarcely made any mention of the changes which take place in the *red corpuscles*, not by any means because I regarded them as unimportant constituents of that fluid, but because as yet remarkably little is known concerning their changes. The whole history of the red blood-corpuscles is still invested with a mysterious obscurity, inasmuch as no positive information has even at the present time been obtained with regard to the origin of these elements. We only know this much with certainty, as I have already (p. 190) had occasion to remark, that a part of the original corpuscular elements of the blood proceed just as directly from the embryonic formative cells of the ovum, as all the other tissues which build themselves up out of them. We know, moreover, that in the first months of the existence even of the human embryo, divisions take place in the cells, whereby an increase in the number of them present in the blood itself is produced. But after this time all is obscure, and this obscurity indeed corresponds pretty exactly with the period at which the corpuscles in the blood of man and the mammalia cease to exhibit nuclei. We can only say that we are acquainted with no fact whatever which speaks in favour of a further independent development, or of a cell-division, in the blood, but that everything points to the probability of a supply from without. The only hypothesis which has in more recent times been advanced with regard to the independent development of the blood-corpuscles in the blood itself, is that of G. Zimmermann,* who assumed that there were little vesicles present in the blood, which gradually grew by intussusception whilst circulating with it, and ultimately constituted the real blood-corpuscles. Now little corpuscles certainly do occur in the blood (Fig. 52, *h*), only, when they are more accurately examined, a peculiarity reveals itself which is unknown in young embryonic forms, namely that they oppose an extraordinary degree of resistance to the most different agencies. In their ordinary state they are of a beautiful dark red, the colour being very intense and frequently nearly black ; if they are treated with water or acids which dissolve the ordinary red corpuscles with ease, it is observed that the little bodies require a very much longer time before they disappear. Upon adding a large quantity of water to a drop of blood, they will be seen to remain for a considerable time after the other corpuscles have disappeared. This peculiarity accords best with what occurs in the changes which take place in the blood, when it is

---

* Zimmermann has recently (' Archiv f. path. Anat. und Phys.,' vol. xviii., pp. 221–242) given us a more explicit statement of his views, and from it we gather that he considers the blood-corpuscles to originate in small, colourless vesicles which are introduced from the chyle into the blood and may be seen in it when its fluidity has been preserved by means of salts. But probably these vesicles are only artificial products, similar to those described nearly ten years ago by Harting (' Nederl. Lancet,' 1851, 3d ser., 1st Jaarg., p. 224).—*From a MS. Note by the Author.*

extravasated or remains for a long time stagnant within the vessels. Such changes undoubtedly lead to a destruction of the corpuscles, so that in the case of the circulating blood also the conclusion may with great probability be drawn, that the bodies in question are not young forms, engaged in development, but on the contrary old ones in process of decay. I agree therefore essentially with Karl Heinrich Schultz's view, who has described these bodies under the name of melanic (melanöse) blood-corpuscles, and regards them as the precursors of the *moulting* of the blood (Blutmauserung)—preparing for the really excrementitious transformations.

There are certain conditions in which the number of these corpuscles becomes extremely large. In very healthy individuals very few of them are found, only in the blood of the vena portæ Schultz believes he has always observed a considerable number. It is certain, however, that there are diseased conditions in which their number becomes so large, that a greater or smaller quantity of them is met with in nearly every drop of blood. These conditions cannot however as yet be classed in definite categories, because but little attention has been excited with regard to them. They are found in slight forms of intermittent fever, in cyanosis after cardiac disease, in typhoid-fever patients, in the fever accompanying ichorous infection after operations, and in the course of epidemic disorders, still always in such diseases as are accompanied by a rapid exhaustion of the mass of blood and give rise to cachectic and anæmic states. This is one of the processes in which clinical observation also might lead to the conclusion that an abundant destruction was going on in the constituents of the blood within the vessels.

In addition to these changes we have precise knowledge concerning another class distinguished by quantita-

tive changes in the number of the corpuscles. These
conditions, of which Chlorosis is the principal representative, offer a certain resemblance to those which are
accompanied by an increase in the number of the colourless blood-corpuscles, to leukæmia in a narrower sense
of the word and the merely leucocytotic states. Chlorosis is distinguished from leukæmia by the circumstance
that the entire number of the corpuscles is smaller.
Whilst in leukæmia colourless corpuscles in some sort
take the place of the red ones and a real diminution in
the number of the cellular elements in the blood is not
produced, in chlorosis the elements of both kinds become
less numerous, without the occurrence of any definite
disturbance in the numerical relation existing between
the coloured and colourless corpuscles. This points to a
generally diminished formation, and, if we may conclude
(as I certainly think one can at the present moment
scarcely help doing), that the red corpuscles also are
brought to the blood from the spleen and lymphatic
glands, all this would indicate that in chlorosis a diminished formation takes place in the blood-glands. Leukæmia is of course much more easily explained, inasmuch
as in it we find representatives of the whole mass of cellular elements and can imagine that a part of them,
instead of being transformed into red corpuscles, are
pursuing their development as colourless ones. In the
history of chlorosis, on the contrary, much obscurity still
prevails, since we cannot positively demonstrate the existence of a primary affection of the blood-glands. Anatomical observations indicate that the foundations of the
chlorotic ailment are very early laid ; for the aorta and
the larger arteries are usually, and the heart and sexual
organs frequently, found imperfectly developed, facts
which lead us to infer that the disposition is either congenital or formed in early youth.

A third series of conditions may here too be mentioned, which, however, do not affect the form of the blood-corpuscles, that, namely, in which the internal constitution of these elements has undergone changes, without the production of any definite morphological effect. Here we have essentially to deal with functional disturbances which are probably connected with more subtle changes in the composition of the blood, changes in the proper *respiratory substance* (respiratorische Substanz). For just as in muscles we find the substance of the primitive fasciculus, the compact mass of syntonine, to be the contractile substance, so in the contents of the red corpuscles do we recognize the presence of the really active, respiratory substance. This under certain circumstances undergoes changes which render it incapable of continuing its functions, a kind of paralysis, if you will. That something of the kind has occurred we see from the fact that the corpuscles are no longer capable of absorbing oxygen, as may be directly proved by experiment. That molecular changes in the composition of the blood are here really at work, we find satisfactory evidence in the action of poisonous substances which, even in extremely minute quantity, so change the hæmatine that it is thrown into a kind of paralysis. To these substances belong a part of the volatile compounds of hydrogen, for example, arseniuretted and cyanuretted hydrogen, and further, according to Hoppe's investigations, carbonic oxide, of all of which comparatively very small quantities are sufficient to diminish the respiratory power of the corpuscles. Analogous conditions have already long since been observed by many in the course of typhoid fevers, in which the capability of taking up oxygen decreases in proportion as the disease assumes a severe and acute character. Microscopically, however, with the exception of a few melanic corpuscles, scarcely anything is to be seen ; chemical experiment and the coarse perception of the naked eye in this instance alone discover the occurrence of peculiar changes. It may therefore be said that in this quarter really the most has yet to be done. We have rather presumptive evidence than facts.

If now we briefly sum up what I have laid before you concerning the blood, we see, either that certain substances find their way into it, which exercise an injurious influence upon its cellular elements and render them incapable of performing their functions ; or that from a definite point, either from sources external to the body, or from some organ, matters are conveyed into it, which thence exercise an injurious influence upon other organs ; or finally that its constituents are not replaced and regenerated in a regular manner. Nowhere in this whole series do we find any one condition, indicating that definite changes once set on foot in the blood itself can be *permanently* maintained, in other words that a permanent dyscrasia is possible, unless new agencies derived from a definite source are continually brought to bear upon the blood. This is the reason why I began by calling your attention to this point of view, which I conceive to be of extreme importance in practice also, namely, that in all forms of dyscrasiæ the chief point is to search for their local origin.

Let us now proceed to the consideration of another subject which comes next in historical importance, namely the *structure and arrangement of the nervous system.*

The great mass of the nervous system consists of *fibrous constituents.* It is to them that nearly all the finer physiological discoveries, which the last fifteen years have brought with them, have reference, whilst the remaining portion of the nervous system, in quantity much smaller, namely, the *grey*, or *ganglionic*, substance, has hitherto opposed difficulties even to histological investigation which are still far from being overcome, so that the experimental examination of this substance has scarcely been able to be taken in hand. It is indeed often maintained that a great deal is now known about the nervous system, but our knowledge is for the most part confined to the white substance, the fibrous portion, whilst we are unfortunately obliged to confess that, both in an anatomical, but more especially in a physiological point of view, we are still involved in the greatest uncertainties with regard to the grey substance, which, as far as its functions are concerned, manifestly holds a much higher position.

As soon as we consider the question of the influence exercised by the nervous system in the different processes of life, anatomically, a single glance suffices to show, that the point of view which neuro-pathologists have been accustomed to set out with, is a very erroneous one. For they fancied they saw in the nervous system an unusually simple whole, from the unity of which resulted the unity of the body in general, of the whole organism. But even though one has nothing but very rough anatomical ideas concerning the nerves, still one ought not to shut one's eyes to the fact that this unity is in a very sorry plight, and that even the scalpel demonstrates the nervous system to be an apparatus composed of an extremely large number of parts of relatively equal value without any single discoverable central point. The more accurately we make our histological investigations, the more do the elements multiply, and the ultimate composition of the nervous system proves to be disposed upon a plan analogous to that which has been followed in all the other parts of the body. An infinite quantity of cellular elements manifest themselves side by side, more or less autonomous, and in a great measure independent of one another.

If in the first instance we exclude the ganglionic substance and confine ourselves simply to the fibrous matter, we have on the one hand the real (peripheral) *nerves* in the narrower sense of the word, and on the other the large accumulations of *white medullary substance,* of which the greater part of the cerebrum, cerebellum, and the columns of the spinal marrow is composed. The fibres of these different parts are indeed on the whole similarly constructed, but disclose in their intimate structure such numerous, and in part, such considerable differences, that there are spots, with regard to which even at this very moment we cannot say with certainty whether the elements we have before us are really nerves, or belong to an altogether different kind of fibres. The greatest certainty has been acquired with regard to the structure of the ordinary peripheral nerves ; in them the following can generally be distinguished with tolerable facility.

All the nerves which can be followed with the naked eye contain a certain number of subdivisions, or fasciculi, which afterwards separate in the form of branches or twigs. On tracing out these individual twigs which keep continually dividing, we find that the nerve under nearly all circumstances retains a fascicular arrangement until nearly its ultimate divisions, so that every fasciculus in its turn comprises a greater or less number of so-called primitive fibres. The term, primitive fibre, which is here employed, was originally selected, because a nerve-fasciculus was regarded as analogous to the primitive fasciculus of a muscle. This notion afterwards became almost obsolete, and Robin was the first who in more recent times again directed attention to the substance which holds the fasciculus together and which he called *perineurium.* It consists of very dense connective

tissue, which upon the addition of acetic acid, it seen to
contain small nuclei, and is different from the looser connective tissue which in its
turn holds the fasciculi together and constitutes the so-
called *neurilemma*.

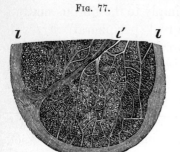

Fig. 77.

ι   ι'   ι

When we use the term
nerve-fibre alone in its histological sense, we always mean
the primitive fibres, and not
the fasciculi which to the
naked eye look like fibres.
These ultimate fibres in their turn possess, one and all,
a special external membrane, which, when it has been
entirely freed from its contents—a matter certainly very
difficult to accomplish, but sometimes occurring spontaneously in pathological conditions, as for example in certain states of atrophy—displays nuclei upon its walls
(Fig. 5, *c*). Within these membranous tubes lie the proper *nerve-contents*, which in ordinary nerves may again
be divided into constituents of two descriptions. These
can scarcely be distinguished apart in a nerve which is
quite fresh ; but in a short time after it has perished or
been cut out, or after the action of any medium upon it,
they at once separate very distinctly from one another,
one of the constituents undergoing a rapid change which
has generally been termed coagulation, and by means of
which it is marked off from the other constituent (Fig.
78). When this has taken place there is distinctly seen
in the interior of the nerve-fibre, the so-called axis-cylin-

Fig. 77. Transverse section through one of the trunks of the brachial plexus.
l, l. Neurilemma, from which one thicker partition *l'* and finer prolongations, indicated by light-coloured lines, run through the nerve and divide it into small fasciculi. These exhibit the dark, punctated, transverse sections of the primitive fibres,
and between them is seen the perineurium. 80 diameters.

der (the primitive band of Remak), a very fine, delicate, pale structure ; and round about it a tolerably firm, dark mass, here and there run-ning together, the *nerve-me-dulla* or *medullary sheath* [white substance of Schwann] ; this fills up the space between the axis-cylinder and the external membrane. But the nerve-tube is generally so tightly filled with its contents that, when viewed in the ordinary way, scarcely anything is seen of the separate constituents, the axis cylinder being always with difficulty visible within the medullary substance. Hence the fact may be accounted for, that its very existence was disputed for years and the view proclaimed by many, that it was also an appearance due to coagulation, produced by a separation of the ori-ginally homogeneous contents into an internal and exter-nal mass. This view is however unquestionably incor-rect : every mode of examination at last discloses this primitive band ; even in transverse sections of nerves the axis-cylinder is very distinctly seen in the interior, with the medulla round about it.

FIG. 78.

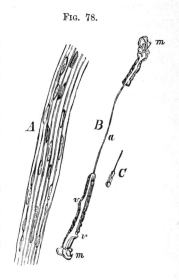

It is the so-called nerve-medulla which gives the nerve-fibres in general their white appearance ; wherever the nerves contain this constituent, they look white ;

Fig. 78. Grey and white nerve-fibres. *A.* A grey, gelatinous nerve-fasciculus from the root of the mesentery, after the addition of acetic acid. *B.* A broad white primitive fibre from the crural nerve : *a* the axis-cylinder laid bare, *v, v* a varicose state of the fibre with its medullary sheath ; at the end at *m, m* the medullary mat-ter (myeline) protruding in convoluted forms. *C.* A fine, white primitive fibre from the brain, with its axis-cylinder protruding. 300 diameters.

wherever it is wanting, they appear translucent and grey. There are therefore nerves which are akin in colour to ganglionic matter, are comparatively transparent and possess a more clear and gelatinous appearance than the others ; and they have thence been called *grey* or *gelatinous nerves* (Fig. 78, *A*).   Between the grey and white nerve-substance therefore there does not exist the difference that the one is ganglionic and the other fibrous, but only this, that the one contains medulla and the other does not.   In general the absence of medulla in a nerve stamps it as one of a lower and more imperfect kind, whilst the presence of this substance announces a more abundant nutrition and a higher development in the part.

Not long ago I made an observation in which a direct illustration of the practical importance of these two conditions was displayed in a very unexpected manner, the usually translucent grey nerve substance having been transformed into an opaque and white matter, namely in the retina. I found namely entirely by accident one day, in the eyes of a man in whom I was looking for changes of quite another kind—round about the papilla of the optic nerve, where the uniformly translucent retina is ordinarily seen—a number of whitish,

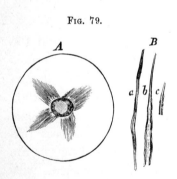

FIG. 79.

A   *B*

a *b* *c*

Fig. 79. Medullary hypertrophy of the optic nerve within the eye (Cf. ' Archiv f. pathologische Anatomie und Physiologie,' vol. x., p. 190). *A*. The posterior half of the globe of the eye, seen from before ; from the papilla of the optic nerve proceed in four directions radiating striæ of white fibres. *B*. Fibres from this optic nerve in the retina, magnified 300 times: *a*, a pale, ordinary, slightly varicose fibre, *b*, one with a gradually thickening medullary sheath, *c*, a similar one with its axis-cylinder protruding.

radiating striæ like those which one sometimes meets
with upon a small scale in dogs, and pretty constantly in
rabbits in different directions. The microscopical examination showed that, like as in these animals, medullated
fibres had developed themselves in the retina, and that
its fibrous layer had become thicker and opaque in consequence of the assumption of medullary substance. On
examining the individual fibres I found, on tracing them
from the fore and middle parts of the retina backwards
towards the papilla, that they gradually increased in
breadth, and at the same time displayed, at first in an
almost imperceptible, but afterwards in a very striking
manner, an investing layer of medulla. This is a kind
of transformation, therefore, which essentially impairs
the functions of the retina, for this delicate membrane
becomes thereby more and more impervious to light, inasmuch as the white substance does not suffer the rays
of light to pass through.

The same change occurs in nerves during their development. A young nerve is a delicate, tubular structure,
provided with nuclei at certain intervals and containing
a pale grey substance. The medulla does not appear
until afterwards, and then the nerve becomes broader
and the axis-cylinder becomes distinctly defined. It may
be said therefore that the medullary sheath is not an
absolutely necessary constituent of a nerve, but is added
to it only when it has arrived at a certain stage in its
development.

Hence it follows that this substance, which was formerly regarded as the essential constituent of a nerve,
according to present views plays a subordinate part.
Those only who do not even now admit the existence of
the axis-cylinder, regard the white substance of course
not only as the greatly predominating constituent, but
also as the really active element of the nerve-contents.

Now it is very remarkable that this same substance is one
which most extensively prevails in the animal body.   I
had, curiously enough, in the first instance in the examination of lungs come across forms which presented very
similar qualities to those which we observe in the medulla of the nerves.   Although this was very surprising,
yet I did not really think there was an actual correspondence, until I was gradually led by a series of further observations which accumulated in the course of several
years, to examine a number of tissues chemically.   The
result showed, that there scarcely exists a tissue rich in
cells in which this substance does not occur in large
quantity ; still it is only in the nerve-fibre that we ob-

 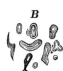

FIG. 80.

serve the peculiarity, that the
substance separates as such, whilst
in all other cellular parts it is
contained in a finely divided state
in the interior of the cells, and is
only set free when the contents
undergo a chemical change, or are subjected to the action
of chemical reagents.   From blood-cells, from pus-corpuscles, from the epithelial cells of the most various glandular parts, from the interior of the spleen and similar
glands unprovided with excretory ducts, this substance
can in every case be obtained by extraction.   It is the
same substance which forms the principal constituent of
the yellow mass of yolk in the hen's egg, whence its taste
and peculiarities, especially its peculiar tenacity and vis-
cidity which are employed for the higher technical purposes of the kitchen, are familiar to every one.   It is this
substance, for which I have proposed the name of *medul-*

Fig. 80. Drops of medullary matter (myeline—according to Gobley, lecithine).
A. Differently shaped drops from the medullary sheath of cerebral nerves, after they
have become swollen up with water.   *B.* Drops from decomposing epithelium from
the gall-bladder in their natural fluid.   300 diameters.

lary matter (Markstoff), or *myeline*, that in extremely large quantity fills up the interval between the axis-cylinder and the sheath in primitive nerve-fibres.

If the nutrition of a nerve suffer disturbance, this substance diminishes in quantity and indeed may under certain circumstances totally disappear, so that a white nerve may be again reduced to the condition of a grey or gelatinous one. This constitutes *grey atrophy*, or *gelatinous degeneration*, in which the nerve-fibre in itself continues to exist, and only the peculiar accumulation of medullary matter has been affected. Herein you may seek for an explanation of the circumstance, that in many cases where, in accordance with the results of anatomical investigation, it was formerly thought one might expect to find a part completely incapable of fulfilling its functions, proof has been afforded by means of clinical observation, aided by electricity, that the nerve is still capable of performing its functions, although in a less degree than normal. Hence too it is manifest that the medulla cannot be the constituent in which lie vested the functions of the nerve as such. To the same conclusion physical investigations also have generally led, and at the present time therefore the axis-cylinder is pretty generally looked upon as the really essential constituent of the nerve, which is also present in pale nerves, whilst in white ones it can only be distinctly isolated by the separation of the investing medullary sheath. The axis-cylinder would therefore seem to be the real *electrical substance* of natural philosophers, and we may certainly admit the hypothesis which has been advanced, that the medullary sheath rather serves as an isolating mass, which confines the electricity within the nerve itself, and allows its discharge to take place only at the non-medullated extremities of the fibres.

The peculiar nature of the medullary matter most fre

quently displays itself in this way, that when a nerve is
torn across or cut (Fig. 78, *m*, *m*), the medulla usually
protrudes from it, presenting, especially after it has been
acted upon by water, a peculiar striated appearance (Fig.
80, *A*).   It takes up water namely, which is a proof that
it is not a neutral fatty substance in the ordinary sense
of the term, but can at most, on account of its great
power of swelling up, be compared to certain saponace-
ous compounds. The longer the action of the water lasts,
the longer are the masses which protrude from the nerve.
They have a peculiar, ribbon-like appearance, keep continually acquiring new streaks and layers, and give rise
to the most singular shapes.   Frequently also fragments
become detached and swim about, forming peculiar, stratified bodies, which in recent times have been confounded
with corpora amylacea, but are distinguished
from them in the most positive manner by their
chemical reactions.

FIG. 81.

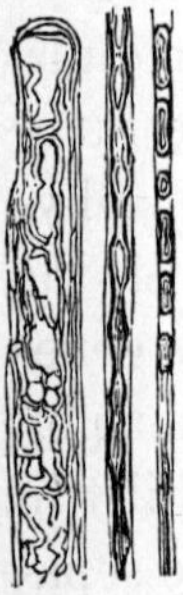

With regard to the histological varieties of
nerves amongst themselves, investigation shows
that in different parts more or less highly developed forms greatly predominate.   On the one
hand, namely, the nerves are essentially distinguished by the breadth of their primitive fibres,
on the other hand, by the presence of medulla.
We have very broad, middle-sized and small
white fibres, and in like manner broad and fine
grey fibres. A very considerable size is generally speaking
but seldom attained by the grey ones, because the size
of a nerve depends more upon the greater or less quantity of medulla it contains than upon the volume of the
axis-cylinder, but still variations present themselves

Fig. 81. Broad and narrow nerve-fibres from the crural nerve with the medullary
substance irregularly swollen up.   300 diameters.

everywhere, so that some nerves are coarser and others finer.

Generally, we may say, that the primitive fibres usually become finer in the terminal portions of nerves, and that the ultimate ramifications of these latter are wont to contain comparatively the finest fibres ; still this is not an absolute rule. In the optic nerve we commonly find from the very moment of its entrance into the eye only very narrow, pale fibres (Fig. 79, *a*), whilst the tactile nerves of the skin present quite up to their terminations comparatively broad and dark bordered fibres (Fig. 83). It has not yet been found possible to arrive at any certain opinion with regard to the import of the different kinds of fibres from their breadth and the proportion of medulla they contain. For a time it was believed that a distinction of this sort could be established between them, namely, that the broad fibres were to be regarded as derived from the real cerebro-spinal parts, the fine ones as parts of the sympathetic ; but this is not found to be borne out by facts, and all that can be said is, that the ordinary peripheral nerves certainly are abundantly provided with broad fibres, whilst the sympathetic nerves contain a comparatively larger portion of fine ones. In many places, as for example in the abdomen, grey, broad fibres predominate (Fig. 78, *A*), with regard to the nervous nature of which doubts are still entertained by some. For the present, therefore, no definite conclusions can be drawn as to any difference in the functions of a nerve from its mere structure, although it can scarcely be doubted that such differences must exist, and that a broad fibre must exhibit other properties, even if only quantitatively different, than a fine one, a medullated fibre others than a non-medullated one. However concerning all this nothing is at present known with certainty ; and since it has been demonstrated by more

18

delicate physical investigations that the nerves, which had been previously assumed only to conduct in the one or the other direction, possess the power of conduction in both directions, I should not, I think, be justified in here advancing any hypotheses with regard to their centripetal or centrifugal conduction.

The great difference, gentlemen, which is to be remarked in regard to the functions of individual nerves, cannot as yet be referred so much to any difference of structure in them, as to the peculiarity of the structures with which the nerve is connected. Thus on the one hand the special function of the central organ from which the nerve proceeds, and on the other, the special nature of its distal termination, afford a clue to its own specific functions.

With reference to the terminations which the nerves present at their peripheral extremities, histology has, I should say, in the course of the last few years celebrated its most brilliant triumphs. Previously it was, as you well know, a matter of dispute whether the nerves ended in loops or in plexuses, or whether their terminations were free, and the one or the other opinion was held with equal exclusiveness. Now, we have examples of most of these modes of termination, but the fewest of that form which was for a time regarded as the regular one, namely the termination in loops.

The most manifest form of termination, though the one whose functions are, singularly enough, even now the least known, is that in the so-called *Pacinian* or *Vaterian** bodies*—organs, concerning the import of which we are still unable to make any statement. They are found in man comparatively most marked in the adipose tissue of the ends of the fingers, but also in tolerably large

* Vater was professor at Wittenberg, and died in 1751.

numbers at the root of the mesentery ; most distinctly and readily, however, in the mesentery of the cat, in which they extend a considerable distance up, whilst in the human body they are situated only at the root of the mesentery, where the duodenum comes in contact with the pancreas in the neighborhood of the solar plexus. Moreover they present great variations in different individuals. Some have very few, others a great number, of them, and it is very possible that certain individual peculiarities result therefrom. Thus I have, for example, on several occasions found a great number of these bodies in lunatics, though I do not wish at present to lay any great stress upon this discovery.

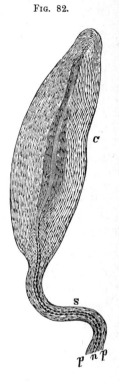

FIG. 82.

A Pacinian body, as seen with the naked eye, is of a whitish colour, usually oval and somewhat pointed at one end, from a line to a line and a half (1—1½‴) long, and firmly attached to a nerve in such a way that a single primitive fibre passes into each body. It presents a comparatively large number of elliptical and concentrical layers, which at the upper end are in pretty close contact, but at the other are separated by a wider interval, and enclose in their interior an oblong space generally some-

Fig. 82. Vaterian or Pacinian body from the subcutaneous adipose tissue of the end of a finger. *S.* The peduncle, consisting of a dark-bordered, medullated primitive nerve-fibre *n*, and the thick perineurium *p*, *p* provided with longitudinal nuclei. *C.* The body itself with the concentric layers of the perineurium which is swollen out into a bulbous shape—and the central cavity, within which the pale axis-cylinder is seen running along and terminating in a free extremity. 150 diameters.

what more pointed towards the upper end. Within
these layers nuclei can be distinctly seen disposed in
regular order, and on following the layers towards the
stem of the nerve, they are there observed finally to pass
into the perineurium which is in this part very thick.
They may therefore be regarded as gigantic developments
of the perineurium, which however only enclose a single
nerve-fibre. Now on tracing the nerve-fibre itself we
observe that its medullated portion usually extends only
up to the beginning of the body, when the medulla disappears and the axis-cylinder is seen continuing its
course alone. It then runs on through the central cavity,
and terminates at no great distance from the upper end
generally simply, yet often in a little bulbous swelling*
and in the mesentery very frequently in a spiral coil.
In rare cases it happens that the nerve divides and several branches pass into the body. But in every case we
seem to have before us a mode of termination. What
these bodies signify, what office they perform, whether
they have anything to do with the function of sensation,
or whether their province is to develop any one of the
properties of the nervous centres, we are as yet entirely
ignorant.

A certain degree of resemblance to these structures is
exhibited by the *tactile bodies* which have been recently
so much the subject of discussion. When the skin and
more especially the sensitive part of it is microscopically
examined, two sorts of papillæ, as was first discovered by
Meissner and Rud. Wagner, are distinguished, the one
narrower, the other broader, though certainly intermediate forms are met with (Fig. 83). In the narrow ones
we constantly find a simple, in broader ones of the same
class a branching, vascular loop, but no nerve. This

* Quite recently Jacubowitsch has, as he thinks, discovered a ganglion cell in
this part.—*MS. Note of Author.*

point is so far of importance, that we have, by means of these observations, been made acquainted with a new nerveless structure. In the other kind of papillæ we very frequently find no vessels at all, but on the other hand nerves, and those peculiar structures which have been designated tactile bodies.

A tactile body manifests itself as an oblong-oval structure, tolerably distinctly marked off from the remainder of the papilla, and has, with some degree of boldness indeed, been compared by Wagner to a fir-cone. It is generally rounded off at the upper and lower end, and does not exhibit a longitudinal striation, as the Pacinian bodies do, but on the contrary transverse nuclei. Now a nerve runs up to every one of these bodies, and from every one of them a nerve returns, or more correctly, we usually see two nervous filaments, generally pretty

Fig. 83.

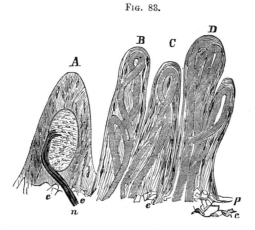

Fig. 83. Nervous and vascular papillæ from the skin of the end of a finger, after the separation of the epidermis and rete Malpighii. *A.* Nervous papilla with a tactile body, up to which ascend two primitive nerve-fibres *n;* at the base of the papilla fine elastic networks *e*, from which fine fibres radiate, between and on which connective-tissue-corpuscles are to be seen. *B, C, D.* Vascular papillæ, with, at *C*, simple, at *B* and *D*, branching vascular loops, and in addition fine elastic fibres and connective-tissue-corpuscles ; *p.* the papillary body running its horizontal course, at *c* fine stellate cells belonging to the cutis proper. 300 diameters.

close to one another, which can be readily traced up to
the side or base of the body. After this point their
course is very doubtful, and in different cases the conditions vary so much that we have not yet succeeded in
making out with certainty the relation of the nerves to
these bodies. In many cases, namely, the nerve is very
distinctly seen to ascend and also to entwine itself
around the body. Sometimes it seems as if the body
really lay in a nervous loop, and thus the possibility of a
more concentrated action on the part of external agencies upon the surface of the nerve was provided for. At
other times again it looks as if the nerve came to a termination much sooner, and buried itself in the body.
Some have assumed, with Meissner, that the body itself
belongs to the nerve which resolves itself into it. This
I do not hold to be correct, and the only point which
seems to me to be doubtful is, whether the nerve ends
in the body or forms a loop around it.

Apart from anatomical and physiological considerations, this example is of great value in the interpretation of pathological phenomena, because we here find
two complete contrasts in parts which in themselves are
quite analogous ; for, on the one hand, we have nerveless but vascular, on the other, non-vascular, papillæ,
yet provided with nerves. The peculiar relations which
the layers of the rete mucosum and epidermis bear to
the two kinds of papillæ, do not appear to present
any essential differences. They are nourished just as
perfectly over the one sort as over the other, and seem
to be just as little provided with nerves over the one as
over the other.

These are facts which indicate a certain independence
in individual parts and furnish distinct evidence that
parts of considerable size and even richly provided with
nerves can subsist, maintain their existence and perform

their functions without vessels, and that on the other hand parts which relatively contain numerous vessels, can absolutely dispense with nerves without incurring any disturbance in the state of their nutrition.

LECTURE XII.

MARCH 31, 1858.

THE NERVOUS SYSTEM.

Peripheral terminations of the nerves—Nerves of special sense—The skin and the distinction of vessel-, nerve-, and cell-territories in it—Olfactory mucous membrane—Retina—Division of nerve-fibres—The electrical organ of fishes—Muscles—Further consideration of nerve-territories—Norvous plexuses with ganglioniform enlargements—Intestines—Errors of the neuro-pathologists.

The great nervous centres—Grey substance—Ganglion- [nerve-] cells containing pigment—Varieties of ganglion-cells; sympathetic cells in the spinal marrow and brain, motor and sensitive cells. Multipolar (polyclonous) ganglion-cells—Different nature of the processes of ganglion-cells.

I RETURN, gentlemen, to-day once more to the skin. The difference which exists between the individual papillæ of the skin seems to me so important theoretically, that I think I must claim your special attention to it. In the greater number of the papillæ we see, as I mentioned to you the last time, a single or, when the papilla is very large, a branched, vascular loop. The majority of these vascular papillæ have no nerves; others again which contain tactile bodies, no vessels. If we imagine the vessels and tactile bodies removed, there remains only a very small quantity of substance in the papilla, but within it there still are morphological elements, and it is easy to convince oneself that connective tissue with its corpuscles (which latter after injection are very easily distinguished from the vessels), is in immediate contact with the cells of the rete mucosum (Fig. 83). The case is especially favourable when, in consequence of any disease, as for example small-pox, a slight tumefaction of the whole thickness of the skin in the parts affected has taken place, and the corpuscles are a little larger than they normally are. In ordinary papillæ it is somewhat more difficult to discover these elements, still upon closer examination they may be seen everywhere, even by the side of the tactile bodies.

Thus, even in the finest of these prolongations of the cutis, it is not an amorphous mass which is found, bearing a constant relation to the vessels and nerves ; on the contrary this mass of connective tissue always manifests itself as the one thing invariably present in the structure, as the real fundamental constituent of the different (vascular and nervous) papillæ, and the individual papillæ do not acquire a different character until in the one case vessel, in the other nerves, are added to this fundamental substance.

We certainly know little concerning the special relations which the vascular papillæ bear to the functions of the skin, still it can scarcely be doubted that an important relation must exist, and that as soon as we are better able to separate the different offices of the skin, greater importance will be attached to the vascular papillæ also. This much however we can even now say, that it is incorrect to imagine that a special nervous branch exists in every anatomical division of the skin : just as physiological experiments* show that considerable sensitive districts exist in the skin, so also more minute histological investigation teaches us that there is a relatively scanty termination of nerves upon the surface. If therefore we think fit to divide the skin into definite territories, those

---

* The allusion is to Weber's experiments with compasses.—*Trans.*

appertaining to the nerves will, as a matter of course, be larger than those belonging to the vessels. But every vessel territory (papilla) also which is marked out by a single capillary loop is divided into a series of smaller (cell-) territories, all of which certainly lie along the banks of the same vessel, but still have an independent existence, each of them being provided with a special cellular element.

In this manner it is very easy to explain how within a papilla a single (cell-) territory may become diseased. Suppose, for example, that such a territory swells up, increases in size, and continually keeps shooting farther and farther upwards, then arborescent ramifications may

Fig. 84.

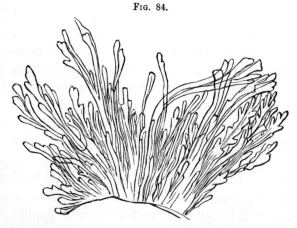

arise (accuminate [spitzes] condyloma*) without the whole papilla's being affected in a like manner. The

Fig. 84. The fundamental substance (connective tissue) of an acuminate condyloma of the penis with freely budding and branching papillæ, after the epidermis and the rete mucosum have been completely detached. 12 diameters.

* The Germans speak of condylomata *lata* and *acuminata*. The condyloma *latum* is *invariably* of syphilitic origin, and is identical with the *plaque muqueuse* of the French, who *never* use the term *condylome* in *this* sense. Condyloma *acuminatum*, on the contrary (by the French termed simply *condylome*), is *not* syphilitic in its nature, but frequently occurs in gonorrhœa, though it is also met with *independently* of this disease.—*From a MS. Note by the Author.*

vessel does not shoot up until later and forces its way into the branches when they have already attained a certain size. It is not the vessel which pushes out the parts by its development, but the first signs of development always show themselves in the connective tissue of the papilla. The study of the conditions of the skin therefore affords special interest to those who wish to devote themselves to the critical examination of the doctrines held concerning general pathology. And first with regard to the neuro-pathological views, it is quite inconceivable how a nerve which lies in the middle of a whole group of nerveless parts, can contrive to force a single papilla from among this group, with which it has not the slightest connection, into a state of pathological activity in which the remaining papillæ of the same nerve-territory take no share. Just as difficult is it, in the diseases of non-vascular papillæ, to find an explanation which shall accord with the views of a humoro-pathologist. Even when in a vascular papilla the different cell-territories attain different states, these would not admit of a ready explanation, if we were to regard the whole process of nutrition in a papilla as directly dependent upon the general condition of the vessel which supplies it.

Similar considerations might be entered upon with regard to all points of the body. Still we have in the skin a particularly favourable example for demonstrating how very incorrect it is to regard all vessels as subject to a particular nervous influence. There are a number of vessels which are entirely removed from the influence of all nerves, and, if we still confine our attention to the skin, the influence which a nerve is in a condition to exercise, is limited to this, that the afferent artery, which supplies a whole series of papillæ in common (Fig. 44) may by its means be brought into an altered condition, so that a contraction or dilatation, and in correspondence with these states a diminished or increased supply of blood to a considerable district, takes place.

If now we return from this digression to our real subject, you will recollect that I had described to you my ignorance concerning the real mode of termination which the nerves have in the tactile bodies. Whether the nerve ultimately forms a loop, or in any manner directly terminates in the internal substance of the body, is not, I think, as yet absolutely decided.

If now we consider other instances of the terminations of nerves, nowhere does any probability manifest itself that they really do form loops. In every case in which more certain knowledge has been acquired, the probability has on the contrary always become greater, that the nerves either terminate in a large plexus or recticular expansion ; or that they end in special apparatuses, concerning which it is still doubtful whether they are peculiar processes of a particular shape, into which the nerves shoot out at their extremities, or whether they constitute peculiar parts, non-nervous in their nature, to which the nerves attach themselves. This latter mode of termination is, it would appear, characteristic of most of the *higher organs of sense*, but in no single instance, in consequence of the extreme difficulty which the investigation of these parts presents, have any views been proposed which have met with universal assent. Notwithstanding the numerous investigations into the structure of the retina and cochlea, the mucous membrane of the nose and mouth, that have been made in the course of the last few years, it must be confessed that the ultimate points of histological detail have not as yet been altogether satisfactorily settled. In nearly all cases there remain two possible ways in which the nerves may terminate. According to some their terminations are connected with special structures which, according to the language

hitherto employed, cannot be regarded as being of a nervous nature, but are peculiar appendages of the nerves,
though they are certainly stated by other observers to
be directly connected with nerve-fibres, as for example
in the nasal mucous membrane. This namely is regularly clothed with cylindrical epithelium, which is plentifully provided with cilia and forms several layers, lying
one above the other, so that there are several rows of
cells covering one another. In these, according to several recent observers, cells are met with, which terminate
in a somewhat long filament, and do not, like other epithelial cells, end upon the surface, but run in an inward
direction, so as to become directly continuous with the
ends of the nerves. According to others, particularly
Max. Schultze, on the contrary, and this view seems to
be the more correct one, peculiar filiform ends of nerves
force their way out between the epithelium. The objects
of smell would therefore according to both views really
come directly in contact with the structures forming the
terminations of the nerves. Similar epithelium-like structures have recently been described as occurring also in
the mucous membrane of the tongue, seated upon peculiar papillæ, which appear to possess a pre-eminently
nervous character.

These structures moreover might lay claim to a certain
resemblance with the ultimate terminations which we find
in the case of the optic nerve in the retina, and in that
of the auditory nerve especially in the cochlea—terminations, which may in the latter case, as far as their external shape is concerned, be compared to long-tailed epithelial cells, whilst those in the retina constitute structures of peculiar delicacy. In the *retina* namely the
optic nerve, after its entrance into the interior of the
globe of the eye, spreads out in such a way, that its fibrous
elements run along on the anterior side of the retina, that

side, namely, which is turned towards the vitreous body
(Fig. 85, *f*) ; posteriorly, there follows a stratum of varying thickness, which belongs to the retina indeed, but in
no wise proceeds from the direct expansion of the optic
nerve.　In this layer we see, where it borders upon the
layer of pigment-cells of the choroid coat, and in immediate contact with these cells, a peculiar stratum which
has been subjected to a strange destiny, inasmuch as it
was for a considerable time transplanted to the anterior

Fig. 85.

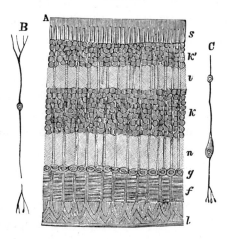

side of the retina—the famous *bacillar layer* (layer of
rods—Stäbchenschicht [membrana Jacobi]) (Fig. 85, *s*).
This layer, which belongs to the most easily injured
parts of the eye, and for this reason in many instances
escaped the notice of earlier observers, consists, when
viewed in profile, of a very large quantity of closely

Fig. 85. *A.* Vertical section through the whole thickness of the retina, after it
had been hardened in chromic acid. *l.* Membrana limitans, with the ascending,
supporting fibres. *f.* Fibrous layer of the optic nerve. *g.* Layer of ganglion-cells.
n. Grey, finely granular layer, with the radiating fibres passing through it. *k.* Internal (anterior) granular layer. *i.* Intermediate, or intergranular, layer. *k'.* External (posterior) granular layer. *s.* Layer of rods and cones. 300 diameters.
B, C (after H. Müller). Isolated radiating fibres.

packed little rods, arranged in a radiated form, and between which at certain intervals appear broader, conical
bodies. When the retina is viewed from behind, *i. e.*,
from the choroid coat, we see regularly arranged between
these cones fine points which correspond to the ends of
the little rods.

Now that which intervenes between this bacillar layer
and the proper expansion of the optic nerve, is likewise
a very complex affair, in which a series of layers following one another in regular succession can be distinguished. Immediately in front of the bacillar layer
comes a comparatively thick stratum, which appears to
be nearly entirely made up of coarse granules, the so-
called external granular layer (Fig. 85, *k'*). Then comes
a thinner layer which generally presents a tolerably
amorphous appearance, the inter-granular layer (Fig.
85, *i*). Then we again have coarsish granules (the internal granular layer) ; these bodies in both layers having
much the appearance of nuclei (Fig. 85, *k*). Next follows a second layer of a more uniform, finely granular or
finely striated appearance, and of a more greyish hue
(Fig. 85, *n*), and then only the tolerably thick stratum
of the optic nerve, which in its turn is bounded by a
membrane, the membrana limitans (Fig. 85, *l*), which is
in close apposition to the vitreous body. Within this
last layer we see, besides the fibres of the optic nerve,
and situated behind them, a number of largish cells,
which have the appearance of nerve-cells (Fig. 85, *g*).

This extremely complex structure in a membrane which
at first sight is so simple and so delicate, readily accounts
for its being extremely difficult to ascertain with certainty all the relations of its individual parts. It was
one of the most important advances towards the knowledge of these relations which was made by the discovery
of Heinrich Müller, that namely from behind, from the

bacillar layer into the most anterior layers, a series of rows of fine fibres could be traced (*radiating fibres*, also called Müllerian fibres), which both receive the granules, and support the cones and rods (Fig. 85, *B*, *C*). This very complicated apparatus is placed as nearly as possible perpendicularly to the course of the fibres of the optic nerve. The greatest difficulty which exists with regard to the anatomical connection of the parts, is to determine whether the radiating fibres, either by bending directly round, or by a lateral anastomosis, become continuous with the optic or ganglionic fibres, and are thus themselves nervous, or whether only an intimate apposition takes place, and so the nerves bear no other relation to the radiating fibres than those of proximity. A tactile body may also, you know, be either regarded as a body formed by a swelling of the nerve itself, or as a special structure up to which the nerve only proceeds or into which it enters. This question (of the connections of the radiating fibres) has not yet been definitively settled. At one time the probability became rather stronger that direct communications existed, at another that nothing more than a mere apposition took place. It can, however, even now no longer be doubted, that this apparatus is essential to the perception of light, and that the optic nerve might exist with all its parts without in any way possessing the power of receiving impressions of light, if it were not connected with this apparatus. It is well known that just that point in the background of the eye, where there are only optic fibres and no such apparatus, is the only one which does not receive impressions of light (the blind spot). In order therefore that the light may be rendered at all capable of acting upon the optic nerve, it unquestionably requires to be collected by means of this apparatus of fibres, and it is therefore an extremely interesting question for delicate physical researches, whether the nerve itself receives at its extreme ends the vibrations of the waves of light, or whether another part exists, the oscillations of which act upon the optic nerve and produce a peculiar excitation in it. At all events there do ascend from the membrana limitans slightly curved fibres (Fig. 85, *l*), probably connective tissue with its corpuscles, which afford a kind of stay or support to the whole apparatus (supporting fibres [Stützfasern]), and are not, I should suppose, freely connected with the rest of it.

We have, gentlemen, by the consideration of these relations brought out the fact, that the specific energy of individual nerves does not so much depend upon the peculiarity of the internal structure of their fibres as such, but that a great deal must be attributed to the special terminal arrangement, with which the nerve is connected, either directly or by contact, and from which the different nerves of sense derive their peculiar powers. If for example we examine a transverse section of the optic nerve external to the eye, it offers no peculiarities as compared with other nerves, which could at all account for this particular nerve's being better able to conduct light than other nerves, whilst on the other hand the peculiar manner in which its extreme ends are distributed sufficiently explains the unusually great sensitiveness of the retina to light.

With regard to the terminations of nerves, there is still one mode to be mentioned ; the *plexiform distribution*. This

FIG. 86.

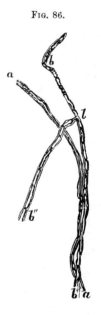

Fig. 86. Division of a primitive nerve-fibre at *t*, where we find a constriction; *b'*, *b''* branches. *a.* Another fibre, crossing the former one. 300 diameters.

is a point to which more recent researches have been principally directed by Rudolph Wagner, inasmuch as this inquirer instituted investigations into the distribution of the nerves in the electrical organ of fishes, and in so doing gave the chief impulse to the doctrine of the *ramification of nerve-fibres*. Up to that time nerves had been regarded as continuous, single tubes, which remained single throughout the whole of their course from a nervous centre to their termination. At present we know that nerves are distributed like vessels. Now seeing that nerve-fibres directly divide, usually dichotomously, and their branches again divide and subdivide, extremely abundant ramifications may in this way in time arise, the import of which is extremely different, according as the nerve is motor or sensitive, and either collects impressions *from*, or diffuses motor impulses *to*, a considerable extent of surface. A truly marvellous instance has lately come to our knowledge in the electrical nerve of the electrical silurus (malapterurus), which has become so celebrated by the interesting experiments of Dubois-Reymond. Here Bilharz has shown that the nerve which supplies the electrical organ is in the first instance only a single microscopical primitive fibre, which keeps continually dividing until it finally resolves itself into an enormously great number of ramifications which spread themselves out upon the electrical organ. Here therefore the nervous influence must all at once diffuse itself from one point over the whole extent of the electrical plates.

In man we are still in want of distinct evidence with regard to this question, because the immense distances, over which individual nerves extend, render it almost impossible to follow any single given primitive fibres from their central origin to their extreme peripheral termination. But it is not at all improbable that in man too analogous arrangements exist in some organs, although perhaps not such striking ones. If we compare the size of the nervous trunks in certain parts with the total number of operations which are effected in an organ, for example, in a gland, it can scarcely appear doubtful that at least analogous arrangements exist there also. This mode of distribution offers peculiar interest in this respect, that many parts which are separated by intervals of space are thereby connected with one another. The electrical organ is composed of a number of plates, but not every plate is supplied with nerves proceeding from the centre and intended only for it. The silurus does not set one or other of its plates in motion, but is obliged to set the whole of them in motion ; it is quite unable to divide the action. It can increase or diminish the intensity, but must always call the whole into operation. If in like manner we consider the arrangements which prevail in certain muscles, we find there is no evidence to justify us in assuming that every portion of a muscle receives special, independent nerve-fibres. On the contrary, a special division of nervous action in muscles only exists to a very limited extent, as we know from our experience in our own bodies. The neuro-pathological doctrines would lead us to infer that *the will, or the soul, or the brain* is able by means of special fibres to act upon every single part, but in reality this is by no means the case, for the nervous centres have mostly only one single path by which they can communicate with a certain number of similar elementary apparatuses.

Now with regard to *nervous plexuses*, we are at the present time acquainted with most extensive arrangements of the kind in man, in the submucous tissue of the intestines, where the relations have recently been more closely investigated, in the first instance by Meissner and after-

wards by Billroth.   The submucous layer of the intestines is therefore, as Willis long ago declared it to be, a

Fig. 87.

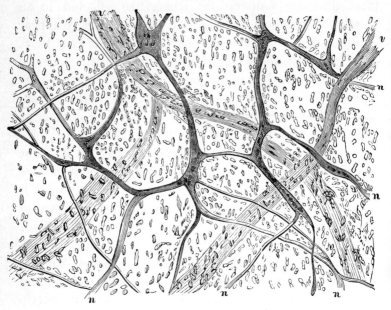

nervous tunic.   On following up the afferent nerves, they
are seen, after having divided, at last to break up into
real networks ; these in new-born infants present at certain points very large nodules, from which the nerve-
fibres spread out into interlacements, so that a certain
resemblance is thereby produced to a network of capillaries.

To what extent such arrangements prevail in the body
generally has not yet been determined ; for these facts
also are almost entirely new, and have only recently
attracted the attention of observers, but probably the

Fig. 87. Nervous plexus from the submucous tissue of the intestinal canal of a
child, from a preparation of Herr Billroth's.   *n, n, n.* Nerves which unite to form a
network, and exhibit at their points of junction glanglioniform swellings abounding
in nuclei.   *v, v.* Vessels, and in the intervals nuclei belonging to the connective
tissue.   Magnified 180 diameters.

number of these nervous membranes will eventually be augmented. In order, however, to avoid any misunderstanding, I must at once add that these plexiform expansions are by no means simple, but that the large nodules I have mentioned have the appearance of ganglions, so that we have here in some sort new nervous centres pre senting themselves, and affording the possibility of a reinforcement of, or obstruction to, the original impulses. For the functions of the part this arrangement is manifestly of great importance, for we should not well be able to explain the peristaltic movements of the intestinal canal, if some contrivance did not exist by which stimuli, that in the first instance were conveyed only to one spot in the canal, could be transferred from network to network and from part to part. The modes of distribution of nerves, with which we were till recently acquainted, were not sufficient to afford anything approaching an explanation of the nature of peristaltic action, whilst these investigations of Meissner's have at once furnished us with a most suitable groundwork for an interpretation of it. So much concerning the general forms which are, as far as we know at present, assumed by the peripheral terminations of the nerves.

On the whole, these results correspond but little with the opinions which were formerly entertained, and with the hypotheses still advanced by the neuro-pathologists. The views of a neuro-pathologist of pure water amount, as is well known, to this, that a nervous centre is able, by means of nerve-fibres, to produce particular effects upon all, even the smallest, particles of the territory under its sway. If a mass of cancer or pus is to spring up in any little spot in the body, or merely a simple disturbance of nutrition to ensue, the neuro-pathologist requires a special arrangement, by means of which the nervous centre is enabled to have its influence conveyed into even the most minute districts of the periphery, and some route along which the messengers can travel who have been appointed to bear the order to the remotest points of the organism. Actual experience teaches us nothing of the kind. At those very spots where we know such an extremely complicated arrangement of the terminal apparatuses to exist, as I have described to you in the organs of sense, the nerves have no connection with the nutrition of the parts, and especially no demonstrable influence upon the elementary structures. In nearly all other places, either whole surfaces, or parts of organs are supplied with nerves in a uniform manner, or from these surfaces and parts of organs collective impressions are conveyed to the centres. In many parts concerning which we can certainly demonstrate that nervous influence is exercised upon them, as for example in middle-sized and small vessels, we do not yet at all know to what extent their individual constituents receive special nerve-fibres. So bad are the anatomical foundations of the neuro-pathological doctrines.

There still remains for us, gentlemen, now that we have discussed the terminal arrangements of the peripheral nerves, to consider the important series of nervous centres, or in a more restricted sense of the term, *ganglionic apparatuses*. As I lately remarked to you, we find these predominating in those parts of the nervous centres in which there is grey matter. Still the mere grey hue of a part is not decisive proof of its ganglionic nature ; and in particular we must not suppose that the ganglion-cells are at all essentially concerned in the production of the grey colour, seeing that we find grey matter in many places where ganglion-cells do not exist. Thus, the most external layer of the cortex of the cerebrum does not contain any well-marked ganglion-cells, although it looks grey ; but we find there a translucent connective substance, pervaded by a large number of delicate vessels, and assuming, in proportion as these are more or less full, at one time more a reddish grey, at another more a whitish grey hue. On the other hand it frequently happens that, where there are ganglion-cells, the substance really does not look grey, but has a positive colour varying between brownish yellow and blackish brown. Thus we find spots in the brain, which have long been known by the names of substantia nigra, fusca, etc., in which the black or brown colour, which we perceive with the naked eye, is dependent upon the ganglion-cells, which form really coloured points.

This coloration appears only in the course of years. The older an individual becomes, the more conspicuously do the colours show themselves ; still under certain circumstances pathological processes also seem to accelerate their manifestation. Thus in the ganglia of the sympathetic it is a striking phenomenon, that certain morbid processes, for example, typhoid fever, appear to exercise a powerful influence in producing an early deposit of pigment. Since the pigment however constitutes a relatively foreign mass in the internal economy of the ganglion-cells, and is not, as far as we know, subservient to their proper functions, but has all the characters of an inert accidental deposit, it may really be quite possible that these conditions should be regarded as a kind of premature senescence in the ganglia. In these cases we discern in the ganglion-cells (Fig. 88, a) in addition to the very distinct, large nucleus with its large, bright nucleolus, the contents properly so-called, which consist of a finely granular substance, and at a certain spot enclose the pigment which is generally deposited excentrically, but sometimes around the nucleus. Under certain circumstances this deposit increases to such an extent that

a great part of the cell is filled up with it. The more
abundant it is, the darker does the whole spot appear to
the naked eye.

Formerly it was imagined that the majority of ganglion-

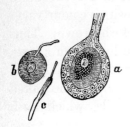

FIG. 88.

cells were merely round bodies, but
the conviction has been gradually
gaining strength, that this form is an
artificial one, and that the real state
of the case is rather, that processes
strike out from the cell in various
directions, and ultimately become
continuous with nerves or other
ganglion-cells. These processes are
in the first instance pale, and even where their transition
into ordinary, darkly-contoured nerve-fibres can be
traced, they are observed (but generally not until a certain distance from the ganglion-cell) to become thicker
and gradually to provide themselves with a medullary
sheath. This circumstance which was formerly unknown
explains how it was, that during so long a period so
much obscurity prevailed with regard to these conditions.
In the first part of their course, therefore, the processes
of the glanglion-cells, especially in the brain and spinal
marrow, are not nerves in the ordinary meaning of the
word, but pale fibres which frequently bear scarcely any
resemblance to the non-medullated fibres I have already
described to you, and have rather the appearance of pale
axis-cylinders (Fig. 88, a, b).

It was long believed that essential differences existed
between the ganglion-cells according as they belonged to
one or other of the three principal divisions of the

Fig. 88. Elements from the Gasserian ganglion.   a. Ganglion-cell with nucleated
sheath, which is prolonged around the efferent nerve-process ; in the interior. the
large, clear nucleus with its nucleolus, and round about it an accumulation of pigment.   b. Isolated ganglion-cell with a pale process proceeding up to it.   c. Delicate nerve-fibre with pale axis-cylinder.   300 diameters.

nervous system, and therefore especially between the cells of the sympathetic and those of the brain and spinal marrow. But in this point also the contrary has proved to be the case, especially since Jacubowitsch has brought to our knowledge the new fact, of the correctness of which I have fully convinced myself, namely, that structures which are perfectly analogous to the ordinary ganglion-cells of the sympathetic, also occur in the middle of the spinal marrow and several parts which are considered to belong to the brain. It may therefore be said, that cells belonging to the sympathetic nerve, concerning which it has already long been known that a great part of its fibres have their origin in the spinal marrow, are really also met with in the spinal marrow, and that in this respect also the cord does not form a simple and necessary contrast to the main trunk of the sympathetic.

If we examine the *spinal marrow*, which affords the clearest representation of the plan of a true nervous centre in the narrowest meaning of the word, a little more closely, we everywhere find in its grey substance (the horns), and indeed in nearly every transverse section, different kinds of ganglion-cells. Jacubowitsch has, and I believe him to be in the main correct, distinguished three different forms, of which he calls the one motor, the second sensitive, and the third sympathetic. These lie generally in separate groups.

I shall revert to this subject when I come to speak more at length concerning the spinal marrow; here I only wish to speak about the different forms of ganglion-cells. The so-called unipolar forms, are, in proportion as the examinations are conducted with more care, continually becoming more and more rare. In the great nervous centres most of the cells possess at least two processes, and very many are multipolar or, more accurately,

Fig. 89.

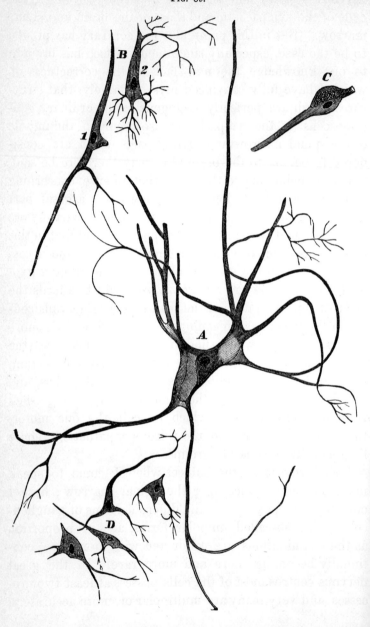

many-branched (*polyclonous*).* A multipolar cell is a body with a large nucleus, granular contents and, if it be particularly large, a spot of pigment, and is provided with processes running in different directions. These processes often divide into twigs and thus commences the condition of which I have already spoken (p. 290), that whole masses of filaments or fibres proceed from one point—a condition which indicates, that, in the first instance indeed according to circumstances, one path or another can be made use of, but that, when once a path has been chosen leading in the direction of the periphery, the impulse must be propagated in a relatively equable manner throughout the whole series of ramifications. These multipolar forms (Fig. 89, *A*) are mostly comparatively large, and lie accumulated in those parts which are subservient to the motor functions! and they therefore may be briefly designated motor cells.

Those forms which correspond to the sensitive spots (Fig. 89, *B*) are usually smaller and do not present such an extraordinary luxuriance of ramification as the larger ones. A large portion of them possess only three, or perhaps, four branches. Those which Jacubowitsch has called sympathetic are, on the other hand again, larger, but have still fewer branches and are distinguished by a greater roundness of shape. These are differences which are certainly not so decided, as to enable us already at once to determine in every single case from the appearance of a ganglion-cell to which category it belongs ; but still, if we consider the individual groups, they are so

Fig. 89. Ganglion-cells from the great nervous centres ; *A*, *B*, *C* from the spinal cord, from preparations belonging to Herr Gerlach, *D* from the cortex of the cerebrum. *A*. Large, many-rayed cell (multipolar, polyclonous) from the anterior horns (motor cell). *B*. Smaller cells with three large processes, from the posterior horns (sensitive cells). *C*. Two-rayed (bipolar, diclonous), more rounded cell, from the neighbourhood of the posterior commissure (sympathetic cell). 300 diameters.

* κλών, ωνός, a shoot, twig.—Tr.

striking, as to incite the observer to reflection upon the
different qualities of these groups.

In the course of time probably further distinctions,
perhaps even in the internal economy of these cells,
will be detected, but at present nothing more can be
stated concerning them. This is a very great and
lamentable void in our knowledge, and a void which
we now particularly feel, because this is just the place
where we should have to discuss the pacific action of
these different elements. But it must not be overlooked
that these conditions are among the most difficult which
are ever submitted to anatomical investigation, and that
one's endeavors to produce specimens of a character to
convince one's own eyes alone, nearly always fail, because
it is scarcely possible to succeed in effecting a real isolation of the cells with all their processes and connections,
and because, on account of the extraordinary fragility of
these bodies, one is nearly always compelled to trace them
out in hardened sections. When sections are made of
structures which to a great extent are composed of fibres
and in which these run in a longitudinal, a transverse, or
an oblique direction, so that an interlacement is always
presented to the view, it depends of course entirely upon
a happy chance whether in a section the course of a single fibre can be followed up over a large space with a
certain degree of distinctness. This difficulty can certainly
be lessened by making the sections in all possible directions and thus increasing the probability of at last stum-
bling upon the direction followed by the divisions of a
branch, but even then the obstacles still remain so great
that one can hardly expect, ever to be able to take in at
one view the whole of the ramifications and connections
of a cell belonging to the great nervous centres, that is
provided with at all a large number of branches.

In this respect also the *electrical organ* of fishes has

become a particularly interesting subject for investigation, inasmuch as the one fibre which supplies the organ has been traced back by Bilharz to a single central ganglion-cell, which is so large that it can be dissected out with the naked eye. This ganglion-cell has also delicate offsets in other directions, but it has not hitherto been possible to determine their ultimate relations any more than we are able to obtain a definite notion of the minute anatomy of the human brain, and especially to discover, to what extent connections take place there between the different cells. By the investigations which have been instituted into the structure of the spinal cord, it has been shown to be extremely probable, that all the processes of the individual ganglion-cells do not become continuous with nerve-fibres, but that a part of them run to other ganglion-cells and thus establish a communication between the cells. Moreover at certain points, especially in several parts of the surface of the *brain*, still finer processes are found, which proceed from ganglion-cells and are connected with peculiar, quite characteristic apparatuses (bacillar layer of the cerebellum and cerebrum), which offer the greatest resemblance to those in the retina, those extremely delicate, vibratory arrangements of the radiating fibres.

The processes of the ganglion cells might therefore, I think, be divided into three categories ; genuine nerve-processes, ganglion-processes, and those of which the import is entirely unknown and which, it would seem, are connected with peculiar and altogether specific apparatuses, concerning which it is for the present uncertain, whether they are to be regarded as the terminations of the nerves, or only as structures placed in apposition to them.

LECTURE XIII.

SPINAL CORD AND BRAIN.

The spinal cord—White and grey matter—Central canal—Groups of ganglion-cells
—White columns and commissures.
The medulla oblongata and the brain—Its granular and bacillar layer.
The spinal cord of the petromyzon and its non-medullated fibres.
The intermediate substance (interstitial tissue)—Ependyma ventriculorum—Neuro-
glia—Corpora amylacea.

THE last time, gentlemen, I laid before you the results
of the most recent observations concerning the nature and
distribution of the ganglion-cells in the great nervous
centres ; allow me now to dwell a moment upon that
organ which serves as a type in the development of the
vertebratæ, and is at the same time the one whose structure we can best take in at one view, namely, the *spinal
cord*.

The spinal cord presents, as is well known, and can
with ease be seen by the naked eye in any transverse
section, in different parts of its course, a different amount
of white matter, though nearly everywhere the white
matter predominates over the grey. This appears in
transverse sections in the form of the well-known horns,
which are distinctly marked off from the pure white of
the rest of the mass by their sometimes pale grey, some-

times reddish grey colour. Wherever then the substance appears white to the naked eye, it is essentially composed of real, medullated nerve-fibres, in which only here and there a few ganglion-cells are imbedded ; and indeed a large proportion of these fibres are of considerable breadth, so that the quantity of medullary matter is at certain points extremely large.

The grey matter of the horns is the real seat of the ganglion-cells, but here too the grey colour is by no means to be entirely ascribed to the accumulation of ganglion-cells ; on the contrary, they never, as you will afterwards see, form more than a small portion of this matter, and the grey hue is chiefly due to there generally being in these parts no separation of that opaque, strongly refractive substance (myeline, medullary matter) which fills the white nerves.

It is in the centre of the grey substance that, as Stilling, especially, has shown, the *central canal* (canalis spinalis) actually exists, which had previously been so commonly supposed to be present, and had also frequently been described as of constant occurrence, but of which nevertheless no one had ever previously been able to furnish a regular demonstration.   In the case of the old observers, as for example Portal, their investigations were in every instance confined to a few pathological specimens, from which they derived all the information they possessed upon the subject, and from which they inferred in a somewhat arbitrary manner that the presence of a canal was the rule.

This central canal is so minute that extremely successful sections are required in order that it may clearly be perceived by the naked eye.   Usually nothing more than a rounded grey spot can be detected, which is distinguished from the surrounding parts by its somewhat greater density.   It is by microscopical examination

alone that we can detect in this spot the transverse section
of the canal in the shape of a minute hole (Fig. 90, *c*, *c*),
which, like nearly all the free surfaces of the body, is invested with a layer of epithelium. It has now taken up
its stand as a really regular, constant and persistent canal. It is continued throughout the whole extent of the
spinal marrow from the filum terminale, where it cannot
at all times be very distinctly demonstrated, up to the
fourth ventricle, where the orifice by which it opens into
the so-called sinus rhomboidalis* is situated in the gelatinous substance of the calamus scriptorius. Here it may

FIG. 90.

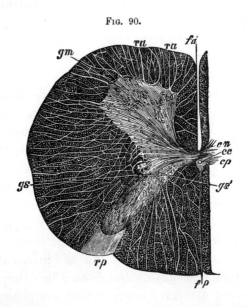

Fig. 90. The half of a transverse section from the cervical part of the spinal marrow. *fa.* Anterior fissure ; *fp*, posterior fissure. *cc.* Central canal with the
central thread of ependyma. *ca.* Anterior commissure with nerve-fibres crossing
one another ; *cp*, posterior commissure. *ra.* Anterior roots ; *rp*, posterior ones.
gm. Accumulation of motor cells in the anterior horns ; *gs*, sensitive cells of the
posterior horns ; *gs'*, sympathetic cells. The black, dotted mass represents a transverse section of the white substance of the cord (the nerve-fibres belonging to the
anterior, lateral and posterior columns) and its lobular divisions. 12 diameters.

* A name given to the floor of the fourth ventricle.

in the first instance be traced as a direct continuation from the floor of the fourth ventricle into a minute funnel-shaped fissure or line.

As for the *ganglion-cells*, they are generally found in the largest number in the anterior and lateral parts of the anterior horns. It is at this spot that we chiefly meet with the large many-rayed corpuscles which we considered the last time—corpuscles, which have in great part been traced into efferent nerves of the anterior root, and therefore give origin to motor nerves.

An analogous, but less distinctly grouped accumulation is found in the direction of the posterior horns, but there the cells are rather the small, many-rayed ones, such as those I lately described to you ; they are connected with the fibres which run into the posterior root, and are therefore probably subservient to the functions of sensation. Besides, there is generally a third, sometimes more closely aggregated, at others more scattered, group of cells to be seen, which in their whole conformation remind us of the familiar cell-forms we meet with in the ganglia (Figs. 89, *C ;* 90, *gs'*). Their special position in the spinal marrow is certainly not so clearly defined as that of the other parts ; perhaps they should be regarded as the origin of the sympathetic roots which run from the spinal marrow to the main trunk of the sympathetic, but this is as yet by no means clearly made out.

In the white substance of the anterior, lateral and posterior columns are found the medullated nerve-fibres, which in general follow an ascending or descending course, so that in transverse sections of the spinal marrow we scarcely gain sight of anything else than transverse sections of the nerve-fibres. Under the microscope therefore we generally see dark points, every one of which corresponds to a nerve-fibre. The whole mass of fibres constituting the columns of the spinal cord is, from

within outwardly, split up into a series of groups or segments chiefly following a radiating arrangement, or in
some sort into wedge-shapes lobules, in consequence of a
sometimes smaller, sometimes larger quantity of connective tissue with vessels pushing its way in between the
separate divisions, which are of a fascicular nature like
those of the peripheral nerves. This connective tissue is
directly connected with the more abundant mass of it
present in the grey matter. Now with regard to the
nerve-fibres themselves, it is probable that a certain number of them proceed throughout the whole length of the
spinal marrow, but it ought certainly not to be assumed
that they are all derived from the brain; a probably
considerable portion no doubt have their origin in the
ganglion-cells of the spinal marrow itself, and then bend
round into the anterior or posterior columns. Besides,
the conviction has more and more gained ground, that,
both between the two halves of the spinal marrow and
between the separate groups of ganglion-cells, direct
communications, *commissures*, exist—fibres passing across
from one cell to another and from one side to the other,
some so as to cross with those of the opposite side (anterior commissure), and some so as to run in a straight and
parallel direction (posterior commissure).

With the help of these anatomical observations a notion, though indeed as yet a very unsatisfactory one, can
be formed of the routes along which the different processes are carried on within the nervous centres. *Every
special function possesses its special elementary, cellular
organs; every mode of conduction finds paths distinctly
traced out for it.* In general too, well-defined peculiarities in the structure of the individual nervous centres
correspond to the differences of function, and particularly
the posterior horns become gradually more and more
strongly developed as we ascend; and in proportion as

this development proceeds, we see the medulla oblongata, the cerebellum and cerebrum, coming into view, whilst the motor parts withdraw more and more into the background and ultimately almost entirely disappear. All nervous centres, the lowest as well as the most highly developed, are disposed upon an analogous plan ; the only thing which, at least as yet, can be regarded as an especially characteristic peculiarity of the encephalon, is the circumstance, to which I called your attention in the last lecture, namely, that in the cerebrum and cerebellum processes from ganglion-cells are connected with particularly complicated apparatuses, which most resemble

FIG. 91.

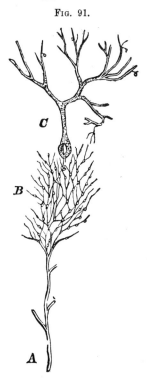

Fig. 91. Diagrammatic representation of the disposition of the nerves in the cortex of the cerebellum, after Gerlach ('Mikroscopische Studien,' plate I., fig. 3). *A*. White matter. *B, C*, grey matter, *B*, granular layer, *C*, cellular layer.

the granular and bacillar layers of the retina (Fig. 91)
which I have brought before your notice. For here too
we find branched, almost arborescent filaments, which
bear upon them minute granules, often in several rows,
and attach themselves to the ganglion-cells in a manner
essentially differing from, and much more delicate than
that observed in the case of the proper nerve-processes.
This kind of ganglion-cells may very likely stand in some
close connection with the psychical functions, but at present we have no accurate information upon the subject,
and it will, I expect, still be a long time before anything
positive can be made out about it, seeing that parts which
are much more accessible to investigation, like the retina,
present the very greatest difficulties to those who seek
to discover the functions of the individual segments.

The conformation which we have found to exist in the
spinal marrow of man is essentially the same throughout
the whole series of vertebrate animals, only that in man
it is generally more complicated, and exhibits a greater
abundance both of nerve-fibres and ganglionic matter. I

FIG. 92.

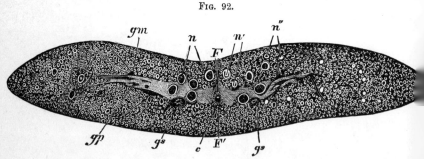

Fig. 92. Transverse section through the spinal marrow of Petromyzon fluviatilis.
F. Anterior fissure, *F'*, posterior fissure, *c*, central canal with epithelium, *gm*, large
many-rayed ganglion-cells with processes in the direction of the anterior roots,
gp, smaller, many-rayed cells with processes running to the posterior roots, *gs*, large,
roundish cells in the neighbourhood of the posterior commissure (sympathetic cells).
n, n. Transverse sections of the large, pale nerve-fibres (Müllerian fibres), *n'*, gaps
out of which the large nerves have gallen ; *n''*, gaps belonging to smaller fibres.
Besides, the cut ends of numerous finer and coarser fibres.

have brought you for comparison a section from the spinal marrow of one of the lowest of the vertebratæ, namely the lamprey (petromyzon). In this animal the spinal marrow forms a very small, flat band which has somewhat of a depression on the surface, and at first sight looks like a real ligament. On making a transverse section of it, it is found to contain the same parts that we see in man, but all only in a rudimentary form. What in ourselves we call grey matter, is also found there on both sides in the shape of a flattened oblong lobe which contains a few scattered ganglion-cells, but only very few, so that perhaps only four or five are met with on each side of the transverse section. In the centre a central canal can likewise be detected, and that too lined with an epithelial layer similar to that which occurs in man. Below and in front of it generally lie a number of largish, round cavities, which correspond to unusually large, non-medullated nerve-fibres (Fig. 93, *a*), which were first seen by Joh. Müller. Farther outwards lie a few other thick fibres, but greatly exceeding these in number a large quantity of very fine fibres which give the transverse section a very diversified, regularly dotted appearance. Among the ganglion-cells three different kinds can here also be distinguished. Towards the outside of the grey matter lie many-rayed cells, larger anteriorly, smaller and more simple posteriorly. More internally and posteriorly on the other hand we find larger, more rounded, seemingly diclonous (bipolar) cells, comparable to the sympathetic forms. These cells communicate across the middle-line by means of real fibres, and besides we find processes which run out from the spinal marrow forwards and backwards and form the anterior and posterior roots. This is the simplest plan we have, displaying these relations; it is the general type of the anatomical structure of these parts.

A circumstance worthy of particular observation here is that in the petromyzon, in the whole substance of the spinal marrow, no medullary matter exists in an isolated form, as is the case in man ; we only find simple, pale fibres, which Stannius has without hesitation pronounced to be naked axis-cylinders. But without taking into account the fact that some of them have an enormous diameter, we find upon more accurate examination, as in the case of the gelatinous grey fibres in man, a membrane very clearly seen in transverse sections, especially after it has been coloured with carmine—and in the centre a finely granular matter, so that they seem rather to correspond to entire nerve-fibres.

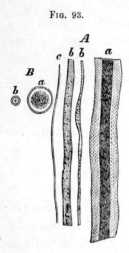

FIG. 93.

Hitherto, gentlemen, in considering the nervous system, I have only spoken of the really nervous parts of it. But if we would study the nervous system in its real relations in the body, it is extremely important to have a knowledge of that substance also which lies *between the proper nervous parts*, holds them together and gives the whole its form in a greater or less degree.

It is by no means very long ago since the existence of such interstitial masses of tissue was really only conceded in the case of peripheral nerves, and since the neurilemma was only traced back as far as the membranes of the spinal cord and brain, such an enveloping tissue being at most allowed to exist within the ganglia and in the sympathetic. In the nervous centres properly so called, and

Fig. 93. Pale fibres from the spinal marrow of Petromyzon fluviatilis. *A*. Broad, narrow, and extremely fine fibres. *B*. Transverse sections of broad fibres with a distinct membrane and granular centre. 300 diameters.

especially in the brain, this interstitial matter of ours was regarded as essentially nervous, for a substance of the kind appeared a natural desideratum, as long as a direct transferrence of impulses from fibre to fibre was admitted to take place, as long therefore as the necessity for a real continuity of conduction within the nerves themselves was not recognized. Thus in the brain a finely granular substance was spoken of as existing, which insinuated itself between the fibres, and though it certainly did not establish a complete connection between them, inasmuch as it occasioned a certain difficulty in the transferrence of impulses, yet nevertheless seemed to render a certain amount of conduction possible, so that when the impulse reached a certain degree of intensity, a direct transferrence from fibre to fibre could take place. This substance is however unquestionably not of a nervous nature, and if inquiry be made as to the relation which exists between it and the familiar groups of physiological tissues, it is impossible to doubt but that the substance in question is a kind of connective tissue; and therefore an equivalent of that tissue with which we became acquainted in the shape of perineurium (p. 265). But the appearance of this substance is certainly very different from that of what we call perineurium or neurilemma. These are comparatively firm, and often indeed hard and tough tissues, whilst the substance in question is extremely soft and fragile, so that it is only with very great difficulty that we can succeed in making out its structure.

I first had my attention directed to its peculiarities in investigations which I many years ago (1846) instituted into the nature of the so-called *lining membrane of the cerebral ventricles* (Ependyma). At that time the view was generally held, which had been put forward first by Purkinje and Valentin, and afterwards especially by Henle, that a real lining membrane did not exist in the ventricles of the brain, but only an epithelial covering, the epithelial cells directly resting upon the surface of the horizontally disposed nerve-fibres. This epithelial layer was what Purkinje called ependyma ventriculorum.* This assumption, it is true, was never shared in by pathologists. Pathological observation held on its course pretty unconcernedly by the side of these histological assertions. However, it appeared desirable that some understanding should be come to on the subject, since in a merely epithelial ependyma an inflammation would scarcely take place, like that which is wont to be attributed to serous membranes. The result of my investigations was, that there certainly does exist a layer beneath the epithelium of the ventricles, which in many parts has quite the character of connective tissue, but in other places possesses great softness, so that it is extremely difficult to give a description of its appearance. Every, even the slightest, traction of the part alters its appearance, and a substance now granular, now striated, now reticulated, now of any other form, is seen.

At first I thought I had succeeded in showing that a tissue analogous to connective tissue did actually exist in this part, and that the presence of a membrane could be demonstrated. But, the more I occupied myself with the examination of it, the more did I become convinced that a real boundary between this membrane and the deeper layers of tissue did not exist, and that a membrane could only be spoken of improperly, inasmuch as the notion of a membrane involves the supposition that it is more or less different from the parts beneath it, and constitutes a separable object. Now in the present

---

* This term has had its signification extended by the Author, who takes it to include the whole of the layer (connective tissue as well as epithelium), which rests upon the nerve-fibres and is interposed between them and the cavity of the ventricles.—*From a MS. Note by the Author.*

instance a separation of a rough kind may certainly not
unfrequently be effected, but a more delicate kind of
separation is altogether impossible. When the surface of
any section of the ventricular wall is examined with a
tolerably high power, the first thing noticed on the surface is an epithelium, sometimes in a better, sometimes
in a worse state of preservation (Fig. 94, *E*). In the
most favourable cases we find cylindrical epithelium with
cilia, extending throughout the whole extent of the
cavity of the spinal marrow (central canal) and of that
of the brain (ventricles). Beneath this layer follows a
sometimes more, sometimes less pure layer of a structure
resembling connective tissue, which at first sight certainly appears to be separated by a sharp outline from

Fig. 94.

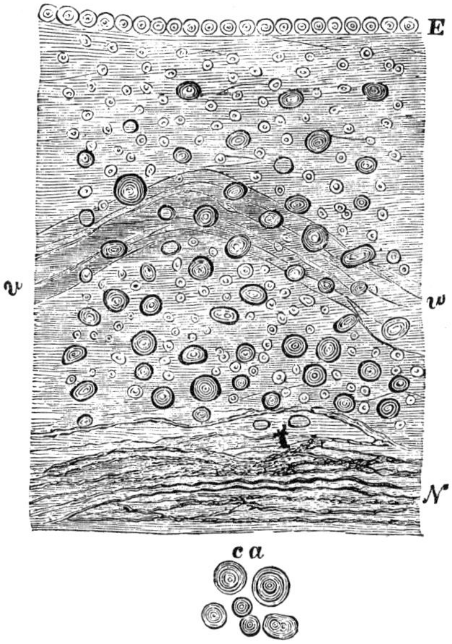

Fig. 94. Ependyma ventriculorum and neuro-glia from the floor of the fourth
cerebral ventricle. *E*, Epithelium, *N*, nerve-fibres. Between them the free portion
of the neuro-glia with numerous connective-tissue-corpuscles and nuclei, at *v* a vessel. In addition, numerous corpora amylacea, which are moreover represented
separately at *ca*. 300 diameters.

the deeper parts, for even with the naked eye, and especially after the addition of acetic acid, an external grey
and translucent layer is very distinctly seen, whilst the
deeper layer looks white.   This white appearance is due
to the presence of medullated nerve-fibres which first
occur singly, then continually become more numerous
and closely aggregated, and as a rule run parallel to the
surface.   Thus it may certainly appear as if a particular
membrane existed here, which could be separated from
the uppermost nerve-fibres.   But now, if we compare
the substance which advances to the surface with that
which lies between the nerve-fibres, no essential difference presents itself ; on the contrary, it turns out that
the superficial layer is nothing more than an extension
upwards, beyond the nervous elements, of a portion of
the interstitial tissue which is everywhere present between them, but in this layer alone is seen in all its
purity.   The connection therefore is a continuous one.

You see from this description that it was a very idle
dispute, when it was discussed for years, whether the
membrane which clothed the ventricles was a continuation of the arachnoid or pia mater, or was a special membrane.   There is, strictly speaking, no membrane at all
present, but it is the surface of the brain itself which
directly meets the eye.   In the case of articular cartilage
also we must call it idle to dispute what kind of membrane invests the cartilage, since the cartilage itself advances right up to the free surface of the joint.   Neither
is there any prolongation from the arachnoid or the pia
mater to the surface of the ventricle ; the last processes
which these membranes send inwardly are the choroid
plexuses and the tela chorioides [velum interpositum].
Beyond these there is no serous covering found investing
the internal surface of the ventricles of the brain.   For
this reason the conditions of the cerebral cavities cannot

be exactly compared with those of ordinary serous sacs. In the tela chorioides or the plexuses, a series of phenomena may certainly manifest themselves, which are parallel to the diseases of other serous parts, but this can never take place in the same manner on the ventricular surface of the brain.

This peculiarity of the membrane, namely, that it becomes continuous with the interstitial matter, the real cement, which binds the nervous elements together, and that in all its properties it constitutes a tissue different from the other forms of connective tissue, has induced me to give it a new name, that of *neuro-glia** (nerve-cement). The view that the substance in question belongs to the class of connective tissues has recently been admitted on nearly all sides, but with regard to the extent to which any isolated structures that occur in it are to be considered as belonging to this substance, opinions are still divided. Even when I instituted my first special investigations into the structure of the ependyma of the brain and spinal cord, it turned out that certain stellate cells which are met with in the middle of the spinal marrow (in the wall of the central canal, the existence of which was afterwards more accurately demonstrated, namely, in what I called the *central thread of ependyma*), and which up to that time had been regarded as nerve-cells, unquestionably belonged to the neuro-glia. Afterwards, and especially by the Dorpat school with Bidder at its head, a series of investigations were published, in which a great number of cells in the spinal marrow were set down as belonging to this connective tissue. Bidder himself was ultimately led to regard all the cells which are found in the posterior half of the spinal marrow, and therefore those sympathetic and sensitive cells also which you have just seen, as connective-tissue-corpuscles. On

* γλία, glue.—*Tr.*

the other hand, Jacubowitsch has utterly denied the occurrence of the cellular elements of connective tissue in
any part of the brain or spinal cord, and has asserted
that the interstitial tissue, which by him too, indeed, is
regarded as connective tissue, is an altogether amorphous,
finely granular or reticulated matter, which nowhere
contains a single corpuscular element. Between these
extremes, I think, we are perfectly justified by experience in steering a middle course. There can, according
to my firm conviction, be no doubt but that the larger
cells which pervade the posterior horns of the spinal marrow are nerve-cells ; but, on the other hand, it must be
maintained with equal positiveness, that, where neuro-
glia is met with, it also contains a certain number of cellular elements. Immediately beneath the surface of the
cerebral ventricles we commonly meet with spindle-
shaped cells lying parallel to it, just like those which are
found in other kinds of connective tissue ; these become
larger under certain circumstances, and, in oblique sections, often display themselves in the form of stellate
cells (Fig. 94).

A substance altogether similar in structure to that,
with which we have already become familiar in connective tissue—especially
as far as its cells are concerned—is also
found between the nerve-fibres of the
cerebrum ; only the cells are so soft and
fragile, that generally nothing but nu-
clei can be perceived, scattered at certain intervals
throughout the mass. On making a careful search, however, even in fresh (not artificially hardened) specimens,
soft cellular bodies of a roundish or lenticular form can

FIG. 95.

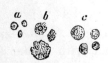

Fig. 95. Elements of the neuro-glia from the white substance of the cerebral
hemispheres of a human subject. *a.* Free nuclei with nucleoli, *b,* nuclei with the
granular remnants of the cellular parenchyma broken up in making the preparation,
c, perfect cells. 300 diameters.

be detected, which possess finely granular contents and large granulated nuclei with nucleoli, and lie, certainly in no very great number, between the nervous elements. At certain spots it has indeed been hitherto impossible to draw a well-defined boundary-line between the two tissues, and especially so at the surface of the cerebellum and cerebrum, between the granules which I have already (p. 307) described to you as connected with large ganglion-cells, and the nuclei of the connective tissue. Wherever the parts are seen severed from their connections, it is not easy to make the distinction, and a positive decision is only possible as long as the parts are viewed in their natural position.

Now it is certainly of considerable importance to know that in all nervous parts, in addition to the real nervous elements, a second tissue exists, which is allied to the large group of formations, which pervade the whole body, and with which we have in the previous lectures become acquainted under the name of connective tissues. In considering the pathological or physiological conditions of the brain or spinal marrow, the first point is always to determine how far the tissue which is affected, attacked or irritated, is nervous in its nature, or merely an interstitial substance. We thus obtain at the very outset the important criterion for the interpretation of morbid processes, that the affections of the brain and spinal marrow may sometimes be rather interstitial, at others rather parenchymatous, and experience shows us that this very interstitial tissue of the brain and spinal marrow is one of the most frequent seats of morbid change, as for example, of fatty degeneration.

Within the neuro-glia run the vessels, which are therefore nearly everywhere separated from the nervous substance by a slender intervening layer, and are not in immediate contact with it. The neuro-glia extends in the peculiarly soft form, which it presents in the great nervous centres and particularly in the brain, only to those parts which must be regarded as direct prolongations of the cerebral substance, namely to the higher nerves of sense. The olfactory and auditory nerves also contain interstitial substance of the same character, whilst in all the rest, and even in the optic nerve itself, an increasing mass of a tougher tissue displays itself, which assumes quite the character of perineurium.

Perineurium and neuro-glia are therefore equivalent parts, the only difference being that the one is of a soft, medullary, fragile nature, whilst the other is akin to the well-known fibrous tissues. The neurilemma stands in the same relation to the perineurium that the membranes of the brain and spinal cord do to the neuro-glia.

Wherever neuro-glia exists, a very singular peculiarity presents itself which it has as yet been impossible to explain either chemically or physically, namely, that in every such case those peculiar bodies may be met with, which even in their structure remind one of granules of vegetable starch, whilst in their chemical reactions they altogether correspond to them—the much discussed *corpora amylacea* (Fig. 94, *ca*). They are found to the greatest extent and in the greatest numbers in the ependyma of the ventricles and spinal canal, and are the more abundant the greater the thickness of the ependyma. In many places but very few of them are found, whilst in others again their numbers increase so greatly, that the whole thickness of the ependyma is filled with them to such a degree, that it looks as if a pavement were before one. They display themselves, however, strangely enough, in pathological conditions also, frequently in great numbers, when, in consequence of some disturbing cause, the quantity of neuro-glia becomes increased in proportion to that of nervous substance, as for

example after atrophic processes. In tabes dorsalis, as
one used to say, or the atrophy of single columns of the
cord, as we now usually interpret the old expression, we
find, in proportion as the atrophy progresses, and the
nerves in certain directions perish—cuneiform segments,
in which the substance up to that time white becomes
from without inwards grey and translucent—there being
apparently a production of grey matter. This degeneration is most frequent in the posterior columns, generally in the immediate vicinity of the posterior fissure,
and here it may go on, and generally does go on, in such
a manner that the wedge penetrates deeper and deeper
and at the same time increases in width. In these parts

Fig. 96.

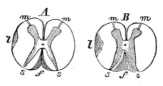

then the whole substance of the medullated fibres gradually disappears, and distinct nerves are no longer discoverable—the whole spot generally consisting of neuro-glia
with an enormous accumulation of corpora amylacea.

Nowhere in the body has there as yet been found anything completely analogous to structures of this sort, excepting, as I have said, in those parts which appear to
be direct protrusions of the cerebral substance, namely
in the higher organs of sense, in the case of which originally a certain quantity of central nervous matter entered
into the sensorial capsules (Sinneskapseln) of the embryo.
In the cochlea too, and the retina, bodies occur, which

Fig. 96. Section of the spinal marrow in partial (lobular), grey or gelatinous atrophy (degeneration). *f.* Posterior longitudinal fissure, *s, s* posterior, *m, m* anterior
nerve-roots, communicating with the grey substance of the horns. In *A* a slighter,
in *B* a more marked degree of atrophy, which is shown in the posterior columns
around the central fissure *f*, and in the lateral columns at *l*. Natural size.

are allied to the corpora amylacea, although the chemical tests have as yet only proved successful in the case of those found in the internal ear.

When these bodies are isolated, they exhibit in every respect such a complete analogy to vegetable starch that, long before I succeeded in discovering the analogy in chemical reaction, Purkinje had already introduced the term corpora amylacea on account of the morphological resemblance. You are no doubt aware, that the chemical correspondence has in many quarters been doubted; the late Heinrich Meckel especially had great doubts upon the subject, and supposed them to have a greater affinity to cholesterine. In more recent times, however, the matter has been investigated even by professed botanists, and every one who has bestowed close attention upon it, has as yet acquired the same conviction which I published as my own. Nägeli pronounces these bodies to be really and truly starch.

Morphologically, they present themselves either as perfectly circular bodies with regular, concentric layers, or their centre is a little on one side; or we find twin bodies; or again the bodies are more homogeneous, pale, with a dim lustre, like fatty substances. When they are cautiously treated with a dilute solution of iodine, they assume a pale bluish, or greyish blue colour, though a great deal certainly depends upon the proper degree of concentration of the test. If afterwards we very cautiously add sulphuric acid, we obtain, when the proper effect is produced, a beautiful blue, which is best shown by allowing the reagent to act very slowly. When sulphuric acid acts violently upon them, a violet tint, which speedily becomes brownish red or blackish, is obtained, presenting a most decided contrast to the neighbouring parts, which become yellow or at most yellowish brown.

LECTURE XIV.

APRIL 7, 1858.

ACTIVITY AND IRRITABILITY OF CELLULAR ELEMENTS. DIFFERENT FORMS OF IRRITATION.

Life of individual parts—The unity of the neurists—Consciousness—Activity of individual parts—Excitability (irritability) as a general criterion of life—Meaning of irritation—Partial death—Necrosis.

Function, nutrition, and formation, as general forms of vital activity—Difference of irritability according to the different forms of activity.

Functional irritability—Nerves, muscles, ciliated epithelium, glands—Fatigue and functional restitution—Stimuli—Their specific relations—Muscular irritability.

Nutritive irritability—Maintenance and destruction of elements—Inflammation—Cloudy swelling—Kidney (morbus Brightii) and cartilage—Neuro-pathological doctrines—Skin, cornea—The humoro-pathological doctrines—Parenchymatous exudation, and parenchymatous inflammation.

Formative irritation—Multiplication of nucleoli and nuclei by division—Multinuclear cells; medullary cells and myeloid tumours—Comparison between formative muscular irritation and muscular growth—Multiplication (new formamation) of cells by division—The humoro- and neuro-pathological doctrines.

Inflammatory irritation as a compound phenomenon—Neuro-paralytical inflammation (Vagus, Trigeminus).

I HAVE given you, gentlemen, a somewhat lengthy sketch of the histological arrangements of the body, in order to make the inference plain to you, which in my opinion must be the starting point of all future considerations that are instituted concerning life and vital activity—that, namely, in all parts of the body a splitting up into a number of small centres takes place, and that nowhere, as far as our experience extends, does a single

central point susceptible of anatomical demonstration
exist, from which the operations of the body are carried
on in a perceptible manner.   And even if we appeal to
the experience which every one daily stores up around
him, we shall find that this is the only view which con-
cedes life to the individual parts of an organism, or
allows it to the plant—the only view which enables us
to institute a comparison both between the collective
life of the developed animal and the individual life of
its smallest parts ; and also between the life of a plant
as a whole and the life of the individual parts of a
plant.

The opposite view which at this very moment is mani-
festing itself with a certain degree of energy—that
namely, which beholds in the nervous system the real
central point of life—is met by this extremely great
difficulty, that, in the very same apparatus, in which it
places its unity, it again finds the same splitting up into
an infinite number of separate centres, which is presented by the rest of the body ; and that in no part of
the whole nervous system it can show the real central
point, from which, as from a seat of government, man-
dates are issued to all quarters.

It may seem very convenient to say that the nervous
system constitutes the real unity of the body, inasmuch
as there is certainly no other system which enjoys such
a complete dissemination throughout the most various
peripheral and internal organs.   But even this wide dissemination and the numerous connections which exist
between the individual parts of the nervous system, are
by no means calculated to show it to be the centre of all
organic actions.   We have found in the nervous system
definite little cellular elements which serve as centres of
motion, but we do not find any single ganglion-cell in
which alone all movement in the end originates.   The

most various individual motory apparatuses are connected with the most various individual motory ganglion-cells. Sensations are certainly collected in definite ganglion-cells, still among them too we do not find any single cell which can in any way be designated the centre of all sensation, but we again meet with a great number of very minute centres.

All the operations which have their source in the nervous system, and there certainly are a very great number of them, do not allow us to recognise a unity anywhere else than in our own consciousness ; an anatomical or physiological unity has at least as yet been nowhere demonstrable. If we really were to set down the nervous system with its numerous separate centres as the central point of all organic actions, even then the thing actually sought for, a real unity, would not have been obtained. If a clear idea is formed of the difficulties which stand in the way of such a unity, it can scarcely be doubted, but that we are continually led astray by the spiritual phenomena displayed in our own persons, in the interpretation of organic processes. Feeling ourselves to be something simple and indivisible, we always start with the presumption that everything else must be regulated by this indivisible principle. But if we trace the development of any given plant from its first germ up to the highest point in its evolution, we meet with a series of processes altogether analogous, without our being able to entertain the supposition for a moment, that such a unity exists in it, as we are led by our consciousness to suppose exists in us. Nobody has been able to detect a nervous system in plants ; in no case has it been discovered that the whole of the fully developed plant was governed from a single point. All the vegetable physiology of the present day is based upon the investigation of the activity of cells, and if violent opposition is still made to the introduction of the same principle also into the animal economy, there is, I think, no other difficulty in the way but the one, that æsthetical and moral scruples cannot be overcome.

It cannot of course here be our business either to refute these scruples or to point out how they might be reconciled with the views I advocate. I have only to show in how great a degree the pathological processes which especially interest us, in all cases conduct us back to the same cellular principle, and how much they are in every case opposed to that notion of a single controlling principle, which is sought to be established by the neuro-pathologists. This opinion of mine has after all really nothing new or uncommon in it. If for thousands of years the life of the individual parts of the body has been talked about, if the position is admitted, that in diseased conditions the death of individual parts, necrosis or gangrene in them may take place, whilst the whole still continues to exist—the inference is, that something of our way of thinking had long been expressed in the views held by the world in general : only people had not formed very clear notions upon the subject. If we speak of the life of the individual parts of a body, we must also know in what way life manifests itself, and whereby it is essentially characterized. This characteristic we find in *activity*, an activity indeed, in which there is displayed by every single part, whilst it contributes its contingent, according to its peculiarities, to the general activity of the body—something identical with the life of the other parts ; for else we should be in no way justified in regarding life as something in every case similar, and derivable from some common origin.

This vital activity is, as far at least as we are able to judge, nowhere, in no part whatever, carried on by means of any cause allotted to it from the very beginning, and entirely confined to it, but we everywhere see that a certain *excitation* is necessary for its production. Every vital action presupposes an excitation, or if you like an *irritation*. The *irritability* of a part, therefore, appears to us the criterion, by which we can judge whether it is alive or not. Whether, for example, a nerve be alive or dead, we cannot immediately determine by an anatomical examination of it, conducted either microscopically or macroscopically. In the outward appearance, in the more obvious structural arrangements, which we are able to decipher by the aid of our auxiliaries, we rarely find sufficient to enable us to come to a decision upon a point such as this. Whether a muscle is alive or dead, we are but little able to judge, inasmuch as we find its structure still preserved in parts which perished years ago. I found in a fœtus, which, in a case of extra-uterine pregnancy, had lain thirty years in the body of its mother, the structure of the muscles as intact as if it had just been born at its full time. Czermak examined parts of mummies, and found in them a number of tissues which were in a state of such perfect preservation, that the conclusion might very well have been come to, that the parts had been taken from a living body. Our notion of the death, decease, or necrosis of a part, is based upon nothing more or less than this, that whilst its form is preserved, and indeed in spite of it, we can no longer detect any irritability in it. This has been most clearly shown quite recently in the course of some investigations into the more hidden properties of nerves. Now that, by the investigations of Dubois-Reymond, activity has been shown to exist in nerves even when in a so-called state of repose, and that it has been discovered, that in a nerve, even when seemingly at rest, electrical processes are continually going on, and that it constantly produces an effect upon the magnetic needle—now we are able, by means of this physical experiment, with certainty to judge when a nerve is dead, for, as soon as death has stepped in, those qualities cease, which are inseparably connected with the life of the nerve.

This peculiarity which we find in some parts exhibited in such a marked degree and so evidently demonstrable, becomes less and less apparent, the more lowly the organization of the part, and our criteria are least to be depended upon in the case of the class of connective tissues ; for we are, indeed, really frequently much puzzled to decide whether a part composed of one of them is still alive or has already perished.

If now we proceed with our analysis of what is to be included in the notion of excitability, we at once discover, that the different actions which can be provoked by the influence of any external agency, are essentially of three kinds ; and I consider it of great importance that you should pay particular attention to this point, as it will greatly assist you in the classification of pathological conditions, and because it is not wont to be set forth with particular distinctness.

When, namely, a given action is called into play, we have to deal with a manifestation either of the *function*, the *nutrition*, or the *formation* of a part. It certainly cannot be denied that at certain points the boundaries between these different processes disappear, and that between the nutritive and formative processes and also between the functional and nutritive ones, there are transitional stages ; still, when they are typically performed, there is a very marked difference between them ; and the internal changes which the individual excited part undergoes, according as it only performs its functions, or is subjected to a special nutrition, or becomes the seat of special formative processes, exhibit considerable differences. The result of an excitation, or if you will, an irritation, may, according to circumstances, be either a merely functional process ; or the effect may be that a more or less increased nutrition of the part is induced without there necessarily being any excitation of its functions ; or a formative process may set in, giving rise to a greater or less number of new elements. These differences manifest themselves with greater or less distinctness in proportion as the individual tissues of the body are more or less capable of responding to the one or other kind of excitation. When, namely, we speak of the functions of parts—in the case of a considerable number of tissues the real functions shrink into a very small compass ; we are on the whole able to say but very little concerning the real functions, in the higher sense of the word, of nearly all the connective tissues, and of the great majority of epithelial cells. We are no doubt able to say what their use under particular circumstances is, still they always rather appear to be relatively inert masses, which scarcely perform any real functions in the ordinary meaning of the word, but rather serve as supports to the body, or as coverings to the different surfaces, or, in other localities, according to circumstances, act as media of union, intervention, or separation.

The case is different, on the other hand, with those parts, which, owing to the peculiar nature of their internal arrangement, are liable to a more rapid change, such as the nerves, muscles, and muscular organs, glands and a few other structures, as, for example, among the epithelia, ciliated epithelium. In all these tissues, which are subservient to important functions, we find that these functions are chiefly due to very delicate changes of arrangement, or if you wish it expressed in more precise terms, to minute changes of place, in the minute particles of the internal matter, the cell-contents. In these cases therefore it is not so much the real cell in its pure form which decides the question, as the specific matters with which it is provided internally ; the chief agent is not so much the membrane or the nucleus of the cell, as the contents. It is these which, when exposed to certain influences, become comparatively rapidly changed, without our being always able morphologically to detect any trace of a change in the arrangement of the contained particles. The utmost that we can observe in the shape of a palpable result is a real locomotion of small, visible particles, but we cannot push our analysis to such an extent, as to enable us to form any opinion as to the internal cause, in virtue of which this locomotion is effected by the ultimate particles which compose the cell-contents. When an excitation takes place in a nerve, we now know that a change in its electrical state is connected with it, a change which, from all that is known to us concerning electrical excitation in other bodies, must of necessity be referred to a change in the position which the individual molecules assume to one another. If we conceive the axis-cylinder to be made up of electrical molecules, we can easily imagine that every two of these molecules take up an altered position with regard to one another at the moment the stimulus is applied. Of these processes we see nothing. The axis-cylinder looks just as usual. If we watch a muscle during its contraction, we remark, it is true, that the intervals which separate the individual so-called discs (p. 82) become shorter ; and as we now know that the substance of the mus-

Fig. 97.

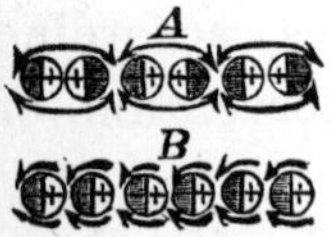

Fig. 97. Ideal diagram of the condition of the molecules of a nerve when it is at rest (in a peripolar state, *A*), or in an electrotonic (dipolar) state, *B*. From Ludwig, ' Physiolog.,' I, p. 103.

cle consists of a series of minute fibrils, which in their turn contain little granules at certain intervals corresponding to these discs, we conclude therefrom with some degree of assurance that really local changes take place in the minutest elements, though they cannot be further referred to any visible or directly recognizable cause. We cannot perceive any definite chemical change, or any alteration in the state of nutrition of the parts ; we only see a displacement, a dislocation of the particles, which, however, probably depends upon some slight chemical change in the molecules composing them.

In the case of ciliated epithelium you see how the fine cilia, which are seated upon the surface of the cells, move in a certain direction, and in this direction exercise a locomotory effect upon the little particles which come near to them. If we isolate the individual cells, we see that every one of them has at its upper end a border of a certain thickness, from which little hair-shaped prolongations run out. These all move in such a way that a cilium which, whilst quiet, stands quite upright, bends forwards and then throws itself backwards. But we are unable to perceive any changes within the individual cilia, by means of which the movement is effected.

Just the same is the case with gland-cells, concerning which we cannot entertain the least doubt that they produce a definite locomotory effect. For since Ludwig has shown in his researches on the salivary glands, that the pressure of the outward current of saliva is greater than that of the inward stream of blood, the only conclusion that is left us is, that the gland-cells exercise a definite motor influence upon the fluid ; and that the secretion is driven out with a definite force, which is not due to the pressure of the blood, or any special muscular action, but to the specific energy of the cells as such. Still we are just as little able to discern in a gland cell, whilst performing its functions, that its constituent particles are engaged in any peculiar material process, as we were in the case of the nerves, or ciliated epithelium.

These facts derive great support from the circumstance that we are able to perceive, that the functional activity of individual parts does experience a certain amount of impairment, if it is continued for too long a time. In all parts certain states of *fatigue* manifest themselves, states, during which the part is no longer able to originate the same amount of movement, that up to that time could be perceived in it. But, in order that they may again become competent to perform their functions, these parts by no means always require a new supply of nutriment, a fresh absorption of nutritive material ; rest alone is sufficient to enable them to resume their activity in a short space of time. A nerve, which has been cut out of the body, and used for experiment, after a certain lapse of time becomes incapable of discharging its functions ; but if it be allowed to repose under favourable circumstances, which prevent it from drying up, it gradually regains its powers. This *restitution of functional power* (functional restitution), which takes place without any proper nutritive action, and in all probability depends upon the circumstance, that the molecules which had quitted their usual position gradually revert to it—we can produce in different parts by means of certain stimuli. According to the views of the neuro-pathologists these stimuli would only act upon the nerves, and through the medium of the nerves upon the other parts ; but with reference to this very point we have some facts which cannot well be explained in any other way than by the assumption, that an influence is really exercised upon the parts themselves.

If we take a single ciliated cell, and, after entirely isolating it from the body, allow it to swim about, and wait until a state of complete repose has declared itself, we can again call forth the peculiar movements of its cilia by adding a small quantity of potash or soda to the fluid, a quantity not large enough to produce corrosive effects upon the cell, but sufficient, upon penetration into it, to induce a certain change in its contents. A peculiarly interesting fact, however, is that the number of substances which will act, as stimuli, upon ciliated epithelium, is limited to these two. This explains how it happened that Purkinje and Valentin (who, it is well known, first made experiments, and those upon a very extensive scale, upon ciliary movement), although they experimented with a very large number of substances, at last, after they had tried all sorts of things—mechanical, chemical and electrical stimuli—came to the conclusion that there was no stimulus whatever, which could provoke the ciliary movement. I had the good fortune incidentally to stumble upon the peculiar fact, that potash and soda are such stimuli. Here we certainly cannot call in any nervous influence to our aid, and such influence appears to be the less admissible for the reason that, in accordance with the well-known experiments, the ciliary movement is maintained in the dead body at a time when other parts have already begun to putrefy. The ciliated epithelium of the frontal sinuses and the trachea is found in human corpses in a state of perfect excitability thirty-six to forty-eight hours after death, when every trace of irritability has long vanished from the remainder of the body.

Much the same is the case with all other excitable parts. We see nearly everywhere that certain excitants act more readily than others, and that many are totally incapable of producing any particular effect. Nearly everywhere do we find *specific relations* or *affinities* to exist. If we cast our eyes upon the glands, it is a well-known fact that there are specific substances, by which we are enabled to act upon one gland, and not upon another ; to rouse the specific energy of one gland, whilst all the rest remain unaffected. In the case of glands it is certainly much more difficult to exclude the influence of the nerves, than in that of ciliated epithelium, still certain experiments are recorded, in which, after the section of all the nerves, say of the liver (G. Harting), it was found possible, by means of the injection of irritating substances into the blood (these being such as experience had shown to bear some intimate relation to the organ), to provoke an increased secretion in the organ.

The discussion of this subject has, as you no doubt are well aware, recently chiefly become centred in the question of the irritability of muscle, a question which has proved so difficult for the very reason that the possession of irritability was restricted by Haller with great exclusiveness to muscle. Haller with the greatest obstinacy combated the opinion that any other part was irritable ; and curiously enough he even contested the irritability of parts, which, as the minuter investigations of later observers have shown, contain muscular elements, as for example, the middle coat of the vessels. Indeed, he made use of tolerably energetic expressions when repudiating the excitability of the vessels, which even then was maintained by others. I have already informed you that there are large tracts in the vascular system (for example, in the umbilical vessels of the fœtus, where they are particularly well marked) in which enormous accumulations of muscular fibres are found, but not a trace of any nerves. Here irritability exists in a high degree ; we can produce contractions of the muscles mechanically, chemically and electrically. Just the same is the case with many other, small vessels, which by no means exhibit nerve-fibres in all their parts. In them too we can at every single point where muscles exist, at once provoke contraction.

The solution of this question has recently, as is well known, been particularly promoted by the fact that, by the employment of certain poisons, especially the woo-rara poison, observers have succeeded in paralyzing the nerves right down to their extreme terminations, or at least as far as these were accessible to the experiment; and this in such a manner, that the objection cannot well be raised, that the excitability of the extreme ter-minations of the nerves contained in the muscle is pre-served. The paralysis produced by the woorara poison is completely confined to the nerves, whilst the muscles just as completely retain their irritability. Whilst the most violent electrical currents were made to act upon the nerve in vain, without the production of the least movement, the slightest mechanical, chemical or electri-cal stimuli are sufficient to throw the muscle experi-mented upon into a state of excitation.

I have mentioned these facts to you, in order that I might not be thought to treat the different divisions of my subject too unequally. The question of function, however, interests us less here. Nevertheless, you will be able to gather from what I have communicated to you, that now-a-days it can no longer be said with any show of reason that the nerves alone are irritable parts, but that we are irresistibly led to consider functional irritabi-lity, at least, as a property belonging to whole series of organs.

Far less known, gentlemen, is that clearly demonstra-ble series of processes in which *nutritive irritability* mani-fests itself—that power possessed by individual parts of taking up, when excited by definite stimuli, more or less matter and transforming it. This constitutes at the same time the first step in the most important processes which we have to follow into the domain of pathologico-anatomical facts.

A part, which nourishes itself, can in doing so either limit itself to a mere maintenance of its existence, or it may, as is especially seen in pathological cases, take up into itself a larger quantity of nutritive material than is wont to happen in the ordinary course of things. If we investigate these processes of absorption more closely, we always find that, as I have already had occasion to remark to you, the number of histological elements remains the same before and after the occurrence of the excitation ; and we thus distinguish simple hypertrophies from the hyperplastic conditions, to which, in their external effects, they often bear so great a resemblance (p. 94, Fig. 27, *B*). It is, however, of extreme importance for the attainment of correct pathological notions, that we should know that a part, which in virtue of some inherent power, takes up a large quantity of material, need not on that account necessarily fall into a permanent condition of enlargement, but that on the contrary, under these very circumstances there often arises subsequently in its internal economy a disturbance which imperils the persistence of the part and becomes the proximate cause of its destruction. There are, as we know from experience, certain limits to the enlargement of every tissue, within which it is able to maintain a regular existence ; if these limits be exceeded, and especially, if suddenly, we always see that obstacles spring up impeding the further life of the part, and that when the process runs a particularly acute course, a weakening of the part sets in, proceeding to a complete destruction of it.

Processes of this kind form a part of that domain which

in ordinary life is assigned to inflammation. A number of inflammatory processes on their first appearance really exhibit nothing more than an increased assumption of material into the interior of the cells, entirely resembling what we find in simple hypertrophy. If, for example, we consider the history of Bright's disease in its ordinary course, we constantly find, that the very first thing which can be detected in a kidney affected with this disease, consists in this, that in the interior of the uriniferous tubules whilst still quite intact, the individual epithelial cells which are, as is well known, even in their normal state tolerably large, become still larger. These epithelial cells which fill up the tubules are not only large, but

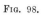

at the same time also present a very cloudy appearance, inasmuch as a larger quantity of material than usual has everywhere been taken up into the cells. The entire uriniferous tubule is thereby rendered broader, and appears even to the naked eye as a convoluted, whitish, opaque body. If we isolate the individual cells, which is somewhat difficult, as the cohesion of the particles compos-

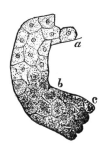

ing them has usually begun to suffer, we find in them a granular mass apparently containing nothing else than the granules which are normally present in the interior of the cells, but which accumulate in greater numbers the greater the energy with which the process is carried on, so that even the nucleus gradually grows indistinct. This is the condition of *cloudy swelling* (trübe Schwellung), as it is met with in many irritated parts, as an expression

Fig. 98. Convoluted urinary tubule from the cortex of the kidney in morbus Brightii. *a.* Tolerably normal epithelium, *b,* state of cloudy swelling, *c,* commencing fatty metamorphosis and disintegration. At *b* and *c* increased breadth of the tubule. 300 diameters.

of the irritation which attends many forms of what is
called inflammation. From these processes backwards to
the phenomena of simple hypertrophy we find no recognizable boundaries at all. We cannot at once say, when
we meet with a part enlarged in this way, and containing a greater amount of matter than usual, whether it
will retain its life or perish ; and therefore it is extremely
difficult in very many cases, when nothing at all is known
concerning the process through which such a change has
been produced, to distinguish simple hypertrophy from
those forms of inflammatory processes which are essentially accompanied by an increased absorption of nutritive material.

In these processes too it is scarcely possible to refuse
the individual elements, when incited by a stimulus
directly applied to them, the power of taking up an
increased quantity of material ; at least it is opposed to
all the results of experience, to assume that such an increased absorption must be due to a special innervation.
If we select a part which, in accordance with all observation, is entirely destitute of nerves, as for example, the
surface of an articular cartilage, we can, as was shown
many years ago by the beautiful experiments of Redfern,
produce altogether similar effects by means of direct
stimuli. In precisely the same way, there are not unfrequently observed, in chronic diseases of cartilage, no-
dular elevations of the surface ; and upon examining
such spots microscopically we find the same thing that I
showed you in a former lecture in a costal cartilage
(p. 48, Fig. 9), namely, that the cells which at other
times are very delicate, small, lenticular bodies, increase
in size, swell up into large, round corpuscles, and in proportion as they take up more matter, enlarge in all directions, so that at last the whole spot forms a little protuberance above the surface. Now in articular cartilage

no nerves at all are found ; the terminal ramifications of those nearest to it are at best situated in the medulla of the bone immediately adjoining, and that, perhaps, is separated from the irritated spot of the surface by an intact, intervening layer of cartilaginous tissue one or two lines in thickness. Now it would indeed be contrary to all experience to conceive that a nerve could from the medulla of the bone exercise a special action upon the cells of the surface of the cartilage, which were the seat of irritation, without a simultaneous affection of the cells lying between the nerve and the irritated spot. If we draw a thread through a cartilage, so that merely a traumatic irritation is produced, we see that all the cells which lie close to the thread become enlarged through an increased absorption of material. The irritation produced by the thread extends only to a certain distance into the cartilage, whilst the more remote cells remain altogether unaffected. Such observations cannot be explained otherwise than by assuming that the stimulus really acts upon the parts to which it is applied ; it is impossible to conclude that it is conducted to the nerve by any channel perhaps more in accordance with the neuro-pathological doctrine, and then only by reflex action conveyed back again to the parts.

There certainly are but few tissues in the body which are so completely destitute of nerves as cartilage, but even when we observe what happens in the parts most abundantly supplied with nerves, we find in every case, that the extent of the irritation, or to speak more accurately, the extent of the irritated area, by no means corresponds to the size of any particular nerve-territory, but that in a tissue in other respects normal the size of the affected area essentially corresponds to that of the local irritation. If we make the experiment with the thread, upon the *skin*, a whole series of nerve-territories are

intersected by it. Still the whole of the territories belonging to the nerves which lie along the thread, are not
thrown into the same morbid condition, but the nutritive
irritation is limited to the immediate vicinity of the
thread. No surgeon expects in operations of the kind,
that all the nerve-territories traversed by the thread,
will become diseased in their whole extent. Great complaints would have to be raised against nature, if every
ligature, every seton were to exercise an irritating influence, beyond the limits of the parts with which it is in
immediate contact, upon the whole extent of the nerve-
districts which it passes through. Thus we see in a tissue in which what takes place in such a case can be very
clearly traced, namely in the *cornea*, that in parts of it
to which no vessels extend, there are certainly still nerves
which possess a reticular arrangement, and leave larger
and smaller districts of tissue between them altogether
devoid of nerves. Now if we apply any stimulus directly
to the cornea, as for example, a red hot needle, or lunar
caustic, the district which is thereby set in morbid action
by no means corresponds to the distribution of any nerve.
It once happened to me with a rabbit that the cautery
lighted precisely upon a nervous filament, but the morbid action remained confined to the immediate vicinity
of this spot, and by no means spread over the whole district appertaining to the nerve.

It is therefore utterly impossible, even if observations,
like those on cartilage which I have laid before you,
are not allowed to have any weight, not to admit that
the phenomena of irritation in parts supplied with
nerves are in no respect different from those which
occur in nerveless parts, and that the immediate effects
essentially depend upon the enlargement and tumefaction of the surrounding elements, so that when there are
many of them, a visible swelling of the whole part is

the result. This is what you observe when a ligature is anywhere drawn through the skin. If on the following day the immediate vicinity of the thread be examined, an active enlargement of the cellular elements is found, quite irrespective of the distribution of vessels and nerves in the part.

There is, as you see, an essential difference between what I here lay down and the opinions which have generally been advanced with regard to the proximate causes of these swellings. According to the old maxim : ubi stimulus, ibi affluxus, it was generally conceived that the first thing which took place was an increased afflux of blood (which was itself referred by the neuro-pathologists to the excitation of sensitive nerves), and then that the immediate consequence of the increased afflux was an increased excretion of fluid from the blood, constituting the exudation which filled the part.

In the first timid attempts which I made to alter this conception, I employed the expression *parenchymatous** *exudation*, retaining the term exudation, out of deference to prevailing opinion. I had, namely, convinced myself that in many places where a swelling had occurred, there was absolutely nothing else to be seen than tissue. In a tissue which consisted of cells, I could, after the swelling (exudation) had taken place, still see nothing

---

* The term Parenchyma was first employed by Erasistratus of Alexandria to designate the mass of tissue *which lies between the vessels of a part*, and in his opinion formed a kind of affusion from them. Thus Galen says (Isagoge s. Introductio, cap. xi.): " Cerebrum ex nullo principali vase compositum esse videtur Erasistrato, eoque nutrimenti parenchyma, *i. e.*, affusio, ipsi esse videtur." In the same way the word is used by Vesalius (De humani corp. fabricâ, lib. V., cap. 7) and by Thom. Bartholin (Anatome, lib. I., cap. 14), for the proper substance of the liver, lying external to, or between, the vessels. It therefore essentially denotes the tissue of which an organ is constituted. In a narrower sense those constituents of an organ which are peculiar to it, and give it its specific character, may be distinguished as its *proper parenchyma*, in contra-distinction to its merely interstitial tissue. In my book the term has been used in both of these senses.—*From a MS. Note by the Author*

but cells; in tissues composed of cells and intercellular substance, nothing but cells and intercellular substance; the individual elements indeed were larger, fuller and filled with a quantity of matter with which they ought not to have been filled, but there was no exudation in the manner in which it had been imagined to exist, namely free, or in the interstices of the tissue. All the matter was contained in the elements of the tissues themselves. This was what I intended to express by the term, parenchymatous exudation, and hence the name, parenchymatous inflammation, is derived—a name which was, indeed, used in former times, but in quite another sense from that I meant—and which is now more generally employed than is perhaps desirable. It is, however, at all events important that you should draw a distinct line of demarcation between this form of irritation as a general standard and the other forms (especially the formative one), inasmuch as in it only the constituent elements of a tissue already existing in the body take up a larger quantity of material, and besides these enlarged elements nothing else is present.

I will immediately send round a preparation to you, in which you will see a very characteristic example of such an inflammation. It is almost the most striking example which for a long time has come before me. It is a specimen from a case of so-called Keratitis, from one of Herr von Graefe's patients, in whom, after violent, diffuse phlegmonous inflammation of the extremities, an extremely rapid inflammatory opacity of the cornea took place. When the cornea was put into my hands, it seemed to me as if it were opaque and swollen in its whole thickness. The vessels of the borders were very full of blood. But when I made a section through the part, it at once became evident, even with a low power, that the opacity extended by no means uni-

formly throughout the whole cornea, but was limited
to a definite portion of the tissue. This portion is so
characteristic in reference to the different explanations
possible, that the case, I think, presents especial interest theoretically.

It turned out namely that the opacity began in the
immediate proximity of the posterior surface and at the
circumference of the cornea, close to the membrane of
Descemet [posterior elastic lamina of Bowman] at the
point where the iris is attached. Thence the opacity,
assuming almost the shape of a flight of steps, mounted
up into the cornea till within a certain distance of the
external surface. Then it proceeded at the same level,
till it descended upon the other side again in a similar
manner. Thus an opaque bow was formed throughout
the whole substance of the cornea, without reaching the
external (anterior) surface and without encroaching
upon the central parts of the posterior surface. If we

FIG. 99.

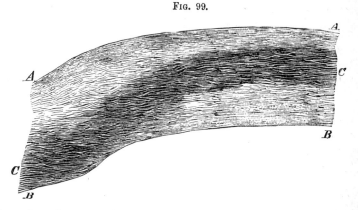

imagine the nutrition of the cornea to proceed from the
aqueous humour, the opacity did not assume the form

Fig. 99. Parenchymatous keratitis. *A*, *A*, Anterior (external), *B*, *B*, posterior
(internal) side of the cornea. *C*, *C*. The clouded zone with enlarged cornea-corpuscles. 18 diameters.

that might have been looked for, for then we should
rather have expected that the hindermost layer would be
the first to undergo the change.   If any influence from
without had been here in operation, the opacity must
have been seated in the most anterior layers ; if again
the opacity were one which essentially proceeded from the
vessels, we might, inasmuch as they chiefly lie along the
border and nearer to the anterior surface, have expected
to find the principal disease there.   Finally, if the
changes had their origin in the nerves, we should have
found the opacity spread in the form of a network on
the surface—and not a bow of this kind.

The substance of the cornea consists, you know, according to general opinion, of lamellæ (plates) which
run in a more or less parallel direction through the

Fig. 100.

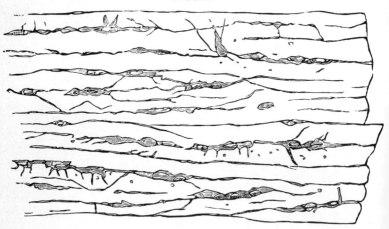

cornea.   Now if this opinion be the correct one, we
should have to deal with a process which, whilst advanc-

Fig. 100. Perpendicular section of the cornea of the ox, for the purpose of showing
the form and anastomoses of its cells (corpuscles).   Here and there are seen the
cut ends of some of the processes of the cells, looking like fibres or points.   500
diameters.   From His, ' Würzb. Verhandl.,' IV., plate IV., fig. I.

ing from lamella to lamella, each time moved a little farther on.   Only the cornea is not composed of perfect lamellæ, but of layers, which certainly are on the whole placed one against the other in a lamellar form, but yet are connected with one another ; they do not lie any how, more or less firmly or loosely upon one another, but there exist direct connections between them.   It is therefore rather a large coherent mass, which is interrupted in certain directions by cellular elements, just as is the case in the very different tissues which we have already specially considered.   A vertical section discloses spindle-shaped cells which anastomose with one another, but at the same time also possess lateral processes ; and in consequence of their being regularly imbedded in the basis substance, this lamellar, foliated or plate-like arrangement of the whole tissue is produced.   When viewed upon the surface, in horizontal section, they show themselves in the form of many-rayed, stellate but very flat cells, which may be compared to bone-corpuscles.

FIG. 101.

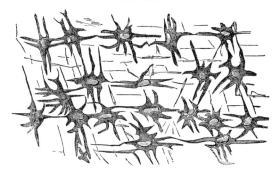

If now in this case of ours we follow the process with a higher power, we discover, what may easily be shown

Fig. 101. Horizontal section of the cornea, parallel to the surface and showing the stellate, flat corpuscles, with their anastomosing processes.   From His, loc. cit., fig. II.

to be the case in every form of keratitis, that the change is essentially seated in the corpuscles or cells of the cornea, and that in proportion as we approach the clouded spot either from without or within, the little narrow cells continually become larger and more cloudy. At last we find them presenting almost the appearance of sacculated canals or tubes. Whilst this enlargement of the elements, this acute hypertrophy, if you will, is going on, the contents of the cells are at the same time becoming more cloudy, and it is this cloudiness of the contents which in its turn occasions the opacity of the whole coat, for the proper basis-substance appears to be altogether unaf-

Fig. 102.

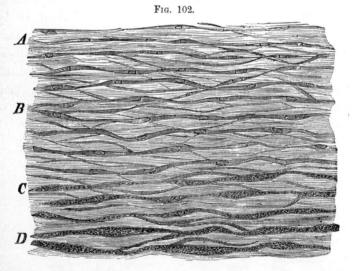

fected. This cloudiness of the contents is in part occasioned by particles which are of a fatty nature, so that the process seems to have begun to assume the character of a degenerative disease. I should have had no hesitation in believing that a destruction of the cornea had here

Fig. 102. Parenchymatous keratitis (cf. Fig. 99), seen with a higher power. At *A* the cornea-corpuscles in a nearly normal condition, at *B* enlarged, at *C* and *D* still more enlarged, and at the same time clouded. 350 diameters.

really set in, but Herr v. Graefe assures me that, from what he has seen, such conditions may, when the disease runs a favourable course, terminate in resolution. And there is really nothing at all in the matter at variance with this possibility ; for, since the cells still exist and the only thing required is that their changed contents be got rid of, a complete restitution may no doubt take place.

Now just this doctrine of a *simply nutritive restitutional power* is of very great importance practically. In such a case as this, where nothing has taken place excepting that the cells, without ceasing to display their activity, have accumulated in their cavities a larger quantity of material than usual, everything is prepared for the process which we call reabsorption ; the cells can transform a certain quantity of the material and convert it into soluble substances, and the material in this form may disappear in the very same way in which it came. The structure in the main remains the same all the while nothing foreign has thrust itself in between the parts the tissue presents throughout its original constituents.

From the phenomena of this nutritive irritation direct transitions to incipient *formative changes* are often seen. If namely, we follow up the higher degrees of irritation which take place in a part, we find that the cellular elements, shortly after they have experienced the nutritive enlargement, exhibit further changes which begin in the interior of the nuclei, generally in such a manner that the nucleoli become unusually large, in many cases somewhat oblong, and sometimes staff-shaped. Then as the next stage we usually see that the nucleoli become constricted in the middle, and assume the form of a finger-biscuit (Bisquit), and a little later two nucleoli are found. This division of the nucleoli is an indication of the impending division of the nucleus itself, and the next stage is,

that about such a divided nucleolus the finger-biscuit-like
constriction, and afterwards the real division, of the nu-

FIG. 103.

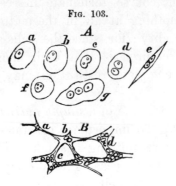

cleus takes place, as we have already seen in colourless
blood- and pus-corpuscles (Figs. 11, *A*, *b*; 56, 63). Here
we manifestly have to deal with something essentially
different from what we had before. In the simple hypertrophy consequent upon nutritive irritation, the nucleus may remain quite intact; here, on the other hand,
we frequently see that the contents display a relatively
slight amount of change, the utmost being that the cells
become larger, whence we infer that a quantity of new
material has been taken up into them.

In many cases the changes are limited to this series of
transformations, of which the division of the nucleus must
be regarded as the conclusion. This may be repeated,
so that three, four or more nuclei arise (Fig. 15, *b*, *c*, *d*).
Thus it comes to pass that we sometimes find cells—not
merely in pathological conditions, but also not unfrequently where the development is altogether normal—
which contain twenty to thirty nuclei or more. Recently
in the marrow of bones, especially in young children,
cells have been observed, where the entire structure is

Fig. 103.   Cells from a melanotic tumour of the parotid gland extirpated in 1851
by Herr Textor.   *A*. Free cells with division of the nucleoli and nuclei.   *B*. Network of connective tissue-corpuscles with division of their nuclei.   300 diameters.

full of nuclei, which often attain the size of the whole original cell. Such formations occur in many tumours in

FIG. 104.

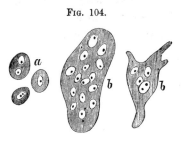

such large quantities, that in England a particular species is thereby distinguished, and on the proposal of Paget a myeloid tumour (medullary swelling) has been received into the classification. This formation is not, however, confined to the medulla of the bones, but occasionally occurs in nearly all situations.

Muscle, upon irritation, exhibits precisely similar forms. Whilst transversely striated muscles are generally provided with nuclei at certain intervals, though in no great abundance, we find, on examining a muscle in the neighbourhood of an irritated part, as for example, a wound, a corroded or ulcerated surface, that a multiplication of the nuclei is going on in it; we see nuclei with two nucleoli; then come constricted, and then divided, nuclei (Comp. Figs. 23, *b*, *c*; 24, *B*, *C*), and so it goes on, until we find in different places whole groups of nuclei lying side by side, in which the divisions have taken place to a large extent, or else whole rows of them, one behind the other. In the most marked cases of this sort the number of nuclei increases to such a degree, that at first sight we can scarcely believe we are looking at muscles; and that fragments of the primitive fasciculi offer the greatest

Fig. 104. Cells from the marrow of bones. *a*. Small cells with single and divided nuclei. *b*, *b*. Large, many-nucleated cells. 350 diameters. From Kolliker, ' Mikr. Anat.,' I., p. 364, fig. 113.

resemblance to those *plaques à plusieurs noyaux* which Robin has described in the marrow of bones. This is something quite peculiar which looks extremely like the commencement of a real new-formation, only that new-forma-tions in the ordinary sense of the word are not limited to sin-gle cell-constituents. Besides we must bear in mind this very important fact, that exactly the same limitation takes place in the earliest embryonic development of muscle, in the course of the first growth of the primitive muscular fasciculi. For this is the manner in which muscle originally grows. If a growing muscle be watched, the same division of the nuclei is wit-nessed, and after groups and rows of nuclei have arisen in it, they are, in the course of growth, gradually thrust farther and farther asunder by the continual increase of the intermediate sarcous sub-stance. Now although a growth in length has not as yet been demonstrated with certainty in a pathologically irri-tated muscle—I say demonstrated, because there really is a probability that something of the kind may yet be proved to be the case—we must still hold the perfect analogy of morbid irritative processes with the natural ones of growth to be a well-ascertained fact. For the formative act of real growth begins with a multiplication

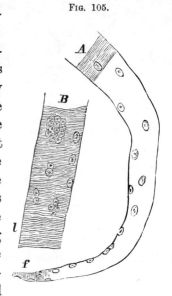

Fig. 105.

Fig. 105. Division of nuclei in primitive muscular fasciculi from the immediate neighbourhood of a cancerous tumour in the thigh. At *A* a primitive fasciculus, the transverse striation of which is not represented all the way down, with its na-tural, spindle-shaped extremity *f*, and incipient multiplication of the nuclei. *B*. Strongly marked proliferation of nuclei. 300 diameters.

of the centres, inasmuch as the nuclei must, as was long since shown by John Goodsir, be regarded as the central organs of the cells.

If now, gentlemen, we advance a step further in these processes, we come to the *new formation of the cells them-selves*. After the multiplication of the nuclei has taken place, the cell may certainly, as we have seen, continue to subsist as a coherent structure ; still the rule is, that even after the first division of the nuclei, the cells themselves undergo division, and that after some time two cells are found lying closely side by side, separated by a more or less straight partition, and each provided with a nucleus of its own (Fig. 6, *b, b*). This is the natural, regular manner in which the real multiplication of cellular ele-ments takes place. Then, the two cells may separate, if the tissue is one which possesses intercellular substance (Fig. 6, *c, d*) ; or may remain lying close to one another, in the case of a tissue simply composed of cells (Fig. 27, *C*). This series of processes, which in their subsequent course lead to a continually proceeding division of the

Fig. 106.

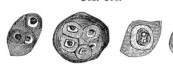

cells, and to the production of large groups of cells from single ones (Figs. 9, 22), occurs in the adult body just as unquestionably as the result of a direct irritation of the tissues, as the class we spoke of before. If, for example, we follow up a little farther the case which we before considered, of the production of a simple mechanical irritation by drawing a thread through the parts, we usu-

Fig. 106. Cells from the central substance of an intervertebral cartilage of an adult. Intra-capsular multiplication of cells. 300 diameters.

ally observe that the swelling is not simply limited to
the enlargement of the existing cells, but that they divide
and multiply. Round about a thread, which we draw
through the skin, a number of young cells generally show
themselves as early as the second day. The same change
may be brought about by the application of a chemical
stimulus. If, for example, caustics be applied to the surface of a part, the first thing that happens is that the
cells swell up and then, when the process follows a regular course, divide, and begin to proliferate more or less
abundantly. Here too we have still to deal with actions
which do not exhibit the slightest difference in the real
mode of their accomplishment, whether the part be provided with nerves, or destitute of them, whether it contain vessels or not.

Accordingly, we cannot say that any part of these
processes appears to be necessarily dependent upon nervous or vascular influence, but, on the contrary, we are
in all these cases referred to the parts themselves. The
relation of the vessels is not by any means to be explained in the way in which it is ordinarily done ; the
absorption of matter into the interior of the cells is unquestionably an act of the cells themselves, for we are
as yet acquainted with no method enabling us to produce this kind of proliferation in the body, by any mode
of experimentation, through the medium of an agency
primarily affecting either the nerves or the vessels. The
circulation may be heightened in the parts as far as it is
possible to heighten it, without the production of such
an increased nutrition of the parts as to give rise to any
swelling or multiplication of the elements themselves.
Those very experiments too upon the section of the
sympathetic nerve which I have already mentioned,
have, as is well known, proved (I myself have very frequently performed this experiment and watched its

effects with this especial object) that an increased afflux of blood may last for weeks—an afflux of blood accompanied by a marked elevation of temperature and corresponding redness, as great, both of them, as we ever meet with in inflammations—without the production of the least enlargement in the cells of the part, or the excitation of any process of proliferation in them. Irritation of the nerves may be combined therewith. But when the tissues themselves are not irritated, when the irritation is not made to act upon the parts themselves, either by the direct application of the irritating matters, or by their introduction into the blood, the occurrence of these changes cannot be relied upon. This is a most important argument, from which I draw the conclusion that these active processes have their foundation in the special action of the elementary parts, an action which does not depend upon an increased afflux of blood or any excitation of the nerves, but which is certainly promoted by them, though it can also continue entirely independent of them, and manifests itself with just as great distinctness in a paralyzed and nerveless part.

In support of these positions I will only add that more recent observations have gradually done away with the whole class of the so-called *neuro-paralytical inflammations*. The two nerves with which we are almost exclusively concerned in the discussion of inflammatory phenomena, are the pneumogastric and the fifth pair, after the section of which, in one case, pneumonia, in the other, those celebrated changes in the eyeball have been observed to declare themselves. These observations have now been explained in this way, that inflammations certainly may come on after such sections, but that the real interpretation to be put upon them is, that they *manifest themselves in spite of the section.** With regard to the pneumogastric it was, as is well known, long since shown by Traube that the paralysis of the rima glottidis, whereby the entrance of the buccal fluids into the air-passages is facilitated, is the principal source of the inflammation ; besides, the more accurate interpretation of the pathological specimens has determined, that a great part of what had been called pneumonia, was really nothing more than atelectasis with hyperæmia of the lungs ; actual pneumonia may with certainty be avoided, if the possibility of the penetration of foreign bodies into the bronchi is cut off. The same has been ascertained to be the case with the inflammations coming on after the section of the fifth pair, and indeed by means of a very simple experiment. After a number of attempts of the most varied kind had been made for the purpose of removing the different disturbing influences affecting the eye that was deprived of its sensibility, a very simple method was at last discovered in Utrecht for providing the eye with a substitute for its sensitive apparatus ; for Snellen sewed before the eyes of animals, in which he had cut the fifth pair, their still sensitive ears. From that time the animals had no more attacks of inflammation, inasmuch as on the one hand a direct protection was afforded to the eye, and on the other the animals were preserved by the presence of a sensitive covering from all traumatic influences. As soon as sensation was re-established, not in the eye itself, but only before the eye, what was really nothing more than a traumatic inflammation was got rid of.†

* For if, as the neuro-pathologists assume, irritation produces inflammation through the medium of the nerves, then, when the nerves are cut, all inflammation ought to be impossible.

† In the text the influence of the section of nerves is perhaps not described with

We can therefore now say, there is no form of disturbance of this kind known which can be traced to the abolition of the action of a nerve. A part may be paralyzed without becoming inflamed ; it may be anæsthetic without becoming exposed to this danger. There is always required in addition some special irritation, either of a mechanical or chemical nature, and proceeding either from without or from the blood, in order to produce the peculiar liability.

In this manner therefore we have, as you see, a series of connecting links between facts eminently pathological and the most common processes of physiological life, facts of which the special import can, however, only be understood and defined, when the distinctions are made to which I called your attention at the commencement of the lecture, that is, when the different kinds of irritation are separated according to their functional, nutritive

sufficient minuteness. According to the author's views, of which a more detailed account may be found in his Handbuch der spec. Pathologie und Ther. Erlangen, 1854 (Vol. I., pp. 31, 50, 80, 276, 314, 319), the section and paralysis of nerves certainly exercise some influence upon the nutrition of the tissues, although perhaps only an indirect one. The states arising from such causes he has classed together under the name of Neurotic Atrophy. Parts which have in this way suffered derangement in their nutrition, and as a consequence have become weakened, are less capable of controlling the disorders by which they are attacked, and accordingly simple irritation in them readily becomes aggravated into inflammation (asthenic inflammation). But in these cases the inflammation is always the consequence of some special irritation, never the direct result of the section of the nerves. Still, as in the case of the fifth pair and the pneumogastric, such section may be the cause of irritants' (foreign bodies and other agents) more readily acting upon the anæsthetic or paralyzed parts. Cl. Bernard has recently declared that the section or irritation of nerves in weakened parts produces effects which cannot be elicited in healthy ones. We have therefore here to deal with a very complicated state of things. The change in the nerve is generally succeeded by a disturbance in the function or circulation of the part, or in both, and when the part is already weakened (i. e., altered in its nutrition) this disturbance may prove a source of irritation to it, and thus the effects be produced which Bernard ascribes to other causes. In quite a similar manner we see that, even when the nervous supply is in its normal state, purely mechanical disturbances in the circulation act upon weakened parts as morbid irritants.—*From a MS. Note by the Author.*

or formative nature. If they are jumbled together, as they have been by the neurists, and especially, if the formative and nutritive processes are not kept apart, then it is impossible to arrive at any simple explanation of the phenomena.

Those states of irritation which we witness in the course of the severer forms of disease—the really *inflammatory kinds of irritation*—never in any case admit of a simple explanation. In inflammation we find side by side all the forms of irritation of which I have given you an analysis. Indeed, we very frequently see, that when the organ itself is made up of different parts, one part of the tissue undergoes functional or nutritive, another formative changes. If we consider what happens in a muscle, a chemical or traumatic stimulus will perhaps in the first instance produce a functional irritation of the primitive fasciculi ; the muscle contracts, but then nutritive disturbances declare themselves. On the other hand in the interstitial connective tissue, which binds the individual fasciculi of the muscle together, real new-formations are readily produced, commonly pus. Here we have to deal with a formative irritation, whilst the inflamed primitive fasciculus commonly produces no pus, any more than it does new muscular substance ; on the contrary we most frequently see, when the irritation has attained a certain height, degenerative processes set in. In this manner the three forms of irritation may be distinguished in one part. Of course there may be in addition also an irritation of the nerves, but this has, at least if we do not take function into account, no connection of cause and effect with the processes going on in the tissue proper, but is nothing more than a collateral effect of the original disturbance. This must, in my opinion, be regarded as the most important result derived from the facts of Special Histology, and it is all the more certain because it can be tested both by experiment and by physiological and pathological experience.

Soon, I will show you how in the study of inflammatory processes a clearer apprehension of their nature may hereby be obtained.

LECTURE XV.

APRIL 10, 1858.

PASSIVE PROCESSES. FATTY DEGENERATION.

Passive processes in their two chief tendencies to degeneration; Necrobiosis (soft
ening and disintegration) and induration.

Fatty degeneration—Histological history of fat in the animal body; fat as a component of the tissues, as a transitory infiltration, and as a necrobiotic matter.

Adipose tissue—Polysarcia—Fatty tumours—Interstitial formation of fat—Fatty
degeneration of muscles.

Fatty infiltration—Intestines; structure and functions of the villi—Reabsorption
and retention of the chyle—Liver; intermediate interchange of matter by
means of the biliary ducts. Fatty liver.

Fatty metamorphosis—Glands; secretion of sebaceous matter and milk (colostrum)
—Granule-cells and granule-globules—Inflammatory globules—Arteries; fatty
usure and atheroma in them—Fatty débris.

WE have, gentlemen, hitherto nearly always spoken
of the *actions* of cells and the processes which manifest
themselves in them, when, in consequence of any external influence, they give signs of their vitality. There
take place in the body, however, also a tolerably large
number of *passive processes*, in which, as far at least as
can be demonstrated, there is no particular activity displayed by the cells. Allow me therefore, before we
proceed farther in the description of the active processes,
to speak a little more in detail concerning these passive
processes. For the history of the affections of cells, as
they are exhibited to us in our patients, is generally

composed of processes, which belong, some of them, rather to the active class, and some of them, rather to the passive one ; and the obvious results are in many cases apparently so similar in both classes, that the ultimate changes which we meet with, after the continuance of the process for a certain time, may very nearly be the same. Here particularly it was for a time, very difficult to define the boundaries, and a great part of the confusion which marked early microscopical efforts, was occasioned by the extraordinary difficulty there was in separating active and passive disturbances.

Passive disturbances I call those changes in cellular elements, whereby they at once either merely lose a portion of their activity, or are so completely destroyed, that a loss of substance, a diminution in the sum total of the constituents of the body is produced. Both series of passive processes, taken together, viz., those which are in the first instance marked by an essential diminution of power, and those which terminate in a complete destruction of the parts, constitute the chief part of the domain of what is called *degeneration*, although—a point that we must hereafter consider more closely—a great part of what must be called degeneration must be transferred to the series of active processes.

It makes of course an extremely great difference whether a vital element continues to subsist as such, or whether it entirely and completely perishes : whether at the conclusion of the process, it still exists, even though in a condition of much diminished functional power, or whether it is altogether destroyed. And here we have the important practical distinction, that in the one series of processes there is a possibility of a repair of the cells, whilst in the other direct repair is impossible, and a regeneration can only take place by means of a substitution of new cells from the neighbourhood. For when a cell

has perished, it is of course impossible for any further
development to originate in it.

This latter category, where the cells are destroyed
during the course of the process, I proposed a few years
ago to designate by a term which has been employed to
express disease generally by K. H. Schultz, viz., *Necrobiosis*.* For we have, namely, always here to deal with
a gradual decay and death, a dissolution, we might almost
say, a necrosis. But the idea of necrosis really does not
offer any analogy to these processes, inasmuch as in necrosis we conceive the mortified part to be preserved
more or less in its external form. Here on the contrary
the part vanishes, so that we can no longer perceive it
in its previous form. We have no necrosed fragment at
the end of the process, no mortification of the ordinary
kind, but a mass in which absolutely nothing of the previously existing tissues is preserved. The necrobiotic processes, which must be completely separated from necrosis,
are in general attended by *softening* as their ultimate result. This commences with a friability of the parts ; they
lose their coherence, at last really liquefy, and more or less
moveable, pulpy or fluid products take their place. We
might therefore without more ado name this whole series
of necrobiotic processes softenings, if a number of them
did not run their course, without the malacia's ever becoming apparent to the naked eye. As soon, namely,
as a process of this sort sets in in a compound organ, as
for example, a muscle, a palpable myo-malacia is certainly produced when all the muscular elements at a
given point are at once affected ; but it happens far more
frequently that, in the course of a muscle, only a comparatively small number of primitive fasciculi are affected,

---

* Necrobiosis is *death* brought on by (altered) *life*—a spontaneous wearing out
of living parts—the destruction and annihilation consequent upon life—natural as
opposed to violent death (mortification.)—*From a MS. Note by the Author.*

whilst the others remain almost intact. Then indeed a
softening really does occur, but such a minute one, that
it is altogether imperceptible to the naked eye and can
only be demonstrated microscopically. In this case we
generally make use of the expression, atrophy of muscle,
although the process which has attacked the individual
primitive fasciculi, does not in any way differ in its nature from the processes which we at other times term
softening of muscle.

This is the reason, why the term softening, which must
be reserved for coarse pathological anatomy, cannot simply be applied to histological processes, and why it is
better to say necrobiosis, when we have to do with these
more delicate processes. The common feature of all the
varieties of the necrobiotic process is, you know, that the
affected part at the close of the process is destroyed, nay
annihilated.

A second class of passive processes is formed by the
simply degenerative forms, in which, at the conclusion of
the process, the affected part is in some condition or other
less fitting it for action, and has generally become more
rigid. This group might therefore be termed *hardenings*
(*indurations*) and thus a group be formed distinguishable
even externally from the necrobiotic processes. Only
the term induration also would easily be misunderstood,
inasmuch as in this class likewise many conditions occur,
in which the hardness of the organ on the whole at least
does not become more considerable, but only isolated,
very minute parts undergo change, so that no very striking effects are apparent to the sense of touch.

Allow me now to hold up to you as types a few of the
processes belonging to this class, which are of the greatest importance in a directly practical point of view.

Among the necrobiotic processes the one which is unquestionably the most widely spread and the most important in the course of all cellular disturbances, is *fatty metamorphosis*, or as it has also long been wont to be called, *fatty degeneration*. This process is attended by a continually increasing accumulation of fat in different organs. Even the old notion of fatty degeneration involved the idea of a continually increasing change of such a nature that pure fat at last took the place of whole parts of organs. It has turned out, however, that this old notion, which is even now retained by many in the language of pathology, includes a great number of completely different processes, and that errors would inevitably be committed if it were sought to interpret the whole group from a pathogenical point of view, in a simple manner.

The history of fat in its relation to the tissues may, generally speaking, be considered under three aspects. We find namely one class of tissues in the body, which serve as physiological reservoirs for fat, and in which the fat is contained as a kind of necessary appurtenance, without however their own permanency being in any way endangered by its presence. On the contrary, we are actually accustomed to estimate the well-being of an individual by the amount of fat contained in certain tissues, and to regard the degree of fulness presented by the individual fat-cells as a criterion of the successful progress of the interchange of matter generally. This forms therefore a complete contrast to the necrobiotic processes, in which the part, in consequence of the accumulation of fat, really altogether ceases to exist.

A second series of tissues do not constitute regular reservoirs for fat, on the contrary fat is found in them only at certain times and transitorily, for after a short time it again disappears from them, without their being on that account left in an altered state. This is the case in the ordinary absorption of fat from the intestinal canal. When we drink milk, we expect in accordance with old experience that it will gradually pass from the intestines into the lacteals, and thence be conveyed into the blood ; we know that the passage of digested matters from the intestines into the lacteals takes place through the epithelium and the villi, and that some hours after a meal the epithelium and the villi are full of fat. Now, with respect to such a fat-containing villus or epithelial cell, we take for granted that in the natural course of events it will at last yield up its fat, and after some time again become perfectly free from it. This is fatty infiltration of a purely transitory character.

Finally, we have a third series of processes, namely, those which lead to necrobiosis and which have of late frequently been regarded as peculiarly pathological ones. But, as it has been shown to be the case in all other conditions that pathological processes are not specific ones, but, on the contrary, that others analogous to them exist in normal life, so also the conviction has been acquired that this necrobiotic development of fat is an entirely regular and typical process in certain parts of the body, nay that it is even met with in very obvious forms in physiological life. The most important types of this process we find on the one hand in the secretion of milk, the sebaceous matter of the skin, the cerumen of the ears, etc., and on the other in the formation of the corpus luteum in the ovaries. In all these parts a development of fat takes place precisely in the same manner that we meet with it in the nocrobiotic fatty metamorphosis occurring from morbid causes, and in what we call sebaceous matter, milk or colostrum we have formations analogous to the pathological masses of fat which constitute fatty softening. If in any person milk is manufactured in the brain instead of in the mammary gland, this constitutes one form of cerebral softening ; the product may morphologically exactly correspond with what in the mammary gland would have been quite normal. The great difference, however, is this, that, whilst in the mammary gland the cells which perish are replaced by a succession of new cells, the disintegration of elements in an organ which is not arranged so as to furnish such a succession, leads to a permanent loss of substance. The same process which in one organ yields the happiest, nay the sweetest, results, brings along with it in another, painful lesions.

If then you picture to yourselves these three different physiological types, we have in the first case an accumulation of fat in the cells in such a way, that at the close of the process every single cell is entirely full of it. This yields us the type of the so-called *adipose cellular tissue*, or simply, *adipose tissue*, as it occurs in such large masses especially in the subcutaneous tissue, where it on the one hand gives rise to beauty, particularly in the female figure, and on the other to the pathological conditions of obesity or polysarcia. Fat-cells always possess a membrane and fatty contents, but the fat so completely fills up the interior, and the membrane is so extremely thin, delicate and tense, that usually nothing else is seen than

FIG. 107.

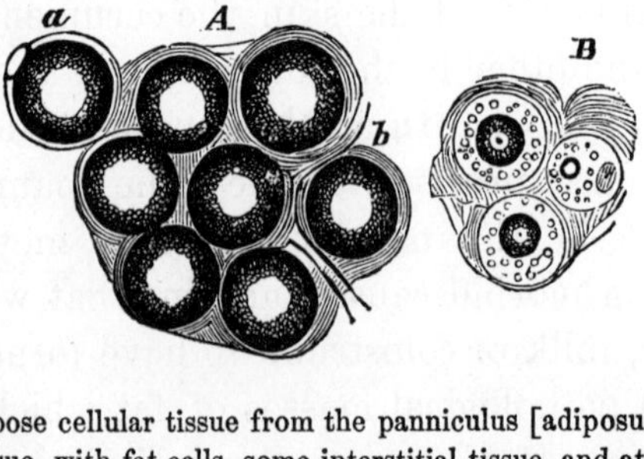

Fig. 107. Adipose cellular tissue from the panniculus [adiposus.]   *A*. Ordinary subcutaneous tissue, with fat-cells, some interstitial tissue, and at *b* vascular loops ; *a*, an isolated fat-cell with membrane, nucleus and nucleolus. *B*. Atrophic fat in phthisis.   300 diameters.

the drop of fat, and thus it was, until very recently, still a matter of discussion whether the fat-cells really were cells. It is in reality very difficult to come to a distinct decision upon the subject, but supporting testimony of a very beautiful character is supplied in the course of natural processes. When a person becomes thinner, the fat gradually disappears, the membrane loses somewhat of its tension, is no longer so thin and delicate, and thus becomes more clearly manifest, being sometimes distinctly separated from the drop of fat, and even provided with a recognizable nucleus (Fig. 107, *A, a*). We have here therefore a real, complete cell with nucleus and membrane, though the contents have been almost entirely supplanted by the fat it has taken up. This so-called adipose cellular tissue is a form of connective tissue (p. 76), and when it undergoes retrogressive metamorphosis, it is clearly seen to be reduced to connective or mucous tissue, for between the cells a small quantity of intercellular substance again becomes apparent (Fig. 107, *A, b, B*).

This species of adipose tissue it is, gentlemen, which under certain circumstances not only gives rise to polysarcia and obesity, from continually increasing quantities of connective tissue becoming involved in this accumulation of fat, but is also the foundation of all anomalous fatty structures, for example, of lipomata. The different forms of these structures, and particularly real fatty tumours, are distinguished from one another only by the greater or less quantity of interstitial connective tissue, which the tumour contains, and upon which their greater or less consistence depends. It is the same form of accumulation of fat which we see appear in morbid conditions in a series of cases which, in compliance with old tradition, are still called fatty degeneration ; and it is indeed particularly the *fatty degeneration of muscles* which in many instances presents nothing else than a more or less advanced development of adipose cellular tissue between the primitive muscular fasciculi. It is a similar process to that which we meet with in the fattening of animals, and which is often exhibited in simply fattened muscles in the human body. Fat-cells insinuate themselves between the primitive muscular fasciculi, and lie of course in stripes in the direction of the muscular fibres, which may remain unchanged. The development in this case has its origin in the interstitial tissue of the muscle. At the com-

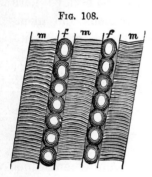

FIG. 108.

mencement of the development, and when it proceeds with very great regularity, it may happen, that single rows of fat-cells lying one behind the other alternate with the rows of muscular elements. In this case, where the primitive fasciculi are forced asunder, and the circulation in the muscle is generally disturbed in consequence of the abundant development of fat, so that the flesh becomes pale—it looks to the naked eye as if there no longer existed any muscular tissue whatever. If, for example, in an inferior extremity, which in consequence of an anchylosis of the knee has remained unexercised, the gastrocnemii are examined, we find nothing but a yellowish mass exhibiting scarcely any striæ and without any appearance of flesh, but upon a more minute examination it is discovered, that the primitive muscular fasciculi still pass, essentially unaltered, through the fat. In this case the fat forms an impediment to the use of the muscle, but the primitive fasciculi still exist and are to a certain

Fig. 108. Interstitial growth of fat in muscle (fattening). *ff*. Rows of interstitial fat-cells; *m, m, m*, primitive muscular fasciculi. 300 diameters.

extent capable of action. This process therefore is essentially different from necrobiosis, where the muscular fibres as such completely perish. Here we have a purely interstitial formation of adipose tissue, ordinary connective tissue becoming converted into adipose tissue, and the term, fatty degeneration, which is so very liable to be misunderstood, should be avoided.

This form occurs pretty frequently, especially in the heart, and may, when it attains a great extent, produce considerable derangement in the motor power of the muscular substance of this organ, but in pathological importance it stands far below real fatty metamorphosis, although this again in its outwardly visible results much resembles it. The hearts described by the old anatomists as fatty were in a great measure only hearts infiltrated with fat; on the other hand, what is meant at the present day when genuine fatty degeneration (metamorphosis) of the heart is spoken of, is not this obesity of the heart, this interlarding of its fibres with fat-cells, but rather a real transformation of its substance, going on in the interior of the fibres (Fig. 23). In the latter case the fat lies *in*, in the former *between* the primitive fasciculi.

The second series of processes consists in the transitory accumulation of fat in certain organs, as we meet with it in a typical form in digestion. When a fatty substance has been eaten, and has passed into the state of emulsion, we find that, when it has reached the upper end of the jejunum, and to some extent even in the duodenum, the villi of the mucous membrane become whitish, clouded and thick, and more minute examination shows, that they are filled with extremely minute granules, much more minute than can be produced by any artificial emulsion. These granules, which are found even in the chyme, come in the first

instance into contact with the cylindrical epithelium
with which every single intestinal villus is invested.   On
the surface of every epithelial cell we find, as was first
discovered by Kölliker, a peculiar border which, when
the cell is seen in profile, exhibits minute and fine striæ ;
when viewed from above, and seen upon the surface,
the cell appears hexagonal and, as it were, dotted over
with a number of minute points (Comp. the epithelium
of the gall-bladder, Fig. 14, and also Fig. 109, *A*).
Kölliker has put forward the conjecture, that these fine
striæ and dots correspond to minute pore-canals, and
that the absorption of the fat is effected by its minute
particles being taken up through these minute pores
upon the surface of the epithelial cells.   But the object
is one which is accessible only to the highest powers of
our optical instruments, and it has therefore hitherto
been impossible to obtain perfectly clear notions as to
whether the striæ really correspond to fine canals. or

Fig. 109.

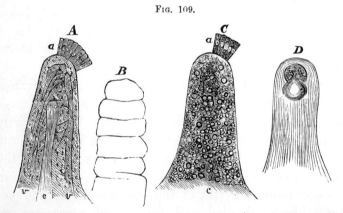

Fig. 109. Intestinal villi, showing the absorption of fat.   *A*. Normal human
intestinal villus from the jejunum ; at *a* the cylindrical epithelium in part still
investing it with the delicate border and nuclei ; *c*, the central lacteal vessel ;
v, v, blood-vessels ; in the rest of the parenchyma the nuclei of the connective and
muscular tissue. *B*. Villus in a state of contraction, from a dog. *C*. Human
intestinal villus during the absorption of chyle, *D*, in a case of retention of chyle ;
at the apex a large fat-drop, emerging from a crystalline envelope.   280 diameters.

whether, as Brücke supposes, the truth is rather that
the whole of this upper border is composed of little
rods or pillars resembling cilia.   I must confess that my
own investigations also have rather disposed me to
adopt this latter opinion, especially as comparative histology shows us real ciliated epithelium to be the equivalent structure in the same parts.   At all events this
much is certain, that, a short time after digestion has taken
place, the fat no longer lies only outside, but is found
also inside, the cells, and first at their outer end ; then
it gradually advances farther and farther inwards in the
cells, and indeed so distinctly in rows, that it might
easily give rise to the impression, that fine canals ran
throughout the whole length of the cells themselves
(Fig. 109, C, a).   But this too is a question which will
not, I think, with our present optical instruments, be so
very speedily settled.   At any rate, the plain fact remains, that the fat passes through the cells, and this
indeed in such a way, that at first only their outer end
is filled with it, then a time comes when they are quite
full of fat, then a little later the outer part again becomes entirely free from it, whilst the inner still contains a little, until at last all the fat entirely vanishes
from the cells.   In this manner its gradual progress may
be followed from hour to hour.   After the fat has advanced as far as the inner extremity of the cells, it
begins to pass into the so-called parenchyma of the
villus (Fig. 109, C).   Whether the epithelial cells have
an orifice below, and whether, as has been quite recently maintained by Heidenhain junior, they are connected with extremely minute canals formed by the connective-tissue-corpuscles, is not quite decided, though it
is very probable.   It is extremely difficult to come to
any definite conclusions with regard to these extremely
minute arrangements of the substance of tissues.   In

the interior of the villi we generally find the network of blood-vessels a little below the surface (Fig. 109, *A*, *v*, *v*), whilst in its axis there is a tolerably wide canalicular cavity with a blunt extremity, the commencement of the lacteal vessel, as far as it can at present be determined with certainty (Fig. 109, *A*, *c*). At the periphery of the villi Brücke has discovered a layer of muscular fibres, which is of great importance in digestion, inasmuch as by its help an approximation of the apex of the villus to its base, a shortening is effected, as may very readily be seen. Upon cutting off villi from the intestine of an animal just killed, they may be seen under the microscope to contract, become wrinkled, thicker and shorter (Fig. 109, *B*); thereby a pressure from without inwards is manifestly produced, which promotes the onward movement of the juices. So far the matter is tolerably clear, only what sort of a structure the rest of the parenchyma has, it is extremely difficult to see. Upon the outer side of the muscular layer, smallish nuclei are seen, which, as I pointed out many years ago, are now and then pretty distinctly enclosed in fine, cellular elements. But whether these parenchymatous cells anastomose with one another so as to form a special network, I am unable to say. During the process of absorption it looks as if the fat which keeps penetrating farther and farther into the interior of the villi, filled up the whole parenchyma.* At last it reaches the central lacteal, and there the regular current of chyle begins.

The whole process therefore presupposes an emulsive condition of the fat, which penetrates through the parts

---

* I have quite recently convinced myself by the examination of transverse sections of villi, filled with chyle, in man, that the fat does not lie scattered in the parenchyma, but forms deposits in the interior of special minute cavities (cells?).— *Note to the Second Edition.*

everywhere in a state of extremely minute division ; in the regular course of events the particles are so extremely minute, that if the chyle is examined when fresh and still warm, scarcely a trace of the solid particles can be detected in it. But every disturbance which occurs in the process of absorption, and impedes the onward movement of the fatty particles, causes them to run together ; larger granules separate in the tissues, drops appear which continually increase in volume, until at length they attain quite a large size. These are found even in the epithelial cells or within the tissue of the villi, and indeed it sometimes happens that the ends of the lacteals grow wider, and swell out into a bulbous form from the great accumulations of fat, so as to be recognized even by the naked eye. Nowhere have they been so frequently witnessed in a striking form, as in cholera, and a good description of these appearances as occurring in this disease was published as far back as 1837 by Böhn. They indicate nothing more than an obstruction to the current of lymph in consequence of the disturbances in the respiration and circulation (Fig. 109, D). Since attacks of cholera are well known to occur with preponderating frequency during digestion and are attended by greatly impeded respiration, which makes itself felt throughout the whole venous system, they must of course also react upon the stream of chyle. Thus the enormous accumulation (retention) of fat in the villi is explained. This is therefore, if you will, a pathological condition, but it only depends upon a transitory obstruction, and we have every reason to suppose that, when the current again becomes free, these large drops of fat are gradually removed. But here we set foot upon other domains, where the boundaries of pathology can only be traced with great difficulty, and this is particularly the case with the liver.

It has been known from of old that the *liver* is the organ, which is by far the most liable to fall into a state of fatty degeneration, and the knowledge of this state has long been derived from popular experiment. The history of the pâtés de foie gras proves this in the most agreeable manner, although M. Lereboullet of Strasburg maintains that the fatty livers of geese are physiological ones, essentially different from the pathological ones which are not eaten, but only observed. However, I must confess that I have hitherto been unable to discover the difference between physiological and pathological fatty livers ; on the contrary, I believe that it is only by admitting the identity of the two that correct notions with regard to the pathological fatty liver can be obtained. We are namely acquainted with a fact which was likewise first observed by Kölliker, that in sucking animals, a few hours after digestion has taken place, a kind of fatty liver is a constant physiological occurrence. When of the same litter of animals some are made to fast, while others are allowed to suck, those which have sucked have a fatty liver a few hours afterwards, whilst the others have not. The fatty liver appears quite pale, though certainly not so white as a goose's liver. This observation led me to examine the question of the relation of the fat to the liver a little more minutely, and I certainly think we may positively conclude that there does exist a close connection between the physiological and pathological forms.

I found, namely, that a short time after the hepatic cells display this repletion with fat, a similar condition is found in the course of the biliary ducts, and that both in them and in the gall-bladder the epithelium presents the same appearances which we have witnessed in the intestinal epithelium during the absorption of fat. You only require therefore to invert the picture we just now considered

(Fig. 109) ; instead of a villus, invested externally with epithelial cells, imagine a canal clothed on the inside with epithelium. The delicate cylindrical epithelium in the gall-bladder has the same striated border as that in the intestine (Fig. 14), and the fat is seen in the same way to penetrate into it from without, to pursue its course downwards and after a time to pass into the wall of the gall-bladder. The same may be said of the biliary *passages* (duct. biliferi, hepat., cystic., choledoch.), which are also provided with cylindrical epithelium of a similar structure. I have watched the same process also in young sucking animals after digestion, and there it is easy to convince oneself that the fat, which for a time is contained in the hepatic cells, is manifestly excreted from them into the biliary ducts, but that in the course of these ducts the fat is reabsorbed and thus a second time returns into the circulation.

Such an *intermediate interchange of matter* as this, where the fat passes from the intestine into the blood, from the blood into the liver, from the liver into the bile, and thence again into the lymphatics, or into the capillaries which conduct the blood back to the hepatic veins and to the heart, presupposes of course, just as absorption in the intestines does, that the conveyance back again must take place under favourable circumstances ; if any disturbing cause arises, a retention will of course ensue, and the place of the fine granules will gradually be occupied by large drops. But this is the mode of proceeding as it can really be traced in the fatty liver.

Upon studying a fatty liver, it is generally seen that the fat is first deposited in that zone of the acini which is immediately contiguous to the capillaries into which the branches of the portal vein break up (Fig, 110. *c, c*). When sections of the organ are carefully examined with the naked eye, it looks in many parts as if one had an

oak-leaf with its ribs and indentations before one ; the
ramifications of the branches of the portal vein correspond
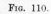
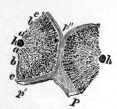
to the ribs, the fatty zone to the sub-
stance of the leaf.　The more abundant the infiltration, the broader does
the fatty zone become, and there are
cases in which the fat fills the whole
of the acini up the central (intralobular) hepatic vein (Fig. 110, *h*) and
every single cell is crammed full of
fat.　In rare cases it certainly happens, that we find just
the reverse, and that the fat lies around the central
vein ; these are cases which are probably to be explained
by supposing that the fat is already in process of excretion and only the last cells still retain a little of it.　Only
we must take care not to confound with this condition a
kind of fatty, necrobiotic atrophy which occurs particularly in chronic cyanosis.*

If now we consider the process in detail, we find that
the manner in which the hepatic cells fill themselves, entirely corresponds to that, in which an epithelial cell in
the intestine becomes filled with fat.　At first we find
fat-granules widely scattered, and indeed very small.
They become more numerous, more closely aggregated,
and after a time larger ; at the same time the cells be-

Fig. 110. The adjoining halves of two hepatic acini.　*p.* A branch of the portal
vein with braches *p′ p″*, corresponding to the interlobular veins.　*h, h.* Transverse
sections of the intralobular, or hepatic, vein.　*a.* The pigment zone, *b* the amyloid
zone, *c* the fat zone.　20 diameters.

* Cyanosis (chronic) is here used to express the general venous congestion which
is consequent upon chronic affections of the lungs and heart.　"Since (as the Author says in a MS. note) it has become known that cyanosis, even when produced
by congenital malformation of the heart, does not arise from a commingling of
arterial and venous blood, but from an obstruction to the venous circulation, it has
seemed reasonable to designate every more general hyperæmia, due to such obstruction, by the same term."　"Acute cyanosis," he adds, "occurs in acute affections of the lungs, as for example, in pertussis."—TR.

come larger, swell up, and larger and smaller drops of fat are found in them (Fig. 27, *B*, *b*), until, when filled to the utmost, they present the same appearance as those of adipose tissue ; scarcely any membrane, and scarcely ever a nucleus is seen, nevertheless they both still continue to exist. This is the condition which is called fatty liver, in the proper sense of the word.

In it too we have what we found to be the case in adipose tissue—a *persistence of the cells*. There is no such thing as a fatty liver in which the cells have ceased to exist ; these constituents of the organs always exist, only they are almost entirely filled with drops of fat instead of with their ordinary contents. It can scarcely be doubted but that even in this condition they still contain a certain amount of matter capable of performing its functions. For in many animals, as for example the cod-fish from which liver-oil is obtained, the functions of the organ are still performed, however large the quantity of oil contained in the cells. In man too, even in the most advanced stage of fatty liver, we still find bile in the gall-bladder. So far therefore these conditions can in no respect be compared to the necrobiotic conditions, which are found in the course of fatty degeneration in so many other parts, and in which the elements perish. In fatty degeneration, in the ordinary sense of the word, we find, in the later stages of the affection, somewhere or other, friable, softened places, where the fat is contained in free drops—in some sort fatty abscesses. It is therefore a fact of extreme importance, and one which I consider to afford very decided indications for the correct appreciation of this form [fatty liver], that in it there is always a persistence of the histological constituents, and that, however much these constituents may become filled with foreign substances, they still continue to exist as cells. Hence it follows, that a fatty condition of the liver may be removed, that it is curable, without any particular regenerative processes being required for the cure. The only requisite is, that the causes of the retention be removed, and the hepatic cells be freed from fat. It is true we have no positive information respecting either the one or the other of these points. We are not acquainted with the states which lead to the retention of the fat, nor with the conditions under which it can again be expelled. However, now that we have got so far, it will probably also be possible to make out the remaining facts. For it is conceivable, for example, that simply the elasticity of the histological elements is of importance ; that when the cell walls become relaxed, they may readily admit a quantity of matter, and tolerate its presence in them, whilst, if they are very elastic, a removal, an expression of their contents, may be more likely to ensue. The state of the circulation also is certainly of importance, and the frequent occurrence of fatty liver in chronic affections of the lungs and heart is certainly in no small degree to be ascribed to the increased pressure to which the venous blood is subjected.

What I was particularly anxious, gentlemen, to render evident to you, was the great difference which this kind of fatty degeneration presents from that which we have previously considered. Whilst there we saw arise between the proper specific constituents of the organ—fat-cells which belonged to the connective tissue, here it is the specific gland cells themselves which are the seat of the fat. On the other hand, you must take into consideration the great difference from the necrobiotic processes of fatty degeneration, in which the cells as such disappear.

We have now, gentlemen, to consider this third series of fatty conditions a little more closely, those, I mean, which are attended by a destruction of the elements, and

of which we have set up the secretion of milk and sebaceous matter as the true types. That these two secretions are analogous to one another, is simply explained
by the circumstance that the mammary gland is really
nothing more than an enormously developed and peculiarly formed accumulation of cutaneous (sebaceous)
glands. In their development both classes are perfectly
analogous. Both are produced, by means of a progressive proliferation, from the internal layers of the epidermis (p. 68, Fig. 18, *A*). To the same category also belong the ceruminous glands of the ear, and the large
glands of the axilla. In all these
cases the fat, which constitutes the
chief constituent of milk, at least as
far as its external appearance is
concerned, and which furnishes the
sebaceous secretion, originates in
the interior of epithelial cells
which gradually perish and set the
fat free, whilst scarcely a trace of
the cells is preserved. The sebaceous glands are generally seated
on the sides of the hair-follicles
at some depth below the surface;
we there find a series of minute lobules, into which a prolongation of the rete mucosum is un-
interruptedly continued. The cells
of this become more numerous and
larger, so as to fill the gland-sacs
with a nearly solid matter. Then the fat begins to be

FIG. 111.

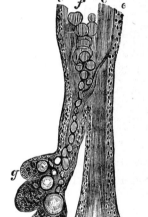

Fig. 111. Hair-follicle with sebaceous glands from the skin. *c*. The hair, *b* its
bulb, *e*, *e*, the layers of cells dipping down from the epidermis into the hair-follicle.
g g. Sebaceous glands in the act of secreting sebaceous matter; at *f*, the secretion
mounting up by the side of the hair and accumulating. 280 diameters.

secreted into their interior, at first in small particles, which soon become larger, and after a short time the individual cells can no longer be distinctly perceived, but only conglomerations of large drops, which rise up out of the gland into the hair-follicle. If we unravel the gland so as to form a flat surface, its layers of cells would have the appearance of epidermis, only that the oldest cells do not become horny, but are destroyed by fatty metamorphosis. The secretion is a purely epithelial one, like the seminal secretion.

This process furnishes us at the same time with an accurate representation of the *formation of milk*. You need only imagine the ducts much lengthened, and the terminal acini greatly developed; the process remains essentially the same: the cells multiply abundantly; the multiplied cells undergo fatty degeneration, and ultimately there remains scarcely any material traces of these cells excepting the drops of fat. The closest resemblance to the manner in which the secretion of sebaceous matter ordinarily takes place, is presented by the earliest period of lactation when the so-called *colostrum* is yielded. A colostrum-corpuscle (Fig. 112, *C*) is the still coherent globule which results from the fatty degeneration of an epithelial cell. The formation of colos-

FIG. 112.

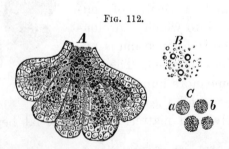

Fig. 112. Mammary gland during lactation, and milk. *A*. Lobule of the mammary gland, with milk issuing out of it. *B*. Milk globules. *C*. Colostrum, *a*, a distinct fat-granule cell, *b*, the same with evanescent nucleus. 280 diameters.

trum and sebaceous matter differs in this respect only, that the fat-granules remain smaller in the former case, and that whilst large drops very soon show themselves in sebaceous matter, in colostrum the last cells which are observed, usually contain only minute fat-granules, very densely aggregated, whereby the whole cell acquires a somewhat brownish appearance, although the fat has no actual colour. This is the granular corpuscle (corps granuleux) of Donné.

For the discovery of this gradual transformation of cellular bodies into fat-granule masses we are indebted to Reinhardt. Still he shrank from extending this important discovery of the formation of colostrum to the history of milk in general, for the reason, that, during the later periods of lactation properly so-called, granulated bodies are no longer met with. It is, however, unquestionable, that between the earlier formation of colostrum-corpuscles and the later one of milk, there is no other difference than this, that in the formation of colostrum the process goes on more slowly, and that the cells maintain their cohesion longer, whilst in the secretion of milk the process is acute and the cells more speedily perish. Perfectly developed colostrum contains an extremely large number of granulated corpuscles, milk nothing more than a number of comparatively large and small drops of fat, mixed up together, the so-called *milk-corpuscles* (Fig. 112, *B*), which are nothing more than drops of fat, and like the majority of the drops of fat that occur in the animal body are surrounded by a delicate, albuminous membrane, called by Ascherson the *haptogenic** membrane (haptogenmembran). But the individual drops (milk-corpuscles) correspond to the drops which we find in the secretion of

---

* *I. e.*, produced by contact.—Transl.

sebaceous matter ; they are produced by the coalescence
of the minute granules which appear in the secretion of
colostrum.

Now that we have seen these types of physiological
transformation, gentlemen, the description of the pathological changes no longer offers any difficulty. With
the exception of very few structures, as for example,
red blood-corpuscles and the nerve-fibres in the great
nervous centres, nearly all other cellular parts may
under certain circumstances undergo a similar metamorphosis, which displays itself in a precisely similar manner, that is, isolated, extremely minute globules of fat
appear in the cell-contents, become more abundant, and
gradually fill up the cell-cavity, without, however, running together into such large drops, as is the case in
fatty infiltration and in the adipose-tissue formations.
Usually, the development of the fat-granules first declares itself at some distance from the nucleus ; very
seldom does it begin at the nucleus. This is the cell
which has long been called the *granule-cell*. Then
comes a stage, in which the nucleus and membrane are
indeed still to be seen, but the fat-granules lie as close
to one another as in colostrum corpuscles ; only at the
spot where the nucleus lay, there is still a little gap
(Fig. 66, *b*). From this stage there is but a short step
to the complete destruction of the cell. For a cell
never remains for any length of time in the state of a
granule-cell, but as soon as it has once entered into this
stage, the nucleus generally disappears at once, and
ultimately the membrane also, probably by a species of
solution. Then we have the simple *granule-globule*, or as
it was formerly called, *inflammatory globule* [exudation-
corpuscle], which Gluge first described under this name
(Fig. 66, *e*).

Gluge in this made one of those mistakes which not

unfrequently marked the early periods of microscopy. He saw, when examining a kidney, bodies of this sort in the interior of a canal, which he took for a blood-vessel; this happening at a time when the doctrine of stasis was most in vogue, he imagined he had before him a vessel with stagnating contents which were disintegrating, and generating inflammatory globules. Unfortunately the blood-vessel was a uriniferous tubule; what he took to be parts of disintegrating blood-corpuscles, was fat; and what he called inflammatory globules, fatty degenerated renal epithelium. One might easily have spared oneself this error in the history of stasis, but at that time there were few people who knew what was the appearance of uriniferous tubules and how they might be distinguished from vessels, and thus some time elapsed before this theory of inflammation was put down.

At present we call the body a granule-globule and regard it as the first distinct proof of degeneration, when the cell no longer retains its existence as a cell, but merely its former shape remains, after the parts which really constitute a cell, namely the membrane and the nucleus, have completely passed away. After this, in accordance with external circumstances, either a complete destruction of the parts ensues, or they may still persist, coherent. If, namely, we have to deal with very soft parts, in which much fluid or juice has been present all along, the granules fall asunder. The medium which bound them together and enabled them to retain the globular form, namely, a remnant of the old cell-contents, is gradually dissolved. The globule breaks up into a crumbling mass, which is often still somewhat coherent in places, but from which one drop of fat after another is detached, so that the correspondence with milk is very beautifully displayed.

This is the manner in which the disintegration of nearly all parts takes place, which essentially consist of cells and naturally contain a good deal of fluid, as for example pus among familiar pathological products (p. 216, Fig. 66). If, on the contrary, the parts are in themselves somewhat more rigid, so that movement in and displacement of, the fatty mass takes place with less facility, the fat remains in the form of the previous cell. Of this we meet with an example in the fatty degeneration of the walls of arteries.

In the aorta, the carotids and the cerebral arteries, changes of the inner coat are often seen with the naked eye of such a nature, that small, whitish spots of a rounded or angular form, occasionally running one into the other, project somewhat above the surface. If an incision is made at these spots, it is found that they are quite superficial, that they lie in the innermost layer of the internal coat and must not be confounded with the really atheromatous condition. If such a spot be cut out, it is found that a fatty degeneration of the connective-tissue-corpuscles of the innermost coat has taken place ; and since they are branched cells, we do not here have granule-cells in their ordinary rounded form, but often very long, fine bodies, which here and there swell up into the form of a spindle or star, and in which the fat-granules lie heaped up like strings of pearls, whilst between there still remains intermediate substance quite intact. It is the cellular elements of the connective tissue which in these cases undergo the change in their totality. Afterwards the intermediate substance also softens, the cellular fat-granule masses fall asunder, and the current of blood carries away the particles of fat with it. In this way a number of uneven places are produced upon the surface of the vessel, which swell up as long as the process continues, afterwards become worn away (usurirt), and acquire a slightly velvety appearance, without there being any ulceration

FIG. 113.

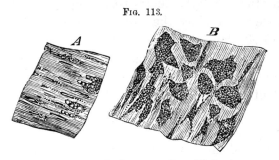

in the proper sense of the word. This is a particular form of *fatty usure* which occurs in many parts, as for example in articular cartilages, and even on the surface of mucous membranes, for example, that of the stomach (Fox). But at no time does the matter accumulate in such abundance as is the case in abcesses which have undergone fatty degeneration. If, on the other hand, a similar process commences beneath the surface, as in the atheromatous process, the fatty degeneration then proceeds from below upwards, and the surface is not reached until the last. By softening, the so-called *atheromatous deposit* (Heerd*) is produced, which contains a softened mass resembling the contents of atheromata [sebaceous,† or epidermic, cysts] of the skin, in which

Fig. 113. Fatty degeneration of cerebral arteries. *A*. Fatty metamorphosis of the muscular cells of the circular-fibre coat. *B*. Formation of fat-granule cells in the connective-tissue-corpuscles of the internal coat. 300 diameters.

* Heerd (hearth) in the sense in which it is here employed, has no precise equivalent in English, although it exactly corresponds to the French *foyer*. " It denotes," says the Author, " the spot, where the fire of the disease burns, but expresses at the same time that this spot is a limited one." I have therefore translated it by various words, such as deposit, dépôt, seat (of the disease), collection, patch (atheromatous), focus, &c.—TRANSL.

† These cysts are wrongly called sebaceous, inasmuch as they are essentially *epidermic*, and are generally derived, not from the sebaceous glands, but from the hair-follicles. The atheromatous matter is in these cases chiefly composed of degenerated and disintegrated epithelium.—*From a MS. Note by the Author.*

the mixture of sebaceous matter and epidermis produces a pultaceous mass. What we find in the arteries
is a mixture of fatty débris with softened intermediate
substance ; and, since the fatty mass is shut off, a kind
of enclosed deposit results—as it were an abscess. It
is only after the softening has proceeded to some extent
that the surface gives way, and matters issue from the
cavity into the vessel, whilst others proceed from the
blood into the cavity.

In this manner *destruction, demolition, ulceration* is
produced, and ultimately the *atheromatous ulcer*, a species
of ulcer very nearly allied to the ordinary forms of ulceration, but indebted for its origin to fatty metamorphosis alone. It is a product of the [atheromatous]
deposit, but it no longer contains any formed elementary
parts. Cholestearine indeed may still be set free, but
we have really and truly to deal with a destructive and
ultimately ulcerative process. It is only in those parts,
in which, as in the mammary and sebaceous glands, there
is a succession of new cells, that the process of fatty
metamorphosis can continue for any length of time
without leading to such an annihilating result. But,
even in these instances, the different cells affected ultimately perish and break up, as in the really fatty degeneration.

LECTURE XVI.

APRIL 14, 1858.

A MORE PRECISE ACCOUNT OF FATTY METAMORPHOSIS.

Fatty degeneration of muscles—Fatty metamorphosis of the substance of the heart
—Formation of fat in the muscles in distortions.

Corpus luteum of the ovary—Fatty metamorphosis of pulmonary epithelium—Yellow softening of the brain—Arcus senilis.

Optical properties of fattily degenerated tissues—Renal epithelium in Bright's disease—Successive stages (cloudy swelling, fatty metamorphosis, fatty detritus [débris], atrophy)—Inflammatory globules—Similarity of the result in inflammatory and non-inflammatory changes.

Atheromatous process in arteries—Its relation to ossification—Inflammatory character of the process; its analogy with endocarditis—Formation of the atheromatous deposit—Appearance of cholestearine—Arterio-sclerosis—Endoarteritis—Calcification and ossification of arteries.

Mixed, activo-passive processes.

TO-DAY, gentlemen, I have sent round a few specimens of fatty degenerations, in part to serve as a supplement to what you saw at the last lecture.

One or two of these preparations are intended to display the fatty degeneration of the substance of the heart. You will observe that, even with the naked eye, certain changes can be recognized in the heart, namely, a discoloration of its whole substance (which no longer presents the red hue of muscle, but wears a pale yellow tint), and besides peculiar spots on the papillary muscles. If you examine these more closely, you will perceive, in the direction of the primitive fasciculi, short, yellowish

streaks which communicate so as almost to present a
plexiform arrangement, and pervade the substance of the
papillary muscles, whilst they offer a striking contrast to
the reddish colour of proper muscular substance.   This
is the perfect form of genuine fatty metamosphoris of the
real muscular substance of the
heart, which differs most essentially
from obesity of the heart, in which
this organ becomes extremely fat
and adipose tissue here and there
so infiltrates its walls, that scarcely
any muscle is to be perceived. Between the two conditions there
always remains the notable difference, that in the former case whole
portions of active substance are
interrupted by parts which are manifestly no longer
capable of action.

FIG. 114.

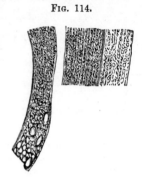

I have besides brought you another specimen of muscle we obtained yesterday at the suggestion of our con-
frère Berend.   A body, namely, with posterior (angular)
and lateral curvature (Kypho-Skoliose) was brought for
post-mortem examination, and, when we examined the
muscles at the point of curvature, we found the longissi-
mus dorsi at the spot where it passed over the projection, converted into quite a flat, thin, pale yellowish
mass.   At one point the muscle has, with the exception
of a membranous layer, entirely disappeared, its red hue
has altogether vanished ; towards the lower part the
muscle also presents an abnormal appearance, but there
it is composed of alternate longitudinal red and yellow
streaks.   This is the form exhibited by most fattily degenerated muscles which we find in distortions of the

* Fig. 114. Fatty degeneration of the muscular substance of the heart in its different stages.   300 diameters.

limbs, as for example, in the different kinds of club-foot. In these it generally turns out, that, in the parts corresponding to the yellow streaks, there is not only a real transformation of the muscular substance, but that an interstitial development of adipose tissue has also nearly constantly taken place there, so that it lies in rows between the primitive muscular fasciculi, and thereby produces a striation which looks yellowish to the naked eye, and is due to an arrangement very similar to that which gives rise to the red striation of genuine muscular tissue.* This is precisely how matters stood in the case I spoke of recently (p. 364, Fig. 108), where we found a row of fat-cells between every two primitive fasciculi ; the yellow that you saw there, was not altered muscle, but a mass of fat which had grown in between the muscular fibres. But in addition to such interstitial adipose tissue there is in the case now before us a parenchymatous degeneration in the same muscle ; the substance of the muscle is also really in a state of fatty degeneration. The degenerated fibres are, however, only to be seen with the naked eye in the lower parts of the muscle, whilst the portion which lay in immediate contact with the greatest projection of the thorax and had been subjected to the greatest tension, to the naked eye presents no trace of muscular tissue. Under the microscope, however, we even there find isolated muscular fibres lying close to one another and still distinctly transversely striated, and others plentifully filled with fat. You see, therefore, that these are two different conditions ; the one form, where the muscle is interrupted in the course of its primitive fasciculi by degenerated places, and where

---

* For, as each row of fat-cells lies between two primitive fasciculi (Fig. 108), the fat (like the substance of the fasciculi, the cyntonine) has a layer of sarcolemma upon each side of it, so that, if the syntonine atrophies, the fat *appears* to have taken its place and to lie *within* the primitive fasciculi, and many well-known authors have taken this to be the case.—*From a MS. Note by the Author.*

therefore the same primitive fasciculus, is, as it pursues
its course, now in a state of degeneration, now preserved
in all its integrity ; the other form in which the disease
sweeps along the primitive fasciculus, and this undergoes
the change in its whole extent at once, and where therefore normal and degenerated fasciculi lie side by side,
and may alternate with one another.

Here is another specimen from a young female (who
died shortly after menstruation in consequence of a burn)
in which you will find a very beautiful corpus luteum in
the ovary. I lay it before you because you will be able
to see, from it, how obviously fatty metamorphosis may
display itself to the unaided eye. The incision into the
ovary has been made perpendicularly to the surface, at a
point where a little prominence and slight rent upon the
surface mark the place at which the ovule has emerged
(Fig. 115, *B*). From the point in the tunica albuginea
where the follicle has burst, the very broad, yellowish

FIG. 115.

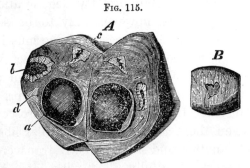

white layer (Fig. 115, *A*, *b*), from which the body derives
its name, is seen running around a red mass. It is this

Fig. 115. Formation of corpora lutea in the human ovary. *A*. Section of an
ovary : *a*, a follicle recently burst and filled with coagulated blood (extravasation,
thrombus), and around it the thin yellow layer ; *b*, a follicle, which had burst at an
earlier period, already corrugated, and provided with a diminished thrombus and
thickened wall; *c*, *d* a still more advanced stage of retrogressive metamorphosis.
B. External surface of the ovary, with the fresh rent caused by the bursting of the
follicle, from the cavity of which the thrombus is seen peeping out. Natural size.

layer which, in a puerperal corpus luteum, is of very great breadth and has a rather reddish yellow tint ; in a menstrual corpus luteum it is narrower, and very distinctly separated on the inner side from the freshly extravasated contents which have filled up the follicle emptied by the extrusion of the ovule. This internal red mass consists entirely of thrombus, or blood-clot. The external layer essentially consists of fattily degenerated cells, and the yellow colour which it bears is occasioned by the refraction produced by the numerous minute particles of fat. This is not a real colour, but a phenomenon of interference.

A similar change you see in a lung which we took to-day out of the body of a man who, after caries of the internal ear, had a thrombosis of the transverse sinus with gangrenous metamorphosis, and, in consequence, gangrene of the lung. The cells we have here to deal with were not taken, however, from the actual seat of the gangrene itself, but from a condensed spot in the neighbourhood, where a very abundant accumulation of masses of proliferating epithelium (catarrhal pneumonia) had taken place. In this case you can see the difference between fat-granule-cells (Fig. 66), and other forms of granule-cells, very prettily shown. For in these masses of epithelium which have filled up the alveoli of the lung, you find extremely numerous pigment-cells, such as in cases like this are brought up in great quantity in the sputa, which are indebted to them for the well-known smoky grey spots (Fig. 11, b). At first sight it is difficult to make a distinction between fat-granule-, and pigment-cells, inasmuch as in both cases apparently the same image is offered to our view. In the one case the cells appear as brownish yellow corpuscles, although their individual particles have no positive colour ; in the other, on the contrary, they contain unquestionable, grey, brown, or black, pigment. The diagnosis of ordinary granule-cells, by which fat-granule-cells are always meant, is, however, very important, because in other parts also, as for example, in the brain, we find both sorts of granule-cells, those containing fat and those containing pigment, side by side ; and even when the affection is limited to very small spots in this organ, it is very important* for the interpretation of the objects found to know whether they belong to the one or the other class. For in the brain also the accumulation of a number of minute particles of fat may on the whole, through the multiplication of the refracting points, occasion an intense yellow colour. The different proportion of fat and the degree of its division produce a greater number of varieties of colour which at last manifest themselves very distinctly to the naked eye, so that the more minute and the more closely aggregated the fatty particles are, the more marked is the production of a pure yellow or brownish-yellow hue even to the naked eye. What we call yellow softening of the brain is also really nothing more than a form of fatty degeneration, where the yellow appearance of the affected spot is owing to the accumulation of finely granular fat. As soon as this is removed, the colour also disappears, although the fat thus extracted is by no means of so deep a hue as the spot whence it was derived. The refraction of light between the extremely minute particles is the chief cause of this phenomenon of colour.

It is self-evident that at every point, where the fatty degeneration attains a high pitch, great opacity will always present itself. A transparent part becomes opaque when it undergoes fatty degeneration ; this we see, for example, in the cornea, the fatty clouding of which may become so marked in arcus senilis, that an en-

* For the pigment would point to apoplexy, the fat to softening.

tirely opaque zone is thereby produced. Even in places, where the parts were originally not transparent, but only translucent, a complete opacity may be seen to declare itself in proportion as the process of fatty degeneration progresses.

Consider, for example, a kidney in the stage of fatty degeneration. I show you here a preparation which does not present the ordinary granular atrophy of Bright's disease, but a more chronic and smooth form. The convoluted uriniferous tubules of the cortex are very much enlarged, and the whole of its epithelium is in a state of fatty degeneration, so that within the tubules there is really nothing else to be seen than a densely crowded mass of fat-granules. If however microscopical sections are very carefully prepared, the fat-granules are in the first instance still seen collected in isolated groups (as granule-cells or granule-globules, Fig. 98) ; but upon slight pressure the mass disperses in such a way, that the whole uriniferous tubule is uniformly filled with finely emulsive contents. Even with the naked eye you can distinctly recognize the change ; and as soon as one has become accustomed to discriminate with some degree of accuracy between these less obvious conditions, there is not the slightest difficulty in discovering from the aspect of such a part the presence of a change in the renal epithelium, and that indeed of this particular kind, for there is no other form of change which could be compared to it. If you examine the surface of the kidney you will perceive that over the rather greyish, transculent ground, upon which the Stellulæ Verheynii* stand out, small opaque spots are scatterred in the most varied manner, most of them forming not real points, but usually small segments of an arc. These will always be found to be parts of

* The stellate veins.—TRANSL.

the convolutions of uriniferous tubules which have
mounted up to the surface. These yellowish, opaque-
looking convolutions correspond to fattily degenerated
uriniferous tubules, or to speak more accurately, to
uriniferous tubules filled with fattily degenerated epithelium. If a section be compared with the surface, the
same markings are very distinctly seen to run through
the whole of the cortex, from the periphery down to the
upper borders of the medullary cones, and to invest the
individual cones formed by the tubuli recti which are
prolonged into the cortical substance—at pretty regular
intervals.

If sections are made in such a case in the neighbourhood of the surface and parallel to it, we readily obtain
a view embracing the fattily degenerated tubules by the
side of more normal ones, and of unaffected glomeruli.
With a lower power and by transmitted light, we see
close to the Malpighian bodies which appear as large,
light, globular structures, the convolutions of the degenerated uriniferous tubules interlacing in various ways,
and the convoluted tubules distinguished by their opaque,
shaded appearance from the straight ones, which are
lighter and more translucent.

I will here call your attention to the circumstance,
that in all fatty parts, where, by reflected light and as we
usually view objects with the naked eye, we see whitish,
yellowish, or brownish-yellow parts—by transmitted
light, as generally employed for microscopes, and especially with the higher powers, either black, or brownish
black, or at least very dark parts, surrounded by
sharply-defined shadows, appear. A granule-globule
which, when lying together with several others, produces a spot white and opaque to the naked eye, will,
when viewed by transmitted light, display a nearly black
appearance.

We have now compared a series of examples of fatty degeneration, and may henceforth confine ourselves to the consideration of genuine *fatty metamorphosis*, in which the normal structure of the part is ultimately destroyed, and the place of the histological elements is gradually occupied by a purely emulsive mass, or, more concisely, *fatty débris*. It makes no difference whether it is a pus-cell, a connective-tissue-corpuscle, a nerve- or muscular fibre, or a vessel which experiences the change ; the result is always the same ; namely, milky débris, an amorphous accumulation of fatty particles in a more or less highly albuminous fluid. But though we hold to the agreement of all cases of fatty metamorphosis in this respect, it by no means, however, follows that the importance of this change as a morbid process is in every case the same. This you may at once infer from the circumstance, that, whilst I have introduced this process to your notice in the category of purely passive disturbances, one of the very structures which we most frequently find in it, the granule-globule, has been re-garded as a specific element of inflammation. For years an inflammatory globule [exudation corpuscle] was looked upon as an essential phenomenon in the process of inflammation, and in fact, the frequency with which cells in a state of fatty degeneration are found in inflamed parts, affords sufficient proof, that in the course of inflammatory processes, which it is impossible we should ever regard as simply passive processes, such transformations must take place. It is therefore very essential to find a means of distinguishing between the two classes. This offers indeed in particular cases very great difficulties, and according to my conviction the only possible method by which clear notions upon the subject can be obtained, consists in examining whether the condition of fatty degeneration is a primary or se-

condary one, whether it sets in as soon as the disturbance can be perceived, or whether it does not occur
until some other perceptible disturbance has gone before.
Secondary fatty degeneration, or that in which this
peculiar transformation occurs only in the second place,
generally succeeds to a first and active stage ; a whole
series of those processes which we do not scruple to call
inflammations run their course in such a way, that a
fatty metamorphosis sets in as the second or third anatomical stage of the change. Here therefore the fatty
degeneration does not arise as a direct result of the
irritation of the part, but where we have the opportunity of more accurately tracing the history of the
changes, it nearly always turns out, that the stage of
fatty degeneration has been preceded by another stage,
namely that of *cloudy swelling*, in which the parts
enlarge and increase in extent and density, in consequence of their absorbing a large quantity of matter
into themselves. Absorbing I say advisedly, because I
hold it to be untrue that the part is in any way forced
by external influences to take up this matter, or that it
is inundated with exudation proceeding from the vessels,
for the same phenomena present themselves also in
parts which have no vessels. It is only when the accumulation has attained such dimensions, that the
natural constitution of the part is thereby endangered,
that a fatty disintegration is set up in the interior of
the elements. Thus we may designate fatty degeneration of the renal epithelium as a stage of Bright's disease (or as I say, parenchymatous nephritis), which has
been preceded by a stage of hyperæmia and swelling,
in which every epithelial cell accumulated a large
quantity of cloudy matter in itself, without there having
been originally a trace of a drop of fat observable.
Thus we see that a muscle under the influence of

agencies which it is universally conceded produce inflammation, as for example after wounds, and chemical corrosions, swells up, that its primitive fasciculi become broader and more clouded, and that as a second stage the same fatty degeneration commences in them, which at other times we see primarily arise.

It may therefore certainly, when quite general terms are used, be said, that there does exist an inflammatory form of fatty degeneration ; still, strictly speaking, this inflammatory form is never anything more than a later stage, a termination, which announces the commencing disintegration of the structure of the tissue, when the part is no longer in a condition to continue a separate existence, but is to such an extent abandoned to the play of the chemical forces of its constituent parts, that the next result is its really complete dissolution. Now inflammatory conditions of this kind are of very great importance, because in all parts whose essential elements become changed in this manner, no immediate restitution is possible. When inflammation takes place in a muscle and in its course the primitive muscular fasciculi fall into a state of fatty degeneration, as a rule they also perish, and we afterwards find a loss of substance in the muscle at the spot where the degeneration took place. The kidney, whose epithelium has passed into a state of fatty degeneration, nearly always shrivels up, and the result is a permanent atrophy. In exceptional cases something perhaps occurs, which reminds us of a regeneration of the epithelium, but usually a collapse of the entire structure ensues. The same thing is witnessed in the brain in yellow softening, no matter how it may have been caused. Whether there have been inflammation or not, a vacuity is formed, which is never again filled up with nervous matter. Perhaps a simple fluid may replace the wanting tissues, but as to any reproduction of a new, functionally active part, that must ever be out of the question.

Herein you must seek the explanation of the circumstance, that conditions apparently very similar, and which from a pathologico-anatomical point of view might be declared to be identical, in a clinical point of view lie widely apart, and that the same forms of changes are met with in analogous parts, without, however the whole process, to which they belong, being the same. When a muscle falls into a state of simple fatty degeneration, its primitive muscular fasciculi may have just the same appearance as if inflammation or permanent tension had acted upon it. Myocarditis generates forms of fatty degeneration in the substance of the heart altogether analogous to those due to excessive dilatation of the cardiac cavities. When one of these, for example, either through some obstruction to the current of the blood, or from insufficiency of the valves, is permanently much dilated, fatty degeneration of the muscular tissue constantly manifests itself in the part which has been most stretched. This form, morphologically speaking, completely resembles the early stages of myocarditis, and in many cases it is utterly impossible to say with certainty in what way the process may have arisen.

I have, in order to clear up to some extent these difficulties, as they are presented by an important, frequent and at the same time much misunderstood process, prepared a series of specimens exhibiting *really atheromatous conditions of the arteries*. For it is particularly in the case of these conditions that the confusion, which has prevailed with regard to the interpretation of the change, has perhaps been the greatest.

At no period in the course of this century has a complete understanding ever been come to as to what was to be understood by the expression atheromatous change in a vessel.   Some have taken the term in a wider, others in a narrower sense, but still it has perhaps been taken in too wide a sense by all.   When, namely, the anatomists of the last century applied the name of atheroma to. a definite change in the coats of arteries, they of course had in their minds a condition similar to that of the skin, to which ever since the days of ancient Greece, the name of atheroma, grit-follicle, (Grützbalg) [sebaceous or epidermic cyst], had been assigned.   It is self-evident, therefore, that the idea of atheroma presupposes a closed sack.   Nobody ever called anything in the skin an atheroma that lay open and uncovered.   It was therefore a curious misapprehension when people recently began to call changes in the vessels atheromata, which were not seated below the surface and shut off from the surrounding parts, but belonged to the surface.   Thus it has come to pass that, instead of an enclosed deposit being, in accordance with the original meaning of the term, called atheromatous, a change has frequently been so termed which commences quite at the surface of the internal arterial coat.   When the matter began to be examined more minutely, and fatty particles (Fig. 113) were found at very different points in the walls of the vessels, both when atheroma was, and was not, present—when at last the conviction was obtained, that the process of fatty degeneration was always the same and was identical with the atheromatous change, it became the custom to unite all the forms of the fatty degeneration of arteries under the designation atheroma.   Gradually, people even came to speak of an atheromatous change in vessels, that only possessed a single coat, for in them too we meet with fatty processes.

At all times there have moreover been observers who

regarded the ossification of vessels as a change belonging
to the same category as atheroma.   Haller and Crell believed that the ossification proceeded from the atheromatous matter, and that this was a juice which, like that
exuding under the periosteum of bone, was capable of
generating plates of bone out of itself.   Afterwards it
was recognized that atheromasia and ossification were two
parallel processes, which, however, might be referred to
a common origin.   Now it would, I think, have been
logical, if in the next place an understanding had been
come to as to what this origin was, from which the atheromatous change and the ossification proceeded.   But,
instead of this, the track of fatty degeneration was pursued, and thus the atheromatous process was extended
to a number of vessels, in which, on account of the thinness and the simple structure of their walls, the formation of any dépôt, which could really be compared to an
atheromatous cyst of the skin, was altogether impossible.

The state of the matter here also is more or less very
simply this, that two processes must be distinguished in
the vessels, which are very analogous in their ultimate
results ; first, the *simple fatty metamorphosis*, which sets
in without any discoverable preliminary stage, and in
which the existing histological elements pass directly into
a state of fatty degeneration and are destroyed, so that a
larger or smaller proportion of the constituents of the
walls of the vessel perishes ; and, in the next place, a
second series of changes, in which we can distinguish *a
stage of irritation* preceding the fatty metamorphosis,
comparable to the stage of swelling, cloudiness, and enlargement which we see in other inflamed parts.   I have
therefore felt no hesitation in siding with the old view in
this matter, and in admitting an inflammation of the inner arterial coat to be the starting point of the so-called
atheromatous degeneration ; and I have moreover en-

deavoured to show that this kind of inflammatory affection of the arterial coat, is in point of fact exactly the same as what is universally termed endocarditis, when it occurs in the parietes of the heart. There is no other difference between the two processes than that the one more frequently runs an acute, the other a chronic, course.

By the establishment of this distinction between the different processes which occur in the arteries, the difference of the course they pursue is at once accounted for. Last time I laid an artery before you, on the inner surface of which you saw little whitish patches, which were due to simple fatty transformation. To-day you see very extensive patches in the aorta, in which the atheromatous change has taken place. But, as is wont to be the case in changes of this kind, in addition to the specific transformation attendant upon the chronic inflammatory processes going on in the deeper parts, you find on the surface also a simply fatty change, so that we have the two processes occurring together. If now we examine atheromasia a little more minutely, for example in the aorta, where the process is the most common, the first thing we see present itself at the spot where the irritation has taken place, is a swelling of larger or smaller size and not unfrequently so large as to form a really hump-like projection (Buckel) above the level of the internal surface. These projections are distinguished from the neighbouring parts by their translucent, cornea-like appearance. In their deeper parts they look more opaque. When the change has lasted for a certain time, the first further metamorphoses do not show themselves at the surface, but just where the internal comes into contact with the middle coat as has been very well described by the old writers. How often have they distinctly contended that the internal coat could be stripped off over the affected spot!

Hence arose the description of Haller, that the pultaceous, atheromatous mass lay in a close cavity, as it were
a little cystic tumour between the internal and middle
coat. The only mistake was, that the tumour was regarded as a distinct body separable from the coats of the
vessels. It is rather the internal coat itself which without
any well defined limits passes into a state of degeneration
within the prominent spot. The farther this degeneration
advances, the more distinctly does an enclosed collection arise out of the destruction of the deepest layers of
the internal coat ; and at last it may be that the swelling
fluctuates, and that upon cutting into it the pultaceous
matter is evacuated, like the pus, when an abscess is cut
into. Now if the mass be examined which is present at

FIG. 116.

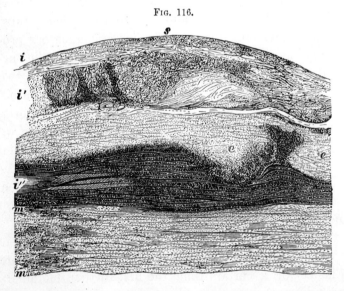

Fig. 116. Vertical section through the walls of the aorta at a sclerotic part in
which atheromatous matter is already in the course of formation. *m m'*. Middle
coat, *i i' i''*, internal coat. At *s* the highest point of the sclerotic part where it projects into the cavity of the vessel, *i* the innermost layer of the internal coat running
over the whole dépôt, *i'* the proliferating, sclerosing layer, preparing for fatty degeneration, *i''* the layer immediately adjoining the middle coat which has already undergone fatty degeneration, and at *e, e,* is in process of direct softening.

the close of this process, numerous plates of cholestearine are seen, which display themselves even to the naked
eye as glistening lamellæ ; large rhombic tablets, which
lie together in large numbers, side by side, or covering
one another, and altogether produce a glittering reflection. In addition to these plates, we find under the
microscope black-looking granule-globules, in which the
individual fat-granules are at first very minute. These
globules are often present in
very large quantity ; some of
them are seen, breaking up,
and falling to pieces, particles of them swimming about,
as in milk. Besides these
there are amorphous frag-
ments of tissue of larger or
smaller size which still cohere,
and are rather due to the softening of the rest of the substance of the tissue which has
not undergone fatty degeneration ; and in them heaps
of granules are here and there imbedded. *It is these
three constituents together, the cholestearine, the granule-
cells and fat-granules, and finally the large lumps of half-
softened substance, which give the atheromatous matter its
pultaceous character*, and really produce a certain degree
of resemblance to the contents of a pultaceous [sebace-
ous, epidermic] cyst (Grützbeutel) of the skin. With
regard to the cholestearine, it is by no means a specific
product, appertaining to this kind of fatty transforma-

FIG. 117.

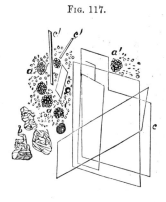

Fig. 117. The pultaceous atheromatous matter from a patch in the aorta. *a a'*. Fluid
fat, the product of the fatty metamorphosis of the cells of the internal coat (*a*),
which become transformed into granule-globules (*a' a'*), then disintegrate and set
free large and small drops of oil (fatty débris). *b*. Amorphous, granularly-wrinkled
flakes of tissue softened and swollen by imbibition. *c*, *c'*. Crystals of cholestearine ; *c* large rhombic plates ; *c*, *c'* fine rhombic needles. 300 diameters.

tion alone. On the contrary, we see in every case,
where fatty products remain stagnant for a considerable
time within a closed cavity in which but little interchange of matter can go on, that the fat sets free cholestearine. All the masses of fat which we meet with
in the body contain a certain quantity of cholestearine
in combination. As to whether the cholestearine which
is set free had already previously existed, or whether a
real new formation of it takes place in the parts, not
a word can as yet be said, inasmuch as no chemical
fact has, it is well known, been made out, which throws
any light upon the manner in which the formation of
cholestearine is effected, or upon the substances, out of
which cholestearine may be formed. This much, however, we must hold fast, that cholestearine is a product
set free at a late period from stagnating, and, particularly,
from fatty matters.

I may take this opportunity to mention the reaction
of cholestearine with iodine and sulphuric acid, which
has recently become important, and is similar to that
which we have already (p. 31) considered when speaking of the cellulose of plants. When, namely, iodine
alone is added to cholestearine, no change is seen any
more than in cellulose, under similar circumstances ;
but when, on the other hand, sulphuric acid is applied
to the iodized mass of cholestearine, its plates become
coloured and assume, particularly at first, a brilliant
indigo-blue tint, which gradually passes into a yellowish
brown, until the cholestearine is converted into a brownish drop. Sulphuric acid alone produces a fatty-looking
substance which is neither cholestearine, nor any special
combination of cholestearine and sulphuric acid, but a
product of the decomposition of the former. Sulphuric
acid alone also produces very beautiful phenomena of
colour with cholestearine.

If now, gentlemen, we trace the development of the atheromatous condition a little further back, we come—anteriorly to the period when the pultaceous matter is found in the seat of the atheroma—across a stage, where nothing more is found than fatty degeneration in its ordinary form of granule-cells, and we distinctly convince ourselves, that the process in this stage absolutely differs in no respect from that which in the case of the heart and kidney we have just declared to constitute the stage of fatty metamorphosis. At this period, immediately before the formation of the dépôt, the state of matters, as seen with a high power, is about as follows. On making a section we see the fatty cells which are interspersed through the tissue becoming larger towards the middle and lying more closely together, but gene-

FIG. 118.

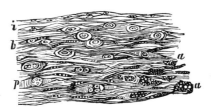

rally bearing the form of cells; but, as we proceed from within outwards they become smaller and less numerous. All these cells are filled with small, fatty granules which strongly reflect the light. Hereby is produced what looks to the eye in a section like a whitish spot. Between these fatty corpuscles runs a meshed

Fig. 118. Vertical section from a sclerotic plate in the aorta (internal coat, inner surface) in process of fatty degeneration; *i*, the innermost part of the coat with round nuclei, isolated, and in groups of several (divided). *h.* The layer of enlarging cells; networks are seen with spindle-shaped cells which enclose sections of cells resembling those of cartilage. *p.* Proliferating layer; division of the nuclei and cells. *a*, *a'.* The layer which is becoming atheromatous; *a*, the commencement of the process, *a'*, the advanced stage of fatty degeneration. 300 diameters.

basis-substance, the really fibrous stroma of the internal
coat, which we plainly see continued towards the exterior into the normal internal coat. This fact, that we
are able to acquire the direct conviction that the fibrous
layer which lies over the dépôt, is continued into the
fibrous layer of the neighbouring normal portions of the
internal coat, is one of especial value in the interpretation
of these processes. In this manner the view which was
for a considerable time defended by Rokitansky also,
that the affection consists in a deposit *upon* the internal
coat, is refuted. In a vertical section it is distinctly
seen that the most external layers run in a curve over
the whole swelling and return into the internal coat, and
the old writers were quite right when they said—speaking of a stage in which the formation of the atheromatous dépôt had already made considerable progress—
that the internal coat over the whole of the dépôt could
be stripped off in a piece. On the other hand, however,
we can convince ourselves, that the inferior layers of
the internal coat run directly into the dépôt, and that
their continuity has been broken by their degeneration,
so that we have not to deal either with an interjacent
deposit (between the internal and middle coat), as the
old writers supposed, but the whole of what we have
before us is degenerated internal coat.

In some particularly violent cases the softening manifests itself even in the arteries not as the consequence
of a really fatty process, but as a direct product of
ınflammation. Whilst at the circumference a fatty
softening takes place, in the centre of the seat of change
a yellowish cloudy appearance is seen to arise, where-
upon the substance almost immediately softens and dis-
integrates, and a mass of coarse, crumbling fragments is
found (Fig. 116, *e, e*) which fills the centre of the atheromatous dépôt.

In the last place, it is a question where the seat of
the fatty degeneration really is. Here too again (as in
the cornea) it may be imagined that the fat is deposited in
spaces intervening between the lamellæ ; and even now
there are still a small number of histologists who will
not admit, that connective tissue contains only cells,
and no empty spaces. But if a section through one of
these (atheromatous) patches be examined from below
upwards, it is seen that the same structure which presents itself in the fatty parts, shows itself also in the
merely horny or half cartilaginous layers. Bands of
fibres, in the intersections of which small lenticular
cavities appear, are found there as they are also in the
normal condition of the internal coat ; but in the cavities
and in the bands of fibres lie cellular elements (Fig.
118). The enlargement which the part undergoes in
consequence of the process and which we call sclerosis,
depends upon this ; the cellular elements of the coat
increase in size and a multiplication of their nuclei
takes place, so that spaces are not unfrequently found
in which whole heaps of nuclei are lying. This is the
mode in which the process sets in. In many cases
division occurs in the cells, and a great number of
young cells are met with. These afterwards become the
seat of the fatty degeneration (Fig. 118, *a, a'*), and then
really perish. Thus we have here an active process,
which really produces new tissues, but then hurries on
to destruction in consequence of its own development.
But one who knows that the fatty degeneration is here
only a termination, and that the process is really a
formative one, inasmuch as it begins with a proliferation
—he can readily imagine the possibility of another termination, namely *ossification*. For here we have really
to do with an ossification, and not merely, as has recently been maintained, with a mere calcification ; the

plates, which pervade the inner wall of the vessel, are
real plates of bone. Since they form out of the same
sclerotic substance from which in other cases the fatty
mass arises, and since a real tissue can only arise out of
a pre-existing one, it follows of course that, when the
process terminates in fatty metamorphosis, we cannot
assume this to consist in a simple dissemination of fatty
particles which has taken place in whatever interspaces
we like to fix upon.

The essential difference which exists in a large vessel,
as for example, the aorta, between this process [athe-
roma] and simple fatty degeneration is therefore this,
that in the latter a very slight swelling arises on the
surface of the internal coat, a swelling, which at once
disappears if the superficial layers be removed by a
horizontal section, and beneath which there still remains
a portion of the coat unaltered. In the other case, on
the contrary, we have in the extreme stage a dépôt
which lies deep beneath the comparatively normal surface, afterwards bursts, discharges its contents and forms
the *atheromatous ulcer*. This commences as a small hole
in the internal coat, through which the thick, viscous
contents of the atheromatous dépôt are squeezed out
on to the surface in the form of a plug; gradually
more and more of these contents is evacuated and
carried away by the stream of blood, until at last there
remains a larger or smaller ulcer which may extend as
far as the middle coat, and indeed not unfrequently
involves it. We have therefore always to deal with
serious disease of the vessel leading to just as destructive results, as we see in the course of other violent
inflammatory processes. You need only apply these
observations to the history of *endocarditis*, and you will
have a correct notion of all that goes on there also.

In the valves of the heart also we find simple fatty

degeneration taking place both at the surface and deep beneath it. The process generally pursues its course so latently that no disturbance is perceptible during life, nor are we able, in the present state of our knowledge, to name any very obvious anatomical change as being the subsequent result of it. On the other hand, what we call endocarditis, what can be demonstrated to arise in the course of rheumatism, and may indubitably appear as a sort of equivalent to the rheumatism of the peripheral parts, begins with a swelling of the deceased spot *itself*. There is, namely, no exudation, but the cellular elements take up a greater quantity of material, and the spot becomes uneven and rugged. Then we see, when the process runs its course somewhat slowly,

FIG. 119

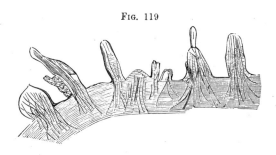

either that an excrescence, a condyloma arises, or that the swelling assumes a more mammillated form, and afterwards becomes the seat of a calcification which may produce real bone. If the process runs a more acute course, the result is either fatty degeneration or softening. The latter gives rise to the ulcerative forms, in which the valves crumble to pieces, drop off, and em-

Fig. 119. Condylomatous excrescences of the mitral valve; simple, granular swellings (granulations) and larger prominences (vegetations), some villous, others branched and putting forth secondary buds; in all elastic fibres running upwards. 70 diameters.

bolical deposits are produced in remote parts (Fig. 73, p. 242).*

Only in this manner, by observing, namely, the earliest stages of the changes, is it possible to form certain and practically useful opinions with regard to pathological processes. Never ought one, basing one's opinion upon the difference of the processes in a clinical point of view, to allow oneself to be induced to regard their ultimate products as necessarily different. The most violent inflammatory processes which run their course in quite a short time, may have the same terminations as those which, in other cases, are brought about more slowly.

It is not my intention to go through the series of the different passive disturbances which may possibly arise in the later stages of irritative conditions, in detail. Else we should be able to discover analogous instances in the history of nearly all degenerative atrophies. In all cases we must discriminate between the conditions in which a part becomes directly the seat of such a retrograde metamorphosis, and those in which it previously underwent an active change.

The description which I have given you of the fatty processes directly applies to the class of *calcifications.* If it be wished to discriminate between ossification and calcification, it is not sufficient to keep the ultimate result in one's eye. A part does not become true bone,

---

* This theory of the detachment of fragments from the valves of the heart, and of the consequent secondary occlusions (embolia) was propounded by me, with illustrations from the histories of patients and the results of post-mortem examinations (Archiv f. path. Anat. und Phys. vol. I., p. 134) as far back as 1847, or five years before Dr. Kirkes, to whom the honour of this discovery is still generally ascribed in England, published his papers on the subject. My observations concerning the detachment of the thrombi in the veins were published a year earlier than this, viz., in 1846, and I then hinted at the occurrence of the same process in the arteries, although I did not give a full account of it until 1847.—*From a MS. Note by the Author.*

because it takes up lime into its intercellular substance and has stellate cells present in it; it may in spite of all this be nothing more than calcified connective tissue. When we speak of pathological ossification, we always presuppose that the mass which ossifies has been called into existence by an active process, an irritation, and not that a previously existing tissue assumes the form of bone, by absorbing calcareous salts. We have therefore calcifications and ossifications in the vessels. In ancient times everything was called ossification. Many of the more recent observers have denied that it ever does occur in vessels. Ossification does however really occur, but so does mere calcification, or, as I will briefly term it, *petrifaction*. The latter is comparatively more frequent in the peripheral arteries, so that the condition which is generally regarded as a special criterion of the atheromatous process and in which the radial artery is felt to be hard and calcareous, and the femoral or popliteal is perceived to have hard and rigid walls, is no proof at all that the process is an atheromatous one. Very frequently this induration has its seat in the middle coat. In this case the calcification really invades the muscular elements, so that the fibre-cells of the circular-fibre coat are transformed into calcareous spindle-shaped bodies. The calcareous matter may in these cases also invade the neighbouring parts, but the internal coat may possibly remain quite unaltered. This is a process therefore, which differs more from what is termed the atheromatous process than periostitis from ostitis. This species of calcification has no necessary connection whatever with an inflammation of the artery, it occurs most commonly in cases where there is a tendency to calcifications generally, and where calcareous salts are set free at other points in the economy and circulate with the juices. This much at least can with certainty be affirmed, that we are as yet acquainted with no stage in these changes, which is at all akin to inflammation.

On the contrary, we see ossification declare itself in the internal coat of vessels in precisely the same manner as when an osteophyte forms on the surface of bone amidst all the phenomena of inflammation. The osteophytes of the inner table of the skull and of the cerebral membranes follow the same course of development as the ossifying plates of the internal coat of the aorta and even of the veins. They always begin with a proliferation of the pre-existing connective tissue, whereby partial swellings are produced, in which the deposition of the calcareous salts does not take place until a late period. As soon as this real ossification exists, we cannot help regarding the process as one which has arisen out of an irritation of the parts, stimulating them to new, formative actions; so far therefore it comes under our ideas of inflammation, or at least of those processes which are extremely nearly allied to inflammation. When a process of this sort is accessible to treatment, we have always other indications for practice, than in those cases, in which our object is, by the agency of stimulating substances, to prevent the occurrence of certain passive disturbances which hinder the part from discharging its natural functions.

What I have said will suffice, I think, to make these, in my opinion, extremely important distinctions clear to you. In the next lecture I will lay before you that one among the degenerative processes which is at the present moment the least clear, namely the lardaceous or amyloid degeneration.

LECTURE XVII.

APRIL 17, 1858.

AMYLOID DEGENERATION. INFLAMMATION.

Amyloid (lardaceous or waxy) degeneration—Different nature of amyloid substances: concentric and laminated amyloid bodies (brain, prostate), and amyloid degeneration properly so-called—Its course—Commencement of the affection in the minute arteries—Waxy liver—Cartilage—Dyscrasic (constitutional)
character of the disease—Intestines—Kidneys: the three forms of Bright's
disease (amyloid degeneration, parenchymatous, and interstitial nephritis)—
Lymphatic glands—Functional disturbances of the affected organs.

Inflammation—The four cardinal symptoms and their predominance in the different
schools: the thermic and vascular theory; the neuro-pathologists, exudations
—Inflammatory stimuli—Lesion of function—Exudation as a consequence of
the activity of the tissues; mucus and fibrine—Inflammation as a complex
irritative process—Parenchymatous and exudative (secretory) form.

I WILL to-day, gentlemen, from among the changes
which must in general be rather ranked with that class
of degenerations which are attended with a diminution
of functional power, introduce to your notice one, which
has recently acquired especial interest, namely that
which has been by some called the *lardaceous* (bacony—
speckig), by others the *waxy*, whilst I have given it the
name of the *amyloid*, change. The term lardaceous
change has again come more into use chiefly through
the instrumentality of the Vienna school. You know
that the term itself is of tolerably ancient date in medicine as a denomination for a firm, compact, homogeneous

appearance of parts.   We find it has been employed for centuries, and even in recent times tumours have been termed lardaceous.   Still the term, lardaceous changes, as now used, has but very little to do with these tumours, and rather refers to things, upon which the old writers, who, I think, were better connoisseurs in bacon than our friends in Vienna, would hardly have bestowed such a name.   The appearance of such organs, namely, as in accordance with Viennese ideas, are said to look like bacon, bears, according to northern notions, a much greater resemblance to wax, and I have therefore now for a long time, like the Edinburgh school, made use of the term waxy change instead.   When we look at a liver or lymphatic gland which constitutes a well-marked specimen of this condition, what strikes the naked eye most, is the translucent, but at the same time, dull appearance which the cut-surfaces exhibit; the natural colour of the parts is also more or less lost, so that a material, at first more of a grey tint, but afterwards perfectly colourless, seems to fill the parts.   The translucent nature of the tissue allows, however, the red of the vessels and the natural hue of the neighbouring parts to glimmer through, so that the altered spots in different organs have rather a yellowish, reddish, or brownish tinge; but this is not a colour belonging to the substance deposited.

The first facts, by the help of which we were enabled to determine more accurately the nature of this substance which had previously been taken, sometimes for a peculiar fatty matter, sometimes for albumen or fibrine, sometimes, finally, for a colloid substance, were furnished by the application of iodine to animal tissues. It will now soon be five years since I first discovered the peculiar reaction of the corpora amylacea found in the nervous centres with iodine, which I have already described to you, and since I had my attention directed to the extraordinary resemblance which these bodies present to vegetable structures—a resemblance such that they have been regarded, now rather as real starch, now rather as analogous to cellulose. The next organ I came across, although there is no close resemblance in external appearance between it and the ependyma, was the spleen and indeed a condition of it, in which its follicles were wholly converted into this translucent, waxy matter (sagoey spleen—Sagomilz). Soon afterwards H. Meckel published his well-known observations which demonstrated the occurrence of this substance in several places, but especially in the kidneys, the liver and the bowels, and we afterwards succeeded in finding it in different other parts, in the lymphatic glands, throughout the whole of the digestive tract, in the mucous membranes of the urinary passages, and finally even in the substance of the muscular organs—the heart, and the uterus—as well as in the interior of cartilages—so that at the present moment there are but few parts of the body that we do not know may undergo this peculiar change.

If we investigate the matter more closely, it seems that two allied, but not identical, substances must be distinguished. In the first place we find bodies which in their chemical properties are more analogous to real vegetable starch, and in form too bear an extraordinary resemblance to vegetable starch-granules, inasmuch as they constitute more or less round, or oval structures, formed by a succession of concentric layers. To this class belong, above all, the corpora amylacea of the nervous system (Fig. 94). Many of the laminated amyloid bodies are of very large size; their diameter may become so considerable, that they may be very distinctly recognized with the naked eye. To this category be-

long, in particular, a part of the laminated bodies, that
are found in the prostate of every adult man and under
certain circumstances accumulate in large quantities, so
as to form the so-called prostatic concretions; and also
rare forms of a similar kind which have been shown by
Frederich to occur in several conditions of the lungs.

These formations vary in size from very small, simple,
homogeneous looking structures up to gigantic bodies, in
which, when they are regularly formed, we see a succession of very numerous layers.   Just as the small
amyloid corpuscles of the nervous system are frequently
composed of two separate ones and constitute twin
structures, it very frequently happens here also, that a
common envelope encloses separate centres (Fig. 120,
d, e).   Nay, in isolated cases this goes on to such an
extent, that whole heaps of smaller bodies are held
together by larger common layers.   These very large

FIG. 120.

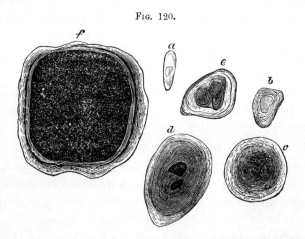

Fig. 120. Laminated prostatic amyloid bodies (concretions); *a*, oblong, pale
homogeneous corpuscle, with a nucleus-like body.   *b*. A larger, laminated corpuscle
with pale centre.   *c*. A still larger corpuscle with several layers and a coloured
centre.   *d, e*. Bodies with two and three centres, in *d* of a deeper colour.   *f*. Large
concretion with a dark-brown, large centre.   Magnified 300 diameters.

though certainly more rare, forms may attain a diameter of two lines, so that they can easily be isolated from the tissue in which they lie, and be subjected to examination even with the naked eye. There seems to be scarcely any doubt, but that in these cases a substance is set free, which gradually adheres to the outside of pre-existing bodies all round, and that therefore we have not here to deal with the degeneration of a definite tissue, but with a kind of separation and precipitation, such as we see occur in the case of other concretions from fluids. It may, with some probability be concluded, that the prostate, through the dissolution of its elements, furnishes a fluid which, by the gradual formation of deposits, produces these particular forms.

Now the peculiarity of these structures is, that by the simple action of iodine they very frequently assume just as blue a colour as vegetable starch does. According as the substance is more or less pure, its colour changes, so that when, for example, there is much albuminous matter mixed up with it, it becomes green instead of blue ; for the nitrogenous substance is rendered yellow by iodine, and the amyloid blue, so that the whole effect produced is green. The greater the quantity of nitrogenous matter, the browner does the colour become, and not unfrequently do we find, side by side in the prostate, concretions, which, after the application of the iodine, present the most varied colours. So far these formations are distinguished from those little amylaceous corpuscles of the nervous system, which, one and all, assume a blue or bluish grey colour on the addition of iodine. It must also be remarked, that many prostatic bodies, though quite analogous in their structure, only become yellow or brown upon the addition of iodine, and consequently differ in chemical constitution.

Essentially different from this separation of starch-like matter, which lies *between* the elements, are the degenerations of the tissues themselves, in which all their constituents (parenchyma and interstitial tissue), as such, become directly filled with a substance also of an amyloid nature, and are gradually infiltrated with it just as tissues become infiltrated with lime in calcification. No two things can be more justly compared than calcification and the amyloid change (lignification). This (amyloid) substance, which produces the real degeneration of the tissue, exhibits the peculiarity, that it never becomes blue under the influence of iodine alone. At least no case is as yet known, in which the substance has yielded this colour with iodine in the parenchyma of tissues. On the contrary, a peculiar yellowish red colour is seen to arise, which it is true in many cases has a slight tinge of reddish violet, so that a certain approximation is manifested to the blue of real starchy matter. On the other hand, it displays pretty regularly a real, either perfectly blue, or violet colour, when the application of iodine is followed by the very cautious addition of sulphuric acid. A certain degree of practice indeed is requisite ; the exact proportion must be hit upon, inasmuch as the sulphuric acid generally destroys the substance very quickly, and either very indistinct colorations are obtained, or the colour manifests itself only for a moment, and then immediately disappears again. Thus this substance is less nearly allied to starch properly so-called and more akin to cellulose, as I have already described it (p. 31). But from cellulose again it is also distinguished by the fact of its becoming coloured upon the application of pure solution of iodine, whilst real cellulose is not at all coloured by iodine alone. Cellulose behaves precisely like cholestearine which remains colourless when treated with iodine, but on the other hand assumes a blue, or under certain circumstances a red, or orange colour upon the addition of iodine and sulphuric acid (p. 400).

Owing to this multiplicity of reactions it is really still very difficult to say with certainty to what class the substance belongs. Meckel has followed up the idea with great care, that we have to deal with a kind of fat which is more or less identical with cholestearine ; but we are as yet unacquainted with any kind of fat which combines in itself the three qualities of becoming coloured upon the addition of iodine alone, of remaining colourless upon the addition of sulphuric acid alone, and of assuming a blue colour when acted upon by iodine and sulphuric acid. Besides the substance itself does not in any way behave like a fatty matter ; it does not possess the solubility which characterizes fat ; and in particular no substance can be obtained from these parts by extraction with alcohol and ether, which possesses the peculiarities of the original one. According to all this there is rather a correspondence with vegetable forms, and the view may still be maintained, that we have here to deal with a process comparable to that which we see set in during the development of a plant, when the simple cell becomes invested with capsular layers, and gradually grows woody.*

---

* The analyses of amyloid spleens recently made by Kekule and Carl Schmidt have yielded such a large proportion of Nitrogen, that both these chemists have come to the conclusion that the amyloid substance is of an albuminous nature. We know, however, from experience, that the results furnished by these analyses of whole organs are very little to be depended upon, so little indeed, that no chemist was ever able to infer from any analyses he had made of the liver, that it was rich in Glycogen. Only when we have discovered the means of isolating the amyloid substance, shall we be able to come to any definite conclusion with regard to its nature.

To Schmidt's analyses of the corpora amylacea of the brain we cannot attach the slightest importance, because his statements concerning them were founded upon an error. He says, namely, he selected for his analyses a choroid plexus (from a human brain) rich in corpora amylacea. But corpora amylacea are never found in

These changes can be best followed in those structures which must on the whole be regarded as the most frequent and the earliest seat of this change, namely the *smallest arteries*. These first undergo the transformation, and only after the constitution of their walls has become changed, is the infiltration wont to extend to the surrounding parenchyma, until at last the whole district of tissue to which the artery leads has experienced the change. If in an amyloid spleen we trace one of these small arteries, whilst it breaks up into so-called penicillus, we see how its wall, in itself already a thick one, becomes thicker in proportion as the change advances, and how at the same time the calibre of the vessel becomes con-

Fig. 121.

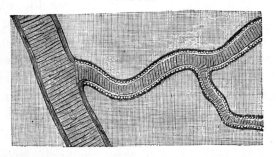

siderably diminished. This accounts for the circumstance, that all organs which experience the amyloid change in a considerable degree, look extremely pale ; an

Fig. 121. Amyloid degeneration of a small artery from the submucous tissue of the intestine, with its trunk still intact. 300 diameters.

large numbers in these plexuses—indeed it seems to me doubtful whether they are ever *formed* there. The concentric corpuscles which Schmidt examined were therefore probably those sabulous bodies (Sandkörper—acervulus cerebri, brainsand) which are nearly always present in the choroid plexuses and so greatly resemble the corpora amylacea in structure, that they were actually taken by Remac to be such. Schmidt, thinking he had the same substance before him in the spleen, published his two analyses with the idea that he was thereby furnishing a doubly strong proof of the albuminous nature of this animal amyloid substance.—*From a MS. Note by the Author.*

ischæmia of the parts is produced by the obstruction which the narrowed vessels oppose to the influx of blood. If now we examine in which of the histological elements of the vessels the substance is first found, it seems to be pretty constantly seated in the little muscles of the circular-fibre coat.   First of all the place of every fibre-cell is occupied by a compact, homogeneous body, in which the centre of the nucleus at first still appears as a hole, but gradually every trace of a cellular structure is lost, so that at last a kind of spindle-shaped flake (Scholle) remains, in which neither membrane, nucleus nor contents can be distinguished.   In the calcification of small arteries exactly the same process takes place ; the individual fibre-cells of the middle coat take up calcareous salts, at first in a granular, afterwards in a homogeneous form, until they are at last transformed into homogeneous-looking calcareous bodies, of a spindle-shaped form, which coalesce and produce plates of a considerable size.   In like manner the amyloid substance pervades whole tracts of tissue, and the walls of the artery are transformed into a mass at last nearly completely homogeneous, compact, shining with reflected light and colourless, which not only does not possess the hardness of calcified parts, but on the contrary exhibits a high degree of friability.

Now when a change of this nature has advanced to a certain height, an analogous change takes place also in the parenchyma of the organs.   This can nowhere be so distinctly traced as in the *liver*.   Here it sometimes happens, that we meet with stages, where nothing else in the whole organ is altered, excepting the minute branches of the hepatic artery.   On making fine sections through the liver, carefully washing them and applying iodine, we sometimes see, even with the naked eye, the small iodine-red lines and points which correspond to the cut branches of the hepatic artery.   In a later

stage, however, it is essentially the hepatic cells which
are affected by the change ; and indeed, what is again
very characteristic, just those hepatic cells, between
which lie the capillary ramifications of the hepatic artery. If namely we picture to ourselves a single acinus
of the liver, we can, in accordance with the pathological changes which may often be recognized even with
the naked eye, distinguish three different zones within
each acinus (Fig. 110). The most external part, which
lies next to the branches of the portal vein, is the chief
seat of fatty infiltration ; the intermediate part, which receives the capillary terminations of the hepatic artery,
belongs to the amyloid degeneration, and the central
part of the acinus around the vena hepatica is the most
common seat of pigmentary infiltration. Even with
the naked eye the pale colourless, translucent and resistant zone of the waxy or amyloid change is sometimes
recognized between the most external yellowish white,
and the most internal yellowish, or greyish brown, layer.

If a single hepatic cell be watched, its previous granular contents, which give every hepatic cell a slightly
cloudy appearance, are seen gradually to become homogeneous ; the nucleus and cell-wall gradually disappear,
and at last a stage sets in in which nothing more can
be perceived than an absolutely homogeneous, slightly
shining body, if you will, a simple flake (Scholle). In
this manner the whole of the hepatic cells in the zone
I have described are sometimes converted into amyloid
flakes, and if the process attains a very high pitch, the
change at last even oversteps this zone, and it may happen, that nearly the whole substance of the acinus is
transformed into an amyloid mass. Thus out of the
hepatic cells there is at last produced in these cases a
kind of corpora amylacea, only they are not laminated
like those we have already spoken of, but form uniform,

homogeneous bodies, in which no internal division, no indication of the peculiar course of their formation can be recognized.

If we take all these facts together, it appears pretty probable, that we have here to deal with a gradual infiltration of the parts with a substance which has been conveyed to them from without. This is a view which derives essential support from the fact, that nearly always when this change declares itself, a considerable number of organs are affected, and that the process is not confined to a single spot, but that many places in the body are simultaneously affected. Hereby the whole process really acquires an essentially dyscrasic appearance. The only place, where, until now at least, an entirely independent development of this change has been observed by me, and where it may therefore with some degree of probability be assumed that the formation is autochthonous and not imported from without, is *permanent cartilage*. The cartilages, particularly in people somewhat advanced in life, assume in various places—as for example, the sterno-clavicular articulations, the symphyses of the pelvis, and the intervertebral cartilages—a peculiarly pale-yellowish hue, and then we may be tolerably certain, that if we try the iodine test with them, we shall obtain the peculiar coloration. These colours are not seen so much in the cartilage-cells as in the intercellular substance, and as cases of the sort do not occur simultaneously with amyloid degeneration of large internal organs, but quite independently, in individuals, who in the rest of their body manifest nothing of the kind—it seems that we really have here to deal with a direct transformation, and not with any importation from without.

But in vain have I hitherto endeavoured to detect any definite change in the blood, from which the inference

might be drawn, that this was really the source of the
deposits. There exists as yet but one single observation, that points to the presence of analogous bodies in
the blood, and this is so strange an one, that we can
scarcely attempt to ground an explanation of the process upon it. A physician of Toronto in Canada had
namely, in compliance with the wish of a patient suffering from epilepsy, examined his blood and discovered in
it peculiar, pale bodies. When then he read of my observations with regard to the coloration of the corpora
amylacea of the brain by iodine, his patient recurred to
his mind, and, I think after the lapse of five years, he
again took blood from him, and again found the bodies,
which are really said to have exhibited the reaction.
In opposition to this observation, it is strange that
nobody else has ever seen anything of the kind, and
as an extremely persistent dyscrasia must here have
been in operation, we should scarcely be justified in
drawing conclusions from this observation, with regard
to the cases we are considering, where the disease attains its height in a much shorter time, and we have in
the blood at least been able to detect nothing of the
kind. Moreover great doubts must be entertained with
respect to the accuracy of the observation. Starch-
granules may very easily find their way into different
microscopical objects, so that (with all due respect for
the observer) as long as matter turns upon a solitary
observation, it must be admitted to be possible that
there was perhaps an error.* I am as yet much more
inclined to admit, that the blood in this disease under-

---

* Dr. Carter of Edinburgh, and after him, M. Luys of Paris, fell into a similar
error, when they imagined they were in a condition to prove that an excretion of
starch took place through the skin. M. Rouget (Journal de Physiologie par
Brown-Séquard, Tom. ii., p. 85) has shown that this starch is derived from external
sources, from articles of food, and that its presence upon the skin therefore is
merely accidental.—*From a MS. Note by the Author.*

goes a chemical alteration in its fluid constituents, than that it contains the pathological substances in a material form.

At all events it is unquestionable, that the amyloid change even now holds a very high place among pathological processes. The inevitable result of the affection is, that the parts which are the seat of it, become totally incapable of discharging their special functions ; that, for example, gland cells which are changed in this manner, are no longer in a condition to perform their special glandular functions, and that vessels can no longer subserve the nutrition of the tissues, or the secretion of the fluids, the duties they had been in the habit of performing.

These considerations afford a ready explanation of the circumstance that clinical disturbances so regularly concur with these anatomical ones. We find, on the one hand, well-marked conditions of cachexia, and on the other, with extreme frequency, dropsy with the whole complex group of changes, which are usually included in the idea we form of Bright's disease. In nearly every instance, in which the amyloid affection reaches an advanced stage, the patients are in a state of great marasmus. There are cases where the whole extent of the digestive tract from the buccal cavity to the anus does not contain a single minute artery, which is not affected with this disease, and wherein every part of the œsophagus, stomach, small and large intestines, the small arteries of its mucous membrane are found changed in this way.

Now this state of things is very apt to escape observation, because this kind of metamorphosis, which exercises such a decided influence upon the functions of the intestines (causing deficiency of absorption, and tendency to diarrhœa), produces scarcely any effect perceptible to the naked eye. The intestines are pale and

have a grey, translucent, sometimes slightly wax-like
appearance ; but this, however, is so little characteristic,
that no inference can with certainty be drawn from it
with regard to the internal changes, and the only possibility of determining the point, when one has no microscope at hand, consists in the direct application of the
test.   One need only brush a little iodine upon the
surface, and a number of densely aggregated, yellow-
ish- or brownish-red spots are soon seen to start up,
whilst the interjacent mucous membrane merely looks
yellow.   These red points are the villi of the intestine,
and if one of them be placed under the microscope, the
walls of the small arteries and even of the capillaries,
which ramify in them, and sometimes also the parenchyma, are seen to be coloured iodine-red.

The most important disturbances of this kind with
which we are as yet acquainted, are those which arise in
the kidney.   A large proportion of the cases of Bright's
disease, especially of the chronic ones, are assignable to
this change, and must therefore be separated from many
other similar forms as constituting a special, altogether
peculiar affection.   Kidneys affected in this way were
called in Vienna, at a time when the chemical reaction
was not yet known, lardaceous kidneys (Specknieren).
I must however again remark that it is impossible to
distinguish immediately with the naked eye, whether
this particular change has taken place or not, and that a
part of the so-called lardaceous kidneys exhibit nothing
more than a kind of induration.   Not until iodine has
been employed can a diagnosis be readily made.   If a
solution of iodine be applied to a quite anæmic cortex,
a number of red points usually first appear which correspond to the glomeruli, and sometines fine streaks also,
which are the afferent arteries ; and next to this, when
the disease is very severe, red parallel lines are also

seen within the medullary cones, lying very close to one another. These are all arteries. The affection of the arteries becomes sometimes so severe, that, after the application of the test, a clear view of the whole course of the vessels is obtained, as if one had a very complete artificial injection before one. But in these very kidneys an injection is hardly practicable. Even the finer materials which we employ as injections, are much too coarse to be able to pass through the narrowed vessels. Upon examining one of these glomeruli microscopically, we see that from the point, where the afferent artery breaks up, the loops are no longer the fine, delicate tubes that they formerly were ; on the contrary they appear compact and nearly solid. Now as these are just the parts which manifestly constitute the real points at which the secretion of the fluid portion of the urine is effected, we can easily conceive that in such cases disturbances in the secretion of urine must arise. Unfortunately we have as yet no completely satisfactory analyses, but it seems that many cases of albuminuria, which are attended with a considerable diminution in the secretion of urea, are connected with these very conditions, and that the excretion becomes more and more scanty in proportion as the disease increases in intensity.* These cases are very frequently complicated

---

* This is what we might expect to take place, wherever we suppose the urea to be secreted. If it is secreted by the epithelium, the epithelium must take it up out of the blood which circulates in the intertubular capillaries. But if the glomeruli only allow a small quantity of blood to pass through them, a small quantity only finds its way into these capillaries, and so but little urea can be taken up and excreted. In those cases in which there is an abundant flow of *watery* urine, the water is chiefly derived from the vessels of the medullary substance, in consequence of the increased (collateral) pressure upon them. Thus the amyloid degeneration of the Malpighian bodies and their afferent arteries has much less influence upon the excretion of water, than upon that of urea. The peculiar views first put forward by the Author concerning the circulation in the medullary substance of the kidney, and the common origin (from the same branches of the renal artery) of the arteriæ rectæ of the medullary cones (pyramids), and of the

with anasarca and with dropsy of the different cavities, and may exhibit in the completest manner all the symptoms of Bright's disease. They differ however essentially from the simply inflammatory form of Bright's disease, which I designate *parenchymatous nephritis*, in this respect, that in the latter the disease has not so much its seat in the glomeruli or the arteries, as in the epithelium of the kidney, and that the change is often for a long time confined to the epithelium, whilst the glomeruli themselves may in such cases still appear unchanged when there is scarcely any epithelium remaining in the substance of the cortex. From these forms a third again must be distinguished, where the *interstitial tissue* is predominantly affected, where thickenings take place around the capsules and uriniferous tubules, constrictions and contractions are effected, and thereby mechanical obstructions to the current of the blood are produced, which must naturally be attended by secretory changes.

It is very important that you should discriminate between these different varieties which exist in what is apparently a single disease, because you will hence see how it is that the facts which have been ascertained concerning the one class cannot forthwith be applied to the other classes, and that neither the same physiological inferences nor the same therapeutical maxims are equally applicable in every one of these several conditions. At the same time, however, it must not be overlooked that these three different forms by no means always appear

---

afferent arteries of the cortex, whereby, in the case of a diminished flow of blood through the latter set of vessels, an increased circulation takes place through the former—will be found in his Archiv. f. path. Anat. und Phys. vol. xii., p. 310, and investigations confirmatory of them have recently been published by Dr. Beale (Arch. of Med., 1859, No. IV., p. 300. According to those (*e. g.*, Bowman) who make all the arterial blood pass through the glomeruli, no such collateral relationship could exist between the cortex and medulla.—*From a MS. Note by the Author.*

unmixed, but that on the contrary frequently two, and sometimes all three, of them exist simultaneously in the same kidney.

Amongst the other preparations which I place before you I have, especially on account of its distinctness, chosen the amyloid disease of the *lymphatic glands*. In these the state of things is much the same as in the spleen. We see on the one hand the small arteries, on the other the essential substance of the glands (*i. e.*, the mass of minute cells which fill the follicles), undergoing the change. You will remember from a previous occasion (p. 208, Fig. 61), that there are follicles lying beneath the proper capsule of the gland, and that these follicles are made up of a

FIG. 122.

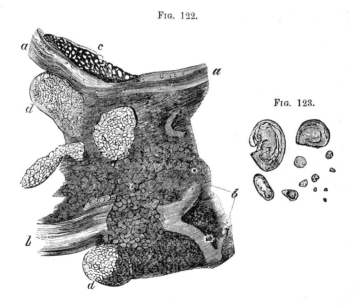

FIG. 123.

Fig. 122.   Amyloid degeneration of a lymphatic gland, from a drawing made by Dr. Fripp of Bristol. *a, b, b.* Vessels with greatly thickened, shining, infiltrated walls. *c.* A layer of fat-cells at the circumference of the gland. *d, d.* Follicles with their delicate reticulum and corpora amylacea.   200 diameters.   Compare Würzburger Verhandlungen, Vol. VII, Plate III.

Fig. 123.   Isolated corpora amylacea of different sizes, some of them ruptured, from the gland represented in Fig. 122.   350 diameters.

delicate network, in which the small cells of the gland are heaped up, cells, which seem to have a double duty to perform, inasmuch as they discharge their own special functions as gland-cells, and at the same time, as we suppose, serve as the starting-points for the development of blood-corpuscles. The arteries run first in the interstices of the follicles, and there break up into capillaries which form a web round the follicles, and sometimes even penetrate into their interior. Now the amyloid disease consists on the one hand in a thickening and narrowing of these arteries, so that they convey less blood, and on the other hand in the conversion of the small cells contained in the individual meshes of the follicles into corpora amylacea, so that afterwards instead of a number of cells in every mesh of the follicle, a single large corpus amylaceum is met with. Thereby the gland acquires even to the naked eye the appearance as if it were sprinkled all over with little spots of wax, and when examined microscopically, it looks as if the contents of the follicles were a pavement of closely set stones.

Concerning the importance of these changes, empirically not much can be affirmed; but, if the contents of the follicles are the essential components of a lymphatic gland, and if from them proceeds the development of the new constituents of the blood, we must, I think, conclude, that this disease of the lymphatic glands and the spleen (in which the follicles are likewise generally affected), must exercise a directly injurious influence upon the formation of the blood; and that the effects therefore produced by the disease are not remote ones, but that the formation of the blood immediately suffers an alteration, so that anæmic conditions must ensue. To the stream of lymph also an obstruction may arise, and in this way again deficiency of absorption, tendency to dropsy, etc., be produced.

If we apply iodine to sections of such glands as these, all the diseased parts become coloured red, whilst every part that retains its normal structure merely becomes yellow. The capsule, which consists of connective tissue, the fibrous trabeculæ between the follicles, the delicate intrafollicular network which separates the different corpora amylacea, and lastly those follicles which contain normal cells, remain yellow. All the other parts assume the iodine-red hue. If we add sulphuric acid, these parts become of a dark reddish brown, or violet red—or if one hits the mark, pure blue ; but if there are still nitrogenous particles present, the colour becomes green or brownish red.

Now, gentlemen, that we have established the classification of morbid disturbances generally according to the difference of action in the tissues, I think of treating more in detail of the process, which the practical physician, according to the ordinary mode of speaking, most frequently meets with, namely *inflammation*.

Our notions of inflammation have undergone an essential change in consequence of the observations, of which you have now heard a certain part. Whilst until quite recently it was the custom to look upon inflammation as a real entity, as a process everywhere identical *in its essence*, after I made my investigations no alternative remained, but to divest the notion of inflammation of all that was ontological in it, and no longer to look upon the process as one differing in its essence from other pathological processes, but only to regard it as one differing *in its form and course*.

In the descriptions given of inflammation by the old writers—as preserved to us in the dogmatical writings of Galen—among the four cardinal symptoms (calor, rubor, tumor, dolor) heat is, as is well known, the most promi nent, for it is the symptom from which the process has acquired its name. Afterwards, in proportion as the question of animal heat in general, and of heat in patho-logical conditions in particular, withdrew into the back-ground, great importance was attached to the redness, and thus it happened that even in the last century, at the time when mechanical theories were in vogue, when especially Boerhaave considered inflammation to consist in an obstruction of the vessels, and in the stasis of the blood consequent upon it, the notion of inflammation was more or less grounded upon supposed conditions of the vessels. After the facts of pathological anatomy had extended their compass, hyperæmia was, especially in France, declared to be the necessary and regular starting point of inflammation. The exclusiveness, with which this view has been maintained even up to our own times, was in a great measure an after-effect of Broussais' views which became the prevailing ones in consequence of the development of the pathologico-anatomical school. Hy-peræmia gradually superseded all the other essential symptoms.

A change in the doctrine on a grand scale has really only been attempted by the Vienna school, for they too, like the French school, grounding their system of patho-logy upon pathological anatomy, have put the products of inflammation in the place of the symptoms of inflam-mation. What, basing their opinion upon their own experience, they especially had in view, and sought to establish as the essence of inflammation, was the product, which, in accordance with traditional notions, was desig-nated as one which had necessarily proceeded from the vessels—as an exudation. In the old classification of symptoms, the swelling, corresponded pretty nearly with the exudation of the Vienna school, and it might there-fore be said that, as previously, first the heat, and then the redness, had held the first place, so now the swelling occupied the foremost rank. It is only in the more speculative views of the neuro-pathologists that the pain is, as is well known, regarded as the essential and original change in the act of inflammation.

There can be no doubt, but that of these different positions the anatomical doctrine of the Vienna school would be the most correct, if it could be demonstrated, that, as the language of most of the physicians of the present day would lead us to believe, an exudation really does take place, in every case of inflammation; that the swelling is essentially occasioned by this exudation; and especially, that this exudation ought to be regarded as a constant and typical one, and the quantity of fibrine contained in it as a criterion of its inflammatory nature.

I have already, in the previous lectures, endeavoured to show you, in what a considerably restricted sense the term exudation must be employed, and how essentially the activity of the elements of the tissues themselves is concerned in the appearance of matters, which we certainly must regard as derived from the vessels and deposited in the parts affected. A good deal is, as we have seen, not so much exudation, as, if I may so express myself, an educt from the vessels in consequence of the activity of the histological elements themselves.

Irritation must, I believe, be taken as the starting-point in the consideration of inflammation, and it is because Broussais and Andral regarded the matter in this light, that I consider the views advanced by them to be the most correct. We cannot imagine inflammation to take place without an irritating stimulus (irritament),* and the

---

* The term *irritament* (Reiz, which, however, sometimes means *irritant*, stimulus) is intended to express the change (mechanical or chemical, palpable (anatomical) or molecular) which takes place in a tissue in consequence of the action of an *irritant*—a change, therefore, which is of a *purely passive* nature (lesion), and which

first question is, what conception we are to form of such a stimulus.

We have already seen that the irritation may in general be traced to one of three different sources, according as it is a functional, nutritive or formative irritation which has taken place. Now there can be no doubt, but that functional stimuli (irritaments) do not play an essential part in inflammation, and for the simple reason, that—a point upon which all the more recent schools at least are agreed—to the four characteristic symptoms *lesion of function* (functio læsa) must be added.

If there be a disturbance of function in inflammation, this presupposes that the inflammatory stimulus (irritament) must be of such a nature as to cause changes in the composition of the part which render it less capable of performing its functions. Nobody would expect a muscle which is inflamed, to perform its functions normally; every one supposes that the contractile substance of the muscle has thereby experienced certain changes. Nobody would expect an inflamed gland-cell could secrete normally, but we should look upon the disturbance of secretion as a necessary consequence of the inflammation. Nobody could expect an inflamed ganglion-cell or nerve to discharge its functions, or normally to respond to stimuli. The conclusion, therefore,

(subsequently) provokes changes in the neighbouring parts not *directly* altered by the irritant—the consequence of which is their *action* or *reaction*. This condition, which is an *active* one, based upon the physiological powers of the parts, represents *irritation* in the proper sense of the word, and as the starting-point in every form of inflammation. See Archiv f. path. Anat. und Phys. vol. xiv., p. i. (Reizung und Reizbarkeit).

The matter will perhaps be rendered clearer by the following familiar illustration : —Suppose three people were sitting quietly on a bench, and suddenly a stone came and injured one of them, the others would be excited, not only by the sudden appearance of the stone, but also by the injury done to their companion, to whose help they would feel bound to hasten. Here the stone would be the *irritant*, the injury the *irritament*, the help an expression of the *irritation* called forth in the bystanders.—*From a MS. Note by the Author.*

that must in accordance with the commonest experience be necessarily drawn from all this is, that changes must have occurred in the composition of the cellular elements altering their natural functional power. Such changes, when they occur after the application of stimuli which are not powerful enough to destroy the parts at once, or to exhaust their functional power, are only possible when the stimuli are either nutritive or formative. And in fact this conclusion is confirmed by what occurs in inflammation. For now-a-days we find the view is already pretty generally spread, that in inflammation we have in the main to deal with a change in the act of nutrition, nutrition being here indeed regarded as embracing the formative and nutritive processes.

If therefore we speak of an inflammatory stimulus (irritament), we cannot properly intend to attach any other meaning to it, than that, in consequence of some cause or other external to the part which falls into a state of irritation, and acting upon it either directly or through the medium of the blood—the composition and constitution of this part undergo alterations which at the same time alter its relations to the neighbouring parts (whether they be blood-vessels or other structures) and enable it to attract to itself and absorb from them a larger quantity of matter than usual, and to transform it according to circumstances. Every form of inflammation with which we are acquainted, may be naturally explained in this way. With regard to every one, it may be assumed that it begins as an inflammation from the moment that this increased absorption of matters into the tissue takes place, and the further transformation of these matters commences.

This view accords to a certain extent, as you no doubt see, with that which has been maintained by the upholders of the vascular theory, according to which the

exudation is regarded as an immediate consequence of
the hyperæmia, and in which it is assumed that inflammation, when it has once declared itself, is characterized
by the presence of a substance more or less foreign to
the natural composition of the part. The only question
is whether the hyperæmia really forms the actual commencement of these processes.

If inflammation were necessarily dependent upon hyperæmia, you can well imagine that it would be logically
impossible to speak of inflammations in parts which do
not stand in an immediate relation to vessels. We could
not imagine an inflammation taking place at a certain
distance from a vessel. It would be completely impossible to speak of an inflammation of the cornea (excepting
as occurring at its border); of an inflammation of cartilage (excepting as occurring in the parts immediately
adjoining the bone); or of an inflammation in the
internal substance of a tendon. But if we compare the
processes which present themselves in these parts with
those which are ordinarily seen in inflamed parts, the
result is unquestionably that the same inflammatory
processes may occur everywhere alike, and that the
changes in the vascular parts can in no essential particular be distinguished from those which take place in the
non-vascular ones.

The term inflammatory (*i. e.*, according to the common
definition, fibrinous) exudation, has, as you are aware,
been somewhat loosely applied, inasmuch as it has been
taken to include different kinds of exudation (fibrinous
and non-fibrinous) furnished by different processes, upon
all of which, however, the common name of inflammation has been bestowed. When, for example, inflammations of mucous membranes are spoken of, it is not
generally supposed, that the mucous membrane will
furnish a fibrinous exudation. We are indeed ac-

quainted with mucous membranes, where fibrinous exudations are of pretty frequent occurrence, for example,
the mucous membrane of the respiratory organs. But
we know also that free (superficial) fibrinous exudations
are scarcely to be met with on the mucous membrane
of the digestive tract, and that they at most accompany
the more serious, and especially the gangrenous and
specific forms. When laryngitis is spoken of, the presence of croup is not immediately inferred. In a case
of cystitis, we do not expect to find the inner surface of
the bladder covered with a fibrinous layer. In the
whole series of so-called gastric inflammations we find,
especially at the commencement of the process, scarcely
anything more than an abundant secretion of mucus.
If therefore we still call these catarrhal inflammations,
inflammations, if we do not wish entirely to cast them
out of the class of inflammations, we must admit that
there may exist a mucous as well as fibrinous exudation
in inflammations, and that the inflammations with a mucous exudation form a special category, appertaining to
certain organs. For, as is well known, we do not find
them in all the tissues of the body, but nearly exclusively
on mucous membranes.

If now you consider the fibrinous exudations a little
more closely, there can be no doubt at all, but that in
this point they entirely agree with the mucous ones.
For we do not meet with fibrinous exudations in all
parts of the body; we know of no form of exudative
encephalitis, for example, which furnishes a fibrinous
exudation. Just as little is there a form of hepatitis
known, in which fibrinous exudations occur. There is
indeed an inflammation of the investing membrane of
the liver (perihepatitis), just as there is an inflammation of the membrane of the brain, in which fibrine
may be set free, but nobody has ever met with fibrine in

a case of genuine hepatitis. Just as little is there
fibrine to be found in the ordinary inflammation of the
substance of the heart (myo-carditis).

On the other hand, you must bear in mind that,
starting with certain preconceived notions, observers
have imagined fibrinous exudations to take place in
many parts, where they are not really to be seen. If
because pus has been obtained from a fibrinous exudation, it is therefore imagined that, wherever pus shows
itself, a fibrinous exudation must be regarded as its
source, no very great power of observation is required
to convince oneself, that this is an error. Take any
ulcerated surface you please, wipe off the pus, and collect what then comes out; you will either have a serous
fluid or pus, but you will not see that the surface you
have wiped becomes covered with a fibrinous layer. If
we confine ourselves to those parts, where inflammations
with real, unquestionable fibrinous exudation do occur,
we have a category nearly as limited as that of the mucous
inflammations. In such a category the first place is
occupied by the serous membranes proper, which even
upon slight inflammatory irritation generally produce
fibrine; the second place is filled by certain mucous
membranes, in which, in a great number of cases,
fibrinous inflammations unmistakably arise, as an aggra-
vation out of mucous ones. Ordinary croup does not
generally at its very outset manifest itself in the form of
fibrinous croup; at the commencement, at a time when
the danger may already be very considerable, there is
often nothing else found than a mucous or muco-purulent
false membrane. Not until after a certain lapse of time
does the fibrinous exudation set in, and then it does so
in such a manner, that we can trace the transitions in
the same false membrane, and see that a certain portion
is manifestly mucous, another manifestly fibrine, whilst

in a third part it can no longer be affirmed with certainty whether the one or the other is present. Here therefore both substances appear as substitutes for one another. Where the inflammatory irritation is more violent, we see fibrine, where slight, mucus, appear.

With regard to mucus, however, we know, that it does not exist in the blood like fibrine. Although a mucous membrane produces incredibly large masses of mucus in a short time, they are nevertheless products of the membrane itself; the membrane is not infiltrated with mucus coming from the blood, but the peculiar mucin matter, the principle of mucus, is a product of the membrane, and is conveyed to the surface by means of the fluid oozing through (transuding) from the blood. In the same manner I have also attempted, as I intimated to you on a former occasion (p. 195), to overthrow the opinion, which is wont to be entertained with regard to the origin of fibrine. Whilst until now fibrine has been regarded as a real transudation from the liquor sanguinis, as the outflowing plasma, I have proposed the explanation, that the fibrine, like the mucus, is a local product of those tissues, on and in which it is found, and that it is conveyed to the surface in the same way as the mucus of the mucous membrane. I then showed you, how we have in this way a most ready explanation of the fact, that in proportion as, in a given tissue, the production of fibrine increases, so also the amount of fibrine in the blood increases; and that the fibrinous crasis is just as much a product of the local disease, as the fibrinous exudation is a local product of the local metamorphosis of matter. Never has any one —any more than it is possible for him by a change of pressure directly to produce mucus from the blood in any place which does not itself produce mucus—been able to produce fibrine by any change in the pressure of the blood; what transudes never consists of anything but serous fluids.

I am accordingly of opinion, that, *in the sense* in which it has usually been assumed to exist, *there is no inflammatory exudation at all*, but that the exudation which we meet with, is essentially composed of the material which has been generated in the inflamed part itself through the change in its condition—and of the transuded fluid derived from the vessels. If therefore a part possesses a great number of vessels, and particularly if they are superficial, it will be able to furnish an exudation, since the fluid which transudes from the blood conveys the special products of the tissue along with it to the surface. If this is not the case, there will be no exudation, but the whole process will be limited to the occurrence in the real substance of the tissue of the special changes which have been induced by the inflammatory stimulus.

In this manner, two forms of inflammation can be separated from one another; the *purely parenchymatous inflammation*, where the process runs its course in the interior of the tissue, without our being able to detect the presence of any free fluid which has escaped from the blood; and the *secretory* (*exudative*) *inflammation* (which belongs more to the superficial organs) where an increased escape of fluid takes place from the blood and conveys the peculiar parenchymatous matters along with it to the surface of the organs. That there are two different forms is clearly shown by the fact that they occur for the most part in different organs. There are certain organs which, under all circumstances, only suffer from the parenchymatous affection, and others again which in nearly every instance exhibit a superficial exudative inflammation.

The distinction into adhesive and purulent forms, which has generally been made in accordance with the example of Hunter, has reference to a much later stage in the process ; the first point to be considered is always, how far the tissues themselves become changed and their products assume a degenerative character, or how far, through the passage of the fluids, the part is again freed from what it has generated in itself, and how far thereby the degeneration of the part is avoided.   Every parenchymatous inflammation has from its outset a tendency to alter the histological and functional character of an organ.   Every inflammation with free exudation in general affords a certain degree of relief to the part ; it conveys away from it a great part of the noxious matters with which it is clogged, and the part therefore appears comparatively to suffer much less than that which is the seat of a parenchymatous disease.

LECTURE XVIII.

APRIL 21, 1858.

NORMAL AND PATHOLOGICAL NEW–FORMATION.

The theory of continuous development in opposition to the blastema- and exuda-
tion-theory—Connective tissue and its equivalents as the most general germ-
store of new formations—Correspondence between embryonic and pathological new formation—Cell-division as the most general starting-point of new
formations.

Endogenous formation—Physalides—Brood-cavities.

Different tendencies of new-formations—Hyperplasia, direct and indirect—Heteroplasia—Pathological formative cells—Difference in their size and in the time
required for their full development.

Description of the development of bone as a model formation—Difference between
formation and transformation—Fresh and growing, in opposition to macerated,
bone—Nature of medullary tissue—Growth in length of tubular [long] bones ;
proliferation of cartilage—Formation of marrow as a transformation of tissue ;
red and yellow, normal and inflammatory marrow—Osseous tissue, calcified
cartilage, osteoid tissue—Bone territories : caries, degenerative ostitis—Granu-
tions in bone—Suppuration of bone—Maturation of pus—Ossification of marrow—Growth of long bones in thickness : structure and proliferation of the
periosteum.

Granulations as analogous to the medulla of bones, and as the starting-point of all
heteroplastic development.

GENTLEMEN,—I propose to-day, in illustration of *formative irritation*, to portray to you the most important features in the history of pathological new-formations, for a knowledge of these will throw light upon a
series of events which present themselves both in the
more complicated formation of tumours, and in the
more simple inflammatory irritative processes. That I

at present entirely reject the blastema doctrine in its original form, you have no doubt already gathered from the previous lectures. In its place I have put the very simple doctrine of the *continuous development of tissues out of one another*. The chief point therefore in individual cases is to determine the particular manner in which the various tissues arise, and by means of definite examples to make oneself acquainted with all the different directions which it is possible this development may follow.

My first observations, in consequence of which I began to entertain doubts with respect to the prevailing blastema and exudation doctrine—as to how far namely, new-formations could be derived from this source—date from researches of mine on *tubercle*.* I found namely that a series of tubercular deposits in different organs, especially in the lymphatic glands, the membranes of the brain and the lungs, never at any time exhibited a discernible exudation, but always, during the whole course of their development, presented organized elements, without its ever being possible to observe either in them, or before they existed, any stage in which amorphous, shapeless matter was present. As long as eight years ago I discerned that the development which takes place in the lymphatic glands upon the occurrence of the well-known scrofulous changes, begins in such a way, that the first conditions met with entirely correspond to those which in other instances are designated by the name of hypertrophy; for nuclei and cells are found in great abundance, though they afterwards break up and directly supply the material for the final accumulation of cheesy substance. The view which I derived

---

* See a paper on tuberculosis and its relations to inflammation, scrofulosis and typhoid fever. Verhandlungen der physikalisch-medic. Gesellschaft zu Würzburg, 1850, vol. i., p. 81.

from these investigations of mine, namely, that a tissue undergoing hypertrophy may supply a completely abnormal, diseased product, appeared to me all the more significant, because I had simultaneously detected an altogether similar series of developmental changes whilst examining an entirely different body, namely, the so-called *typhous matter* (Typhus-masse). At that time the view of the Vienna school had been universally adopted, that, in the different typhous processes, an exudation of an albuminous nature and soft, medullary character filled the parts, and that thereby swellings of a medullary appearance were produced. But whether the typhous matter be examined in the lymphatic glands of the mesentery, or round about the follicles of Peyer's patches, no exudation capable of organization is at any time met with, but always a directly continuous development from the pre-existing cellular elements of the glands, the follicles and the connective tissue, to the typhous matter.

These observations were of course as yet insufficient to justify me in setting about effecting a general change in the existing doctrine, because we see organic elements arise at numberless points, where at that time at least cellular elements were altogether unknown to exist as normal constituents, and there was therefore scarcely any other explanation possible than that new germs were formed by a kind of generatio æquivoca [spontaneous generation] out of the mass of blastema. The only places besides the glands, where such a development arising out of previously existing elements might have been inferred with some degree of probability to take place, were the surfaces of the body with their epithelial elements. Then it was, that my investigations into the nature of the connective tissues, with which I have already so much plagued you, proved entirely decisive. From the moment that I was able to maintain that there was scarcely any part of the body which did not possess cellular elements—that I could show that bone-corpuscles were real cells, and that connective tissue in different places contained, now a larger, now a smaller, number of really cellular elements—from that moment germs in abundance were supplied from which new tissues might possibly be developed. In fact, the more the number of observers increased, the more distinctly was it shown, that by far the greater number of the new-formations which arise in the body proceed from connective tissue and its equivalents. From this rule comparatively few pathological new-formations are excepted, and these belong on the one hand to the class of epithelial formations, and on the other are connected with the more highly organized tissues of a specific, animal (p. 55) nature, for example, the vessels. We may therefore, with trifling restriction, *substitute for the plastic lymph, the blastema of the earlier, the exudation of the writers, connective tissue with its equivalents as the common stock of germs* (Keimstock) *of the body*, and directly trace to it as the general source the development of new-formations.

If we take a definite internal organ, for example, the brain or the liver, it was scarcely possible, as long as people saw nothing more than nervous matter in the brain, and admitted the existence of nothing more than vessels and hepatic cells in the liver, to imagine the occurrence of a new-formation in them without the intervention of a special formative matter. For it was of course easy to convince oneself that new-formations do not in the liver usually proceed from the hepatic cells or the vessels. And that in the substance of the brain, the nerves as such do not give rise to new-formations, has been known ever since the microscope has been em-

ployed, for since that time it has been known that
medullary cancers are not due to the proliferation of
nervous matter, but consist of cellular elements of
another kind.   In fact, the body appears to us at the
present day, as Reichert was the first to note, to be
made up of a more or less continuous mass of connective tissue-like constituents, in which at certain points
other things, such as muscles and nerves, are imbedded.
Now it is in this more or less connected frame-work,
that, according to my investigations, genuine new-formation goes on, and that in accordance with the same law,
which regulates embryonic development.

This law of the correspondence between embryonic
and pathological development was, as you know, laid
down by Johannes Müller, who continued the investigations commenced by Schwann.   But at that time the
contents of an ovum were placed on a level with
blastema ; it occurred to no one that the whole process
of development in the ovum took place within the limits
of a cell, but it was concluded simply, that there was
a certain quantity of organizable material in the ovum,
which—in virtue of a peculiar power innate in it, by
means of some organizing force, or as those would
have it who regard the matter from a " higher " point
of view, impelled by an organizing idea—transformed
itself into this or that particular shape.   But here too
the conviction has been gradually acquired, that the
matter in question is a cellular substance, and if what
has been most rigidly maintained by Remak is correct,
namely, that the cleavage of the yolk also is due to a
visible division of cells, to the growing in of membranous partitions into the interior of the ovum, and
their coalescence, we have not here to deal with a free
organizing impulse taking place within the yolk, but
with progressive acts of division on the part of the

originally single cell.   But long before this simple view
of the process of the cleavage in the yolk had been
arrived at, it had been very distinctly perceptible that in
pathological processes a comparison between plastic exudations, or blastema, with the matters contained in the
ovum, was obviously inadmissible, and that, where really
formed parts were found, they had proceeded from a
pre-existing part, a cell.

The mode of origin of new formations is, as it seems,
a double one.   We have, namely, either to do with a
simple division, such as we discussed when treating of
irritation (p. 346).   We then see the whole series of

Fig. 124.

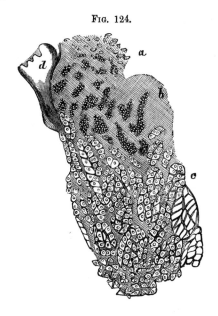

Fig. 124. Proliferation of the growing cartilage of the diaphysis of the tibia of
a child.   Longitudinal section.   *a.* The cartilage-cells on the border of the epiphysis, some of them simple, some of them in a state of commencing proliferation.
b. Groups of cells that have arisen from the repeated division of simple cells.
c. Groups of cells lying near the calcifying border of the diaphysis, and considerably developed through the growth and enlargement of the individual cells; the
intercellular substance growing continually more and more scanty.   *d.* Section of a
bloodvessel.   150 diameters.

changes from the division of the nucleolus to the final division of the cell. If an epithelial cell acquires two nuclei, divides and this process is repeated, a long series of developmental changes may, by means of a continual repetition, be produced. If the skin becomes irritated in consequence of continued friction, and the irritation is increased to a certain point, the epithelium will thicken, and if the proliferation is very energetic, it may lead to the production of tolerably large tumour-like formations. The same mode of development which is presented by layers of epithelium, we meet with also in the interior of organs. In cartilage, for example, where the individual cellular elements are inclosed in an intercellular substance, the place of each of them is at last occupied by an accumulation of numerous cells, the whole group, like the cell from which it proceeded, being shut off from its neighbors by the intercellular substance. This mode of development, therefore, is one which, though very simple in itself, may, since it originates in dissimilar parts, produce very different results.

But we have besides another class of new-formations

FIG. 125.

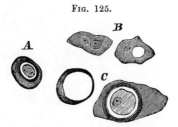

Fig. 125. Endogenous new formation; cells containing vesicles (physaliphores). *A*. From the thymus gland of a new-born infant together with epithelioid cells: in the interior of a vesicle which has a double contour (more distinctly marked in *C*) and is besides surrounded by a cell-like border, lies a perfect nucleated cell. *B*. *C*. Cancer-cells (Cf. Archiv. für pathol. Anatomie, Vol. I., Pl. II., and Vol. III. Pl. II.) *B*, one with two nuclei; *C*, one with a physalid which nearly fills the whole cell and another, where the physalid (brood-cavity) again encloses a perfect nucleated cell. 300 diameters.

in the body which are indeed much less well known, and of which the special peculiarities cannot as yet be seized with such great precision. These are processes, where we see *endogenous* changes set in in the interior of pre-existing cells. In a simple cell a vesicular cavity forms, which, contrasted with the somewhat cloudy and generally slightly granular contents of the cell, presents a very clear, bright, homogeneous appearance. In what manner cavities of this first kind, which I class together under the name of *physalides*, arise, is not yet altogether certain. The greatest probabilities are in favour of the nuclei being, in certain forms, likewise the starting-point of these formations. For, beside these cells, others are seen with two nuclei, one of which, in several of them, has become somewhat larger and brighter than usual, though still preserving the character of a nucleus. Subsequently, this vesicle becomes so large that the cell is gradually almost entirely filled with it, and its former contents with the nucleus only look like a little appendage to the vesicle. So far the process is tolerably simple. But besides these vesicles, thus growing and filling the cells, others are met with, in the interior of which elements of a cellular nature are enclosed. This is of pretty frequent occurrence in cancerous tumours, but also in normal parts, for example in the thymus gland. This form seems to indicate, that in fact by means of a process which cannot be directly traced to any division of the pre-existing cells, and indeed in peculiar vesicular cavities (which I have named *brood-cavities* (or -vesicles —Bruträume),) in the interior of cellular elements, new elements of a similar kind may be developed. However, this is at all events a condition which plays but a subordinate part in the whole history of new-formations ; the regular form is the one first described. There are only a few pathological new-formations, in the history of which this endogenous development plays any distinct part, whilst in nearly all forms cell-division is met with to a great extent.

The essential points of difference between the several modes of development of cells are therefore these : in one class of formations the divisions proceed with a certain regularity, so that the ultimate products from their very beginning exhibit a complete correspondence with the parent structures, and the young structures at no time deviate in any remarkable degree from the parent-cells. Such processes are in ordinary life mostly designated as hypertrophies, but I have, in order to express the nature of the change more accurately, proposed the name of *hyperplasiæ*, inasmuch it is not an increase in the nutrition of existing parts that takes place, but a real formation of new elements (p. 94).

In another class the development proceeds in such a way, that divisions certainly also do take place, but make very rapid progress and produce cells which gradually decrease in size, and ultimately in some instances become so small, that they can scarcely be distinguished to be cells. The proliferation may cease at this point, and then the cells severally begin to grow, and to become larger ; and under certain circumstances a structure may in this case again also be produced analogous to that in which the development originated. This, however, is not usually the case ; generally, the young cells pursue a somewhat different course of development, and a heterologous structure begins to form.

The mode of development, which I here describe to you, may also run its course in such a way, that the cells do not at once begin to divide, but the nuclei first greatly multiply, becoming continually more numerous and at the same time smaller. We find something similar to this in pus, in which a division of the nuclei very rapidly takes place, and generally in such a way, that the originally single nuclei at once divide into a considerable number of smaller ones, which at first remain coherent. But in pus it is not certain whether the division of the nucleus is succeeded by a real division in the cell, whilst in other new-formations this is certainly the case—only the complete division, or if you will, the cleavage, of the cells is delayed for a long time, and this intermediate stage of the mere division of the nuclei continues for a disproportionately long period, and seems to occur in some sort independently.

These two plans are the ones regularly followed by all those kinds of new-formations which do not *directly* lead to hyperplasia ;* the normal condition is here in the first instance interrupted by an intermediate state, in which the tissue appears essentially changed, without one's being able straightway to determine whether a growth of a benignant or malignant nature will be developed out of it. This is a stage of seemingly absolute indifference ; from the appearance of the individual elements it cannot at all be inferred what their real destiny is ; they behave exactly like the so-called formative cells of the embryo, which also at first exactly resemble one another, no matter whether a muscular or nervous element, or anything else, is about to proceed from them. Nevertheless I regard it as very probable that delicate internal differences do really exist, which to a certain extent determine beforehand the subsequent metamorphoses—not merely potential differences in the formative cells, but really material differences, only of so

---

* There are processes which begin with Hyperplasia and end with Heteroplasia, and others again, which begin with Heteroplasia and end with Hyperplasia. The new formation of vessels, for example, never begin straightway with the formation of vessels, but first of all cells are formed (heteroplasia), and afterward vessels (hyperplasia) are developed out of these cells.—*From a MS. Note by the Author.*

delicate a nature, that we are not as yet able to demonstrate them.

In the development of the embryo a phenomenon has been known for years which positively indicates the existence of such differences in the formative cells, inasmuch as the different segments of the ovum run through their phases of development with different degrees of rapidity, and especially those parts which are destined to form the higher organs, run through their individual stages with much greater celerity than those whose lot it is to form the lower tissues. In the size of the cells also differences seem to exist. In a similar manner we frequently see that in pathological formations also differences occur in reference to the time occupied in their development. Whenever the development of the cells takes place with great rapidity, we may be sure it is a more or less heterologous development. An homologous, hyperplastic formation always presupposes a certain tardiness in the processes which give rise to it; the cells generally remain of a larger size, since the divisions do not usually proceed until very small forms are produced.

Though so extremely simple in nature and in theory, these modes of development are certainly extremely difficult of demonstration in individual places. The parts which apparently ought to be the most conveniently situated for the purpose of investigation, and in which Henle indeed, as long as twenty years ago, all but made the discovery of such a development, are the epithelia. Here, where a development often so abundant takes place upon the surface of a membrane, one would suppose it must be extremely easy to trace its course accurately in the individual cells. Henle, you know, endeavoured to show that mucus-corpuscles, and indeed many forms which belong to pus, were produced on the

surface of mucous membranes along with the epithelium
in such a way, that no real difference was to be perceived between the two classes in their earliest stages,
and that the mucus-corpuscles must therefore in some
sort be looked upon as epithelial cells that had gone
astray, as children that had turned out ill, that had been
impeded in the progress of their development by some
early disturbance, but really were intended to become
epithelial cells. Unfortunately the notion was then and
long afterwards prevalent, that epithelium like all other
tissues was normally developed out of a blastema. It
was, you know, imagined that on the surface of every
mucous membrane in the first instance there transuded a
plastic fluid from the vessels running to the surface, and
that the epithelial cells were formed out of it. Schleiden's theory was steadfastly adhered to, that nuclei first
form in a fluid, and that membranes do not develop
around them until afterwards. At present, however
much the different surfaces presented by the skin and
the mucous and serous membranes are examined, the
conviction is everywhere unmistakeably acquired, that
the cellular elements extend down to the very surface of
the connective tissue, and that there is nowhere a spot,
where free nuclei, blastema or fluid exist, but that on
the contrary it is especially the deepest layers which
contain the most densely crowded cells. If, at the time
when Henle made his investigations, it had been known,
that no blastema ever exists in these parts, and that no
development de novo ever takes place there, but that
the epithelial cells there present must have been developed either from old cells or from the connective tissue
underneath them, he too would certainly also have
come to the conclusion, that mucus- or pus-corpuscles
which are not furnished by an ulcerating surface (which
would of course be destitue of epithelium) must be

derived by direct descent from pre-existing epithelial
cells.

So nearly, even at that time, had correct views upon
the subject been obtained, but the blastema theory
enthralled men's minds, and we all stood under its influence. Besides, it appeared impossible to point out
everywhere in the interior of the tissues the requisite
antecedent structures. Not until cellular elements had
been shown to exist in connective tissue did it become
possible to produce a germinal tissue (Keimgewebe)
which is at present everywhere, and from which in the
most various organs similar growths may be developed.
Now that we know that connective tissue—or tissues
equivalent to it—exists in the brain, the liver, the kidneys, in muscle, cartilage, skin, etc., now there is of
course no longer any difficulty in conceiving how the
same pathological product may arise in all these apparently so dissimiliar structures. No specific blastema of
any sort, deposited in all these parts, is at all required,
but only the application of a similar stimulus to the connective tissue of the different localities.

Now with regard to the details of this doctrine, allow
me in the first place to bring to your notice a concrete
example of normal development, which will perhaps be
the best calculated to supply you with a picture of the
often so complicated processes with which we are here
concerned. I choose as my example that organ, in
which the process of development is in itself best
known, and which at the same time on account of the
peculiarity of its structure least admits of misinterpreta-
tion, namely the *bones*. They are too hard and thick
for any one to talk about the presence of blastema or
exudation in their proper parenchyma. The growth of
the bones at the same time affords us direct standards
wherewith to compare the different new-formations,

which may occur in the bones in morbid conditions, for every one of these new-formations finds a certain prototype in the normal development of bone.

All the larger bones grow, as is well known, in two directions. This is most simply shown in the long bones, which gradually increase in length and thickness. The growth in length takes place from cartilage, that in thickness from periosteum. But a flat bone also is invested on the one hand with cartilaginous parts or their equivalents (sutures) and on the other with membranes which correspond to periosteum. A growth from cartilage and a growth from periosteum can therefore be distinguished in every bone. This furnishes us with a plan of the development of long bones, which is found even in the writings of Havers, and according to which the new layers of bone incapsulate the old ones, and every more recent layer is not only wider but longer than that next above it in age. Every new layer of osseous substance which is formed out of periosteum is longer (higher) than the one immediately preceding it, inasmuch as new layers of perichondrium are being continually converted into periosteum. At the same time every new layer of osseous substance which grows out of cartilage is broader (thicker) than that which went before it, inasmuch as every new layer of the (growing) cartilage which proceeds to ossification surpasses its predecessor in breadth (thickness). The growth from cartilage, however, can only take place in the direction of the extremities of the bone, inasmuch as the cartilage of its diaphysis is, at a very early period of intra-uterine life, so completely ossified,* that no cartilage remains ex-

---

* This complete ossification in long bones is not confined to intra-uterine life, but every new layer of cartilage which grows out of the terminal cartilage up to the age of puberty ossifies (when matters follow a normal course) throughout its whole thickness, so that no cartilage remains at the circumference of the bone.—*From a MS. Note by the Author.*

cepting at the two ends. Now a tissue once ossified
ceases (save under exceptional circumstances) to grow,
so that any increase of thickness in the diaphysis must
be wholly due to a development out of periosteum, in
which growth proceeds much more slowly than in cartilage. This is the reason why the shaft of a long bone
is narrower than its extremities.* Whilst in this way
parts which were previously either connective tissue or
cartilage, are converted into bone, the development of
the medullary tissue is going on within the bone. The
original bone is extremely dense, a very solid and relatively compact mass. Subsequently the substance of
the bone disappears more and more, one part of it after
another is dissolved, and the medullary cavity [canal]
arises, the size of which is not in any way restricted to
that of the original osseous rudiment, but often considerably exceeds it. Thus the development of bone, when
taken as a whole, does not consist merely in the gradual
apposition of a succession of fresh osseous layers derived
from periosteum and cartilage, but also in the continual replacement of the innermost layers of the bone by masses
of marrow.

In the interpretation of these facts the blastema theory was long appealed to as the great authority. Havers
and Duhamel, who made excellent investigations into
the history of bone, started with the supposition that a
nutritious juice (succus nutritius) was secreted, from
which the new masses arose. The development of the
marrow was imagined to consist in a formation of
cavities, into which first a viscous juice and then a fatty
matter was secreted—cavities which were invested by
the medullary membrane, and whose contents varied

---

* For a diagram of the growth of long bones, see Havers (Osteologia nova.
Francof. 1692, Tab. I., fig. 1), and Kölliker (Handbuch d. Gewebelehre, 3d edit.,
Leipzig, 1859, p. 259).

with age. However, as I have already pointed out to you, there are no sacs in the areolæ of the bones, but a continuous tissue, the medullary tissue, which fills the medullary spaces [cancelli] and cavities and belongs to the class of connective tissues, although it considerably differs from ordinary connective tissue. We have therefore here to deal, as you see from this simple fact, with a substitution of tissues. As osseous tissue* is formed out of periosteum and cartilage, so marrow is formed from osseous tissue, and the development of a bone consists not merely in the formation of osseous tissue, but it presupposes that the series of transformations goes beyond the stage of bone, and that medullary tissue is then produced. Medullary tissue therefore constitutes in some sort the physiological termination of the formation of bone as an organ.

However simple this view may be, still it furnishes us with a picture of the growth and history of bone different from the traditional one. Formerly, observers nearly always contented themselves with viewing the matter much in the same light that osteologists are wont to do; they took a macerated bone, examined it when divested of all its soft parts, and built up the processes accordingly. It is, however, necessary that the relations should be traced in the moist, living healthy or diseased bone, and that one should pay attention not only to the development of bone upon the outside from the growing layers of the cartilage and periosteum, but also to that of the medulla on the inside, as the ultimate product of the development in this class of tissues, even if it be not the noblest one. The most important and really

---

* *Osseous tissue* (tela ossea, tissu osseux) = bone corpuscles + calcified inter-cellular substance. *Bone* as an *organ* = osseous tissue + medullary tissue + peri-osteum + vessels + nerves. *Osseous substance* is sometimes taken to mean a por-tion of bone considered as an organ.—*From a MS. Note by the Author.*

decisive point, through which the whole subject of bone acquires another aspect, is, I consider, this, that the bone in the formation of marrow is not simply dissolved and its place taken by some exudation or blastema, but that the dissolution of the osseous substance is a transformation of the osseous tissue, and that the dissolution results from a transformation of the intercellular substance of the bone into a soft mass of tissue which is no longer in a condition to retain the calcareous salts. If therefore you ask whence the new elements come which arise in the midst of osseous tissue, or how a cancer or collection of pus can form in the middle of the compact cortex of bone, I return you the very simple answer, that they arise in precisely the same manner, that in the course of the natural and normal development of bone the marrow arises. In no part does the osseous tissue first dissolve, then an exudation, and next a new-formation, follow, but the existing tissue is directly converted into the succeeding one. The existing osseous tissue is the matrix of the succeeding cancerous tissue, the cells of the cancer are the immediate descendants of the cells of the bone.

If now we consider the course of the formation of bone a little more in detail, we find, as we have already in part seen, that the cartilage prepares for ossification in such a way, that its cells in the first instance become larger ; that divisions then take place in them, first in the nuclei and afterwards in the cells themselves ; that these divisions then proceed with great rapidity, so that we obtain larger and larger groups of cells, and in a comparatively short time the place of a single cell is occupied by a relatively very large group of cells (Fig. 124). You will remember from my first lecture (p. 33), that a cartilage-cell is distinguished from most other cells by its secreting a special membranous capsule in which it is inclosed. This membranous capsule, on the division of the cells which it contains, sends in septa between them, which serve as new envelopes for the young cells, yet in such a way, that even the gigantic groups of cells, which proceed from each of the original cells, are still enclosed in the greatly enlarged parent capsule.

It is manifest, that the greater the number of cells which undergo this change, the larger the cartilage will become, and that the height to which any one of us

FIG. 126.

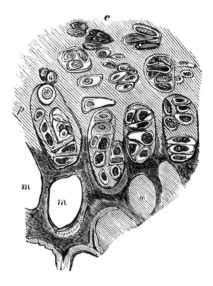

Fig. 126. Vertical section through the ossifying border of a growing astragalus. *c.* Cartilage with smallish groups of cells, *p,* the layer where the proliferation and enlargement are the most marked along the line of calcification. In the cartilage-cavities are seen, partly complete nucleated cells, partly shrivelled, angular and granular looking bodies (artificially altered cells). The dark mass advancing into the intermmediate substance represents the deposition of calcareous salts, behind which the formation of medullary spaces (*m, m, m*) and osseous trabeculæ [spicula] is here beginning with unusual rapidity. The marrow has been removed; round the cavities which lie farthest back, the trabeculæ are surrounded by a lighter border of young osseous tissue (produced from marrow.) 300 diameters.

attains, essentially depends upon the extent to which growth occurs in the individual groups of cartilage-cells. Whether we ultimately become tall or short, is, if I may say so, left entirely to the discretion of these elements. When the growth of the proliferating cartilage has reached this point, the cellular elements are very close together, so that a comparatively trifling quantity of intercellular substance lies between them (Fig. 124). The farther the development advances, the more does the appearance of the cartilage alter, and at last it looks almost like dense-celled vegetable tissue. The cells themselves however are difficult to be seen, because they are extremely sensitive ; they readily shrivel up upon the addition of the mildest fluids and then appear like angular and jagged corpuscles, almost analogous to those of bone, with which however they have at this time nothing to do.

The cells which have sprung from this excessive proliferation of the originally simple cartilage cells, constitute the parent structures from which proceeds all that afterwards arises in the longitudinal axis of the bone, and especially the osseous and medullary tissue. The cartilage-cells may be converted by a direct transformation into marrow-cells and continue as such ; or they may first be converted into osseous, and then into medullary, tissue ; or lastly they may first be converted into marrow and then into bone. So variable are the permutations of these tissues in themselves so nearly allied, and yet in their external appearance so completely distinct. When a direct transformation into marrow is the first effected, the old intercellular substance of the cartilage at the border next to the bone begins first of all to grow soft ; then some of the adjoining capsules usually also very soon experience this change, so that the cellular elements come to be more or less set free in a softer basis-substance. Simultaneously with the occurrence of this softening the chemical reaction of this tissue also becomes altered, and we always obtain the distinct reaction of mucin. At the same time divisions begin to take place, and this not in the same way as previously, when the cellular elements at once separated into two new analogous cells (hyperplasia), but rather in such a way, that a number of little nuclei arise in them (physiological heteroplasia). Subsequently, in proportion as this process of transformation reaches a higher and higher pitch, and fresh portions of the intercellular substance are continually being converted into this more homogeneous and soft matter, the cells generally divide, and we obtain a number of smaller ones, which are very minute in comparison to the large cartilage-cells, from which they proceeded, and contain either a single nucleus with a nucleolus, or sometimes also, like pus-corpuscles, several nuclei. Thus gradually arises a tissue extremely rich in cells, *the young, red, medullary tissue*, as we generally find it in the marrow of new-born infants. If the process stops here, the size of the transformed spot indicates at the same time the extent of the subsequent medullary space. Subsequently, these little cells may take up fat, and then it appears, first in small granules, but by degrees in large drops, and at last to such an extent that the cells are entirely filled with them. Thereby the original medullary tissue is transformed into adipose tissue ; the fat, however, is always contained in the interior of the marrow-cells, as it is in the cells of the panniculus adiposis. But this *yellow, fatty* marrow does not occur in all bones. In the bodies of the vertebræ we almost always find the small cells. In the long bones of the adult the fatty marrow always occurs normally, but in pathological conditions it may very rapidly yield up its fat, the elements may divide and we then again have red, but inflammatory, marrow.

In this whole series of allied processes from the first development of marrow out of cartilage until the production of inflammatory marrow—the last disturbance which manifests itself in injured bones (as we see in amputations)—there at no time exists any amorphous substance, blastema or exudation; we can always trace the descent of one cell from another; every one of them has been directly developed from an earlier one, and will have as long as the proliferation continues, a direct progeny of cells.

The second series of transformations in the longitudinal axis of the cylindrical [long] bones is furnished by the osseous tissue, which may arise out of marrow and cartilage. In the one case the marrow-, in the other, the cartilage-cells, become the subsequent bone cells. This act of real ossification, the production of the osseous tissue, is extremely difficult to observe, chiefly for the reason, that what first takes place in the course of these processes, is not the production of real osseous tissue, but only the deposition of calcareous salts. Generally, namely, there first of all takes place in the immediate vicinity of the border of the bone a calcification of the cartilage, which gradually advances, first along the borders of the larger groups of cells, and then around the individual cells, always following the substance of the capsules, so that every individual cartilage-cell is surrounded by a ring of calcareous substance. But this is not yet bone, it is nothing more than calcified cartilage, for, upon dissolving the calcareous salts, the old cartilage is again brought into view—and indeed it offers no analogy to bone in any other respect excepting in the presence of calcareous salts.

Now, in order that this calcified cartilage may become

FIG. 127.

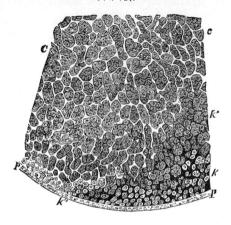

FIG. 128.

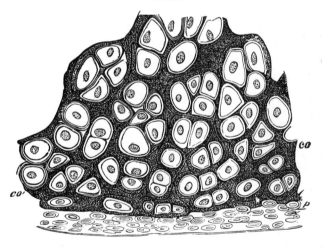

Fig. 127. Horizontal section through the growing cartilage of the diaphysis of the tibia of a seven months' fœtus. *C c.* The cartilage with groups of cells that have undergone proliferation and enlargement; *p p*, perichondrium. *k.* Calcified cartilage, in which the individual groups of cells, and cells, are enclosed in calcareous rings; at *k'* larger rings, at *k''* progress of the calcification along the perichondrium. 150 diameters.

Fig. 128. Right corner of Fig. 127, more highly magnified. *co.* Calcified cartilage *co'* commencement of calcification, *p* perichondrium. 350 diameters.

real bone, it is necessary that the cavity in which every cartilage-cell lies, be converted into the well-known, radiated, jagged bone-cavity [lacuna]. This process is so extremely difficult to obtain a sight of, because on making sections the masses of lime crumble away before the knife, and furnish débris within which it is impossible to see well what really is present. In this circumstance you must seek for an explanation of the fact, that up to the present time there are still, and probably still will be for several years, continual disputes with regard to the mode of origin of bone corpuscles. I hold that view to be correct, according to which the bone-corpuscles* in certain places directly originate out of the the cartilage-corpuscles, and indeed in this way, that in the first place the cavity of the capsule which invests the cartilage-cell, becomes narrower, manifestly because fresh capsular matter is deposited on the inside. But in proportion as this takes place, the inner border of the capsular cavity begins to assume a distinctly indented appearance† (Fig. 133, c') and the space occupied by the original cell is thereby considerably diminished. In rare

---

* Cartilage-corpuscle = capsule + cartilage-cell; bone-corpuscle = bone-cell.— *Transl.*

† The lacunæ may be said really to have no existence in *living* bone (or osteoid tissue) ; they are merely the gaps (holes) in the intercellular substance in which the bone- (or osteoid-) cells lie, and are normally so entirely filled by these cells, that it is impossible to give the outlines of both in a drawing. The outline of the cell is the outline of the lacuna. Who, in drawing a deal-board, would ever think of giving a second contour to every knot, in order to represent the outline of the gap which would result from the falling out of the knot! Hence Authors have come to speak of the *nuclei* of lacunæ, whereby of course they mean the nuclei of the cells which fill the lacunæ, but which, thanks to the deeply rooted but erroneous impression left upon their minds by microscopical sections of *macerated* bone, they have failed to recognize, or have not even sought for, taking for granted they had lacunæ before them. In the preparation of sections, however, the cells frequently shrink, so that an interval is left between them and the walls of the lacunæ.

What is here said of the lacunæ of course equally applies to the canaliculi. Both represent the margins of the calcified intercellular substance, where it comes into contact with the bone-cells and their processes.—*Based upon MS. Notes by the Author.*

cases, we still succeed in finding cartilage-corpuscles, in which the capsular cavity has (without the occurrence of calcification) become diminished in consequence of the deposition of new capsular matter, so as to assume the form of a bone cavity (lacuna)—which it generally assumes only after ossification—whilst the old cellular element (the cartilage-cell with its nucleus) still remains in it. After this—still without the occurrence of any calcification—the boundary disappears which originally existed between the capsules of the cartilage-cells and the basis-substance, and we find jagged elements* (the future bone-cells) in an apparently entirely homogeneous substance—in other words, a tissue still soft, though in structure like bone (osteoid tissue, Fig. 133, *o*). Usually this process is concealed by means of the early calcification of the cartilage and only certain processes, for example, rickets, give us the opportunity of seeing the osteoid transformation take place in just the same manner in those parts of the cartilage also which are beginning to calcify.

But the old limits of the capsule still represent the real district which is under the sway of the bone-corpuscle, and, as I pointed out to you at the commencement of my lectures (p. 41) with an especial reference to this point, in pathological conditions this district comes again not only in force but also into view. Within these limits we see the bone-corpuscle accomplish its peculiar destinies. If, for example, the bone is by any cause impelled to enter

* The cartilage-cells (and the same holds good of the marrow-cells) during ossification throw out processes (become jagged) in the same way that connective-tissue corpuscles, which are also originally round, do, both physiologically and pathologically. These processes—which in the case of the cartilage-cells are generally formed after, but in that of the marrow-cells frequently before, calcification has taken place—bore their way into the intercellular substance, like the villi of the chorion do into the mucous membrane and into the vessels of the uterus, or like the pacchionian granulations (glands) of the pia mater of the brain into (and occasionally *through*) the calvarium.—*From a MS. Note by the Author.*

upon new transformations, one bone-corpuscle after another with its territory experiences the change. At the border of necrosed portions of bone, when the line of demarcation forms, we may distinctly observe, that the surface of the bone, when viewed along the edge, becomes marked with excavations, the extent of which corresponds to the original cells. Upon the surface vacuities are observable, which in some instances run together and form holes. The bone-corpuscle which formerly occupied the site of the hole has, in proportion as it under-

FIG 129.*

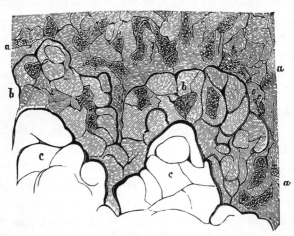

Fig. 129. Line of demarcation in a piece of necrosed bone from a case of pædarthrocase ; † a, a, a the necrosed bone with very much enlarged osseous corpuscles and canaliculi ; here and there slight indications of excavations upon the surface. b, b. The vacuities, which have taken the place of the cell-districts of the bone (Cf. Fig. 134), seen at the side of the object on a different level ; here and there enlarged bone-corpuscles still to be seen through a layer of basis-substance which covers them. c, c. Completely empty cavities. 300 diameters.

* The drawing was made from a somewhat thick preparation, and does not represent one level surface, but three different planes which form, as it were, terraces, one above the other. Of these c is distinctly in focus ; b is on a lower (or higher) level, and is less distinctly seen ; a is lower (or higher) still, and is therefore still more out of focus. Hence it is that the canaliculi (which besides are badly represented), are not clearly seen.—*From a MS. Note by the Author.*

† Necrosis (scrofulous) of the fingers in children.

went transformation itself, also determined the surrounding parts to enter upon the change. These are the processes, without the aid of which it is impossible to comprehend the history of caries. For the whole essence of caries consists in this : the bone breaks up into its territories, the individual corpuscles undergo new developmental changes (granulation, suppuration), and remnants * composed of the oldest basis-substance remain in the form of small, thin shreds in the midst of the soft substance. I traced this out again only to-day in a stump, in which, a fortnight after amputation, periostitis with slight suppuration and incipient peripheral caries was found to exist. When in such a case the thickened periosteum is stripped off, we see, at the moment it quits the surface and the vessels are drawn out from the cortex of the bone, not, as in normal bone, mere threads, but little plugs, thicker masses of substance ; and if they have been entirely drawn out, there remains a disproportionately large hole, much more extensive than it would be under normal circumstances. On examining one of these plugs you will find that around the vessel a certain quantity of soft tissue lies, the cellular elements of which are in a state of fatty degeneration. At the spot where the vessel has been drawn out, the surface does not appear even, as in normal bone, but rough and porous, and when placed

---

* In ossification (in cartilage) there is a portion of the original intercellular substance of the cartilage—that, namely, which lies between the large groups of cartilage-cells (secondary cells—Tochterzellen)—which, though it belongs to the groups as wholes, yet when these, in the course of ossification, are transformed into a number of isolated bone-cells, becomes, comparatively speaking, almost entirely independent of these cells individually (which have their own *immediate* intercellular substance to attend to, and from most of which it must be separated by a considerable interval), and therefore escapes the changes which befall them. It is this portion (well shown in Fig. 126, where it is represented by the trabeculæ separating the medullary spaces *m*), which remains behind in caries, whilst the *secondary* intercellular substance perishes. In other processes, however, which run a more chronic course (in cancer, for example), everything is destroyed.—*Based upon MS. notes by the Author.*

under the microscope, you remark those excavations, those peculiar holes, which correspond to the liquefying bone-territories. If it be asked therefore in what way bone becomes porous in the early stage of caries, it may be said that the porosity is certainly not due to the formation of exudations, seeing that for these there is no room, inasmuch as the vessels within the medullary canals (Figs. 32, 33) are in immediate contact with the osseous tissue. On the contrary, the substance of the bone in the cellular territories liquefies, vacuities form, which are at first filled with a soft substance, composed of a slightly streaky connective tissue with fattily degenerated cells. If round about a medullary canal the territory of one bone-corpuscle after another liquefies, you will after a time find the canal bounded on all sides by a lacunar structure. In the middle of it the vessel conveying the blood still remains, but the substance around about is not bone or exudation, but *degenerate tissue*. The whole process is a *degenerative ostitis*, in which the osseous tissue changes its structure, loses its chemical and morphological characters, and so becomes a soft tissue which no longer contains lime. The tissue, which fills the resulting vacuity in the bone, may vary extremely according to circumstances, consisting in one case of a fattily degenerating and disintegrating substance (the bone-corpuscles perishing), and in another of a substance rich in cells and containing numerous young cells ; this latter is formed by the division and proliferation of the bone-corpuscles, and the newly produced substance is very analogous to marrow. Under certain circumstances this substance may grow to such an extent, that—if we again borrow our illustration from the surface of the bone, where a vessel sinks in—the young medullary matter sprouts out by the side of the vessel, and appears as a little knob, filling one of the pits in the surface. This we call a *granulation*.

When we examine granulations for the purpose of comparing them with medullary tissue, we find that no two descriptions of tissue more closely correspond. The marrow of the bones of a new-born infant could at any time, both chemically and microscopically, be passed off as a granulation. Granulations are nothing more than a young, soft, mucous tissue, analogous to marrow. There is an inflammatory osteoporosis, which, as has been correctly stated, merely depends upon an increased production of medullary spaces, so that the process which is quite normal in the interior of a medullary cavity, is met with also more externally in the compact cortex. It (the osteoporosis) is distinguished from granulating peripheral caries only by its seat. If you go a step further and suppose the cells, which in osteoporosis are present in moderately large numbers, to become more and more abundant, whilst the intercellular substance constantly becomes softer and diminishes in quantity, we have *pus*. The pus is here no special product, separable from the other products of proliferation and formation ; it is certainly not identical with the pre-existing tissues, but its origin can be directly traced back to the elements of the pre-existing tissue. It is not produced by any special act, by any creation de novo, but its development proceeds from generation to generation in a perfectly regular and legitimate manner.

We have therefore before us a whole series of transformations ; the bone first produced and proceeding from cartilage may undergo a transformation into marrow, then into granulation-tissue, and finally into nearly pure pus. The transitions are here so gradual, that the pus which is in immediate contact with the granulations, constitutes, as is well known, a more mucous, stringy, and tenacious matter, which really contains mucin like the granulation-tissue, and only when we proceed farther outwards, exhibits the properties of completely developed pus. The perfect pus of the surface gradually passes, as we descend, into crude pus, the mucous, tenacious, immature pus of the deeper layers, and what we call *maturation* depends simply upon the gradual conversion of the mucous intercellular substance of the originally tenacious pus, which is allied in structure to granulations, into the albuminous intercellular substance of pure pus. The *mucus* dissolves and the creamy fluid is produced. *The maturation is therefore essentially a softening of the intercellular substance.* So direct is the connection which subsists between development, and retrograde metamorphosis, physiological and pathological conditions.

In just the same manner that the cartilage-cell may become a bone corpuscle, the marrow-cell also may become a bone-corpuscle. In the medullary spaces of bone those marrow-cells which are situated at the circumference, generally assume at a later period a more oblong form, and take a direction parallel to the internal surface of the medullary spaces, and the medullary tissue in this situation has a more fibrous appearance and has indeed been regarded as a medullary membrane, but it should not be separated from the marrow in the centre of the spaces, and only constitutes the most compact layer of the medullary tissue. Now as soon as osseous tissue is about to form, the nature of the basis-substance alters. It becomes firmer, more cartilaginous, and the individual cells appear to lie in largish cavities. Gradually they become jagged, from sending out little processes, and then nothing more is required than that calcareous salts should deposit themselves in the basis-substance—and the bone is complete. Thus here again also the osseous tissue is formed by a very direct transformation ; and by the deposition of one such osteoid * layer after another

* Osteoid I call the tissue which, when it takes up calcareous salts, becomes bone,

from the medulla, a compact substance is produced, like that of the cortex, which is always characterized by the lamellar deposition of osseous tissue in the previously existing medullary spaces. The original bone is always pumice-stone-like, and porous ; its porosities become filled by the subsequent development of osseous lamellæ from the layers of the marrow, the process continuing until the vessel, which does not admit of ossification, alone remains.

Now with regard to the development of bones in *thickness*, the process is in itself much simpler, but it is also at the same time very much more difficult to see, because ossification here proceeds very rapidly, and the proliferating periosteal layer is so thin and delicate, that extremely great care is required in order to catch sight of it at all. Pathology furnishes us with an incomparably better opportunity for studying the process than physiology. For it is just the same whether the bone grows physiologically in thickness, or pathologically in consequence of periostitis ; the difference is only one of quantity and time.

When fully developed, the periosteum consists for the most part of a very dense connective tissue which contains an extremely large quantity of elastic fibres, and in which the vessels ramify, before they pass on into the cortex of the bone itself. Now when the growth of the bone in thickness commences, we see that the most internal, vascular layer (of the periosteum) increases in thickness and swells up, and then it is said an exudation has taken place, it being taken for granted, that every swelling proves the occurrence of an exudation, and that the exudation here lies between the periosteum and the bone. But if you set to work and

—in other words, soft, uncalcified, osseous tissue.—*From a MS. Note by the Author.*

analyze the substance deposited, no trace of any plastic exudation is found ; the swollen spot appears on the contrary organized in its whole thickness from without inwards, and this most distinctly close to the bone, whilst towards the surface of the periosteum the structural relations can be less readily unravelled. This swelling may under certain circumstance increases to a very considerable extent. In periostitis we do not unfrequently see, you know, regular nodes formed, and one need only recall the more physiological history of callus after fracture. In either of these cases we seek in vain for an exudation. If the thickened layers are traced in the direction of that part of the periosteum which still remains unthickened, we can very distinctly see what Duhamel long ago exhibited in a very beautiful manner, but is forgotten over and over again, namely, that the layers which constitute the thickening are ultimately all of them continued into the layers of the periosteum. As little as the periosteum is unorganized, so little are the thickened layers without organization. Microscopical examination shows at the surface of the bone a slightly striated basis-substance, and in it, numerous,

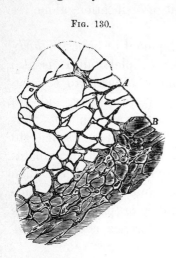

Fig. 130.

Fig. 130. Vertical section through the periosteum and periosteal surface of a parietal bone from a child. *A*. The proliferating layer of the periosteum with anastomosing networks of cells and division of nuclei. *B*. Formation of the osteoid layer by means of the sclerosis* of the intercellular substance. 300 diameters.

* Sclerosis signifies thickening with condensation.—*From a MS. Note by the Author.*

small, cellular elements ; the farther we recede from the bone, the more do divisions of cells occur, and at last we meet with the simple, very small connective-tissue-corpuscles of the periosteum. The division follows the same course as in cartilage, only that the dividing cells of the periosteum are very delicate. The greater the irritation, the greater also the proliferation, and the more considerable the swelling of the growing spot.

The cells which thus result from the proliferation of the periosteal corpuscles are converted into bone-cor-puscles exactly in the way I described when speaking of the marrow. In the neighbourhood of the surface of the bone the intercellular substance grows dense and becomes almost cartilaginous, the cells throw out pro-cesses, become stellate, and at last the calcification of the intercellular substance ensues. If the irritation is very great, the corpuscles grow very considerably, and then real cartilage is produced ; the corpuscles enlarge to such an extent that they grow into large, oval or round cells, and each of these forms a capsule around itself by secretion. In this manner cartilage may arise in the periosteum also, by means of a direct transforma-tion of its proliferating layers, but it is by no means necessary that real, true cartilage should be produced ; generally only the osteoid transformation takes place, when the intercellular substance becomes sclerotic and at once calcifies.

Thus it is, that on the surface of every growing bone, as Flourens particularly has shown, new bone is continu-ally deposited layer after layer, and that the new layers grow round the old bone in such a way, that a ring, which is early put around the bone, after a time lies inside it, enclosed by the young layers which have formed outside around it. These are connected with the old bone by means of little columns which give the

whole a pumice-stone like appearance, and here too the
subsequent condensation into cortical substance is accomplished by means of the formation—within the
individual cavities bounded by the little columns—of
concentric layers of osseous substance out of the periosteal marrow.

These are the normal and pathological processes which
we recognize in the formation of bone. From them you
may gather, that we have in them to do with a series of
permutations or substitutions, which lead in one case to
a higher, in another, to a lower form of structure, but
are however constantly connected with one another,
and, according to the conditions which operate upon the
parts, assume sometimes one aspect, sometimes another.
It is in our power to incite individual portions of cartilage to ossify, or to transform themselves into a soft
tissue. In this whole series the marrow stands alone as
the type of the heterologous forms, inasmuch as it contains the smallest and least characteristic cells. The
young medullary tissue presents the same structure as
the young formations, with which all heterologous
tissues begin, and since, as I have already hinted, it at
the same time constitutes the real type of all granulations, it may be said that, *wherever new-formations are
about to arise on a large scale, a substitution analogous to
the type of young medullary tissue (granulation) also takes
place ;* and that, no matter how great the solidity possessed by the old tissue, *a kind of proliferation nevertheless always takes place, which produces the germs of the
subsequent elements.*

LECTURE XIX.

APRIL 24, 1858.

PATHOLOGICAL, AND ESPECIALLY HETEROLOGOUS NEW-FORMATION.

Consideration of some forms of pathological formation of bone. Soft osteoma of the maxillæ—Rickets—Formation of callus after fracture.

Theory of substitutive new-formation in opposition to exudative—Destructive nature of new-formations—Homology and heterology (malignity)—Ulceration—Mollities ossium—Proliferation and luxuriation—Medulla of bones, and pus.

Suppuration—Its two forms: superficial, occurring in epithelium; and deep, in connective tissue—Eroding suppuration (skin, mucous membrane): pus and mucus-corpuscles in their relations to epithelium—Ulcerative suppuration—Solvent properties of pus.

Connection of destruction with pathological growth and proliferation—Correspondence of the first stage in pus, cancer, sarcoma, etc.—Possible duration of the life of pathologically new-formed elements, and of pathological new-formations considered as wholes (tumours)—Compound nature of the larger tuberous* tumours (Geschwulstknoten), and miliary character of the real foci (Heerde)—Conditions of growth and recurrence: contagiousness of new-formations and importance of the anastomoses of cells—Cellular pathology in opposition to the humoral and neuristic—General infection of the body—Parasitism and autonomy of new-formations.

GENTLEMEN,—I will to-day begin by laying some pathological preparations before you, for which I remained in your debt last time.

I begin with an interesting object which has lately come into my hands, and exhibits with a distinctness

---

* Tuberous, in contradistinction to infiltrated, tumours (infiltrations).—*From a MS. Note by the Author.*

which I have rarely had occasion to witness, the transitions from periosteal connective tissue into osteoid tissue, and this too with a peculiar modification, inasmuch as calcification has not taken place in large portions of the parts which already possess a structure of bone. The preparation comes from a tumour in the jaw of a goat, and contributes towards our knowledge of the transitions from connective tissue into osteoid tissue about the same information, that the history of rickets has supplied us with concerning the transformation of cartilage. The tumour which affected the superior and inferior maxillæ, but each separately, has such little density, that it can be cut with great facility, and only in a few places does the knife meet with greater resistance. On making thin sections, we see, even with the naked eye, that the more and less dense portions alternate with each other, so that the whole has a reticular appearance. When examined under the microscope with a low power,

FIG. 131.

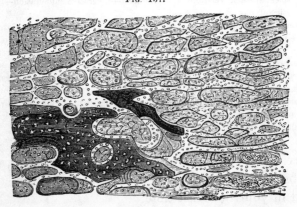

Fig. 131. Section from the soft osteoma from the jaw of a goat—showing the characters of periosteal ossification. Networks of osteoid trabeculæ with jagged cells enclose primary medullary spaces, filled with fibrous connective tissue. The dark parts represent calcified and completely developed osseous tissue. 150 diameters.

it is at once perceived that the disposition of the constituent parts is entirely that of a bone, for (primary*) medullary spaces and trabecular networks alternate with each other, just as if the observer had before him the medullary spaces and trabeculæ of a spongy bone. The substance which forms the trabecular networks, is on the whole dense, and is therefore readily distinguishable, even with a low power, from the more delicate substance which is enclosed by the trabeculæ and fills the cavities of the meshes. This latter substance presents, when more highly magnified, a finely striated fibrous appearance. The bands of fibres in part run parallel to the borders of the trabeculæ. In these latter the same structures can be seen with a high power, that are usually presented by the bone, namely jagged corpuscles, distributed with great regularity.

This structure exactly corresponds to that which we have seen in the development of bone from periosteum ; it is, in short, the plan followed in the growth of bone in thickness. Wherever young periosteal deposits are examined, there is found in the meshes of the network, formed by the osteoid substance, this primary marrow containing fibres, but no cells, as is the case at a later period. This primary marrow consists of the remains of the periosteum itself (after its proliferation), which have not yet undergone the transformation. The transformation into osteoid tissue advances into the proliferating periosteum in the first instance always in such a way,

---

* The *primary* medullary spaces formed out of *periosteum* are subsequently all filled with compact bone, and it is by the conversion of this into true mucous medullary tissue, abounding in cells (which afterwards take up fat) that the *secondary* medullary spaces are formed. Of the primary medullary spaces formed out of *cartilage*, however, a considerable number do not pass through any such intermediate stage as that just described as occurring in periosteal ossification, but become *at once* filled with true medullary tissue and are therefore equivalent to the ordinary, *secondary* medullary spaces.—*From a MS. Note by the Author.*

that the fibrous tissue becomes condensed (sclerotic),
though only partially so, the condensation beginning at
the bone and proceeding outwards in certain directions ;
in this way there arise, at first resting like columns upon
the bone, hardish cones * which are united by transverse
bands, parallel to the surface of the bone, and thus con-

Fɪɢ. 132.

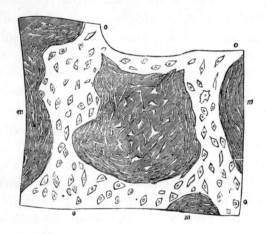

stitute this network. If now acetic acid be applied to
these parts, we see at once that the whole fibrous mass
which fills the alveoli, contains the most wonderful connective-tissue-corpuscles, which are so arranged, that
next to the trabeculæ all around they lie in concentric
rows, whilst in the most internal parts of the marrow
they constitute stellate corpuscles which anastomose with
one another, as you have already seen on many occasions.
But that in some parts the trabeculæ have already
become true bone, one may very beautifully convince

Fig. 132. A portion of Fig. 131, more highly magnified. o, o. The osteoid trabeculæ ; m, m, m the primary medullary spaces with spindle-shaped and reticulating
cells. 300 diameters.

* These are the little columns mentioned in p. 110 as being perpendicular to the
long axis of the bone, and as intervening between the Haversian system—*Transl.*

oneself at the spots, where calcareous salts are really deposited in them. Whilst the periphery of such calcified trabeculæ (Fig. 131) offers a brilliant, almost cartilaginous appearance, in their middle an opaque, finely granular matter presents itself which pervades the intercellular substance, and towards the interior of the trabeculæ passes into a nearly homogeneous, calcareous layer, in which at intervals the osseous corpuscles may be recognized. Here we have therefore already a complete osseous network, and at the same time an exact picture of the regular growth of bone in thickness.

If, however, the spots are very carefully examined, where the borders of these trabeculæ and bands of bone come into contact with the fibrous substance of the meshes, it is seen that no perfectly defined limit exists there, but that the intercellular substance of the osteoid tissue is gradually lost in the intercellular substance of the fibrous marrow, so that here and there a few of the connective-tissue-corpuscles of the fibrous connective tissue are included in the sclerotic substance of the trabeculæ. Hence you may infer, that the formation of the real osseous substance from connective tissue is essentially effected by the gradual change of the intercellular substance, and that this loses its originally fibrous nature and becomes converted into a dense, shining, cartilaginous mass, without its ever really attaining however to the structure of cartilage. Here there is never a stage exactly corresponding to any of the known forms of cartilage, but it is out of connective tissue that we see the osteoid substance directly arise, which in cartilage also and marrow is the first to arise when they become bone. This is so far very important, that you can from all these instances acquire the conviction that people have been mistaken in speaking of the cartilage of bone (Knochenknorpel). Cartilage as such can only calcify ; when it is to become bone, a transformation of its tissue must take place, the chondrine-containing basis-substance must become converted into a gelatine-yielding intercellular substance.

I have, moreover, gentlemen, made a series of preparations from ricketty bones for you—on the one hand, because rickets above all offers an especially favourable opportunity for obtaining an insight into several processes of the normal growth of bone, which in other cases are obscured by the presence of calcareous salts—and on the other hand, because you will thus form some idea of the peculiarity of this process, as such.

Rhachitis, has, as you are aware, by more accurate investigation been shown to consist not in a process of softening in the old bone, as it had previously generally been considered to be, but in the non-solidification of the fresh layers as they form ; the old layers being consumed by the normally progressive formation of medullary cavities, and the new ones remaining soft, the bone becomes brittle. But besides this essential feature of the non-occurrence of calcification in the parts, there is displayed also a certain irregularity in growth, so that stages in the development of bone which, when the formation is normal, ought to set in late, set in at a very early period. In normal growth, the pointed processes, in which shape the calcareous salts shoot up into the cartilage, form, along the margin of calcification, such a completely straight line, that it should almost be described as mathematically regular. This condition ceases to obtain in rickets, and the more so, the greater the severity of the case ; interruptions occur in such a way, that in some places the cartilage still reaches a long way down, whilst in others the calcification has mounted up to a considerable height. These uncalcified parts sometimes become so completely separated from one another, that they remain forming specks of cartilage in the midst of the bone, and surrounded on all sides by it—and that cartilage is still found at points where the bone ought long since to have become transformed into medullary tissue. The farther the process advances, the more, however, do we also meet with isolated, scattered masses of lime in the cartilage, in many instances to such a degree, that the whole of the cartilage on section appears dotted with white points. The irregularity of the process is further shown in this, that whilst in the normal course of things the medullary spaces should begin to form only at a short distance behind the margin of calcifiation (Fig. 126), they here exceed these limits, and in many cases a series of connective cavities extends far beyond the border of calcification, which are filled with a soft, slightly fibrous tissue, and besides have vessels running up into them. Medullary spaces and vessels are therefore met with, where normally and properly not a single medullary cell, and scarcely a single vessel ought to be found.

In this manner there may at all times be found side by side in the parts, where the process has attained its height, a whole series of different histological conditions. Whilst in other cases we find at a certain definite point cartilage, at another calcification, at a third, bone, or medullary tissue, here everything lies in the greatest confusion; in one place, medullary tissue, above it osteoid tissue, or bone, by its side calcified cartilage, and below it, perhaps, cartilage still retaining its original condition. The whole of the rhachitic portion of the diaphysal cartilage—and it may extend for a considerable distance—of course acquires no real firmness, and this is one of the chief causes of the liability to distortion, which ricketty bones exhibit, not in the continuity of the diaphyses, but at the articular ends. This is in many cases extremely considerable and is the sole cause of many a deformity, as, for example, in the thorax. The curvatures in the continuity of the

bones are always infractions,* those of the epiphyses are
due to the proliferation of the cartilage and constitute
simple inflexions; and it is easy to conceive that parts,
which are so entirely deprived of their regular development (as they are in rickets), and ought, properly, to be
densely impregnated with calcareous salts, must retain
great mobility.

FIG. 133.

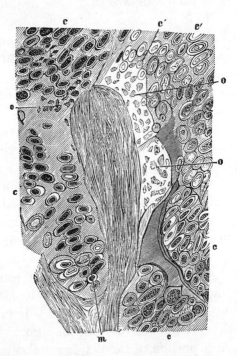

Fig. 133. Vertical section of cartilage from the diaphysis of a ricketty, growing
tibia from a child two years old. A large conical process of medullary tissue, sending out a lateral band on the left side, extends from *m* up into the cartilage; it consists of fibrous basis-substance with spindle-shaped cells. At the circumference, at
c, c, c the cartilage in a state of proliferation with large cells and groups of cells;
at *c′, c′* commencing thickening and internal indentation of the cartilage-capsules
which at *o, o* coalesce and form osteoid tissue. 300 diameters.

* By infraction I understand an incomplete fracture (solution of continuity) *within*
the periosteum, which remains intact.—*From a MS. Note by the Author.*

The enlargement and multiplication of the individual cells takes place in the same manner, as in the cases we have already considered ; but inasmuch as at a later period individual parts in the cartilages, that properly ought to have become bone, do not calcify, and especially a formation of medullary spaces often takes place a long way up above the border of calcification—in many of these rhachitic parts the whole history of the development of bone is clearly revealed in a connected form. Large and often very vascular conical processes of fibrous medullary tissue are seen extending upwards from the bone into the cartilage, and it may be very distinctly perceived, that these processes do not force their way into the cartilage from without, but that they owe their origin to a fibrillation of the intercellular substance of the cartilage itself. It is around them chiefly that the osteoid transformation of cartilage also can best be seen, and particularly that the gradual conversion of a cartilage-corpuscle into a bone-corpuscle can very distinctly be witnessed. Out of the cartilage-corpuscle which has a moderately thick capsular membrane, arises a structure, provided with a capsule continually increasing in thickness, within which the space for the cell constantly grows smaller, and which, when it has attained a certain degree of thickness, acquires indentations on its inner wall, like the so-called dotted canals of vegetable cells. Such is the mode in which the first rudiments of the bone-corpuscle are traced, after which a fusion of the capsule with the basis-substance very generally ensues, and with the production of anastomosing processes from the cells the formation of the bone-corpuscle is completed. At times isolated osteoid cartilage-corpuscles calcify alone without the occurrence of any fusion ; and whilst between them lies the ordinary intercellular substance of cartilage, the capsules of the osteoid corpuscles fill themselves completely with calcareous salts. In other places on the contrary the fusion of the capsules with the intercellular substance takes place very rapidly ; the new intercellular substance formed by this fusion assumes a coarsely fibrous appearance, and in the place of several groups of cartilage-cells we see a fibrous mass, containing jagged osseous (bone-), or osteoid corpuscles. There is therefore no sharply defined boundary in the tissue, but the condensed or fibrous substance, which surrounds the jagged bodies, is directly continuous with the translucent substance which holds the cartilage together. Essentially, however, it is the same structure.*

This isolated transformation of single cartilage-cells into bone corpuscles is obviously of the greatest impor-

Fig. 134.

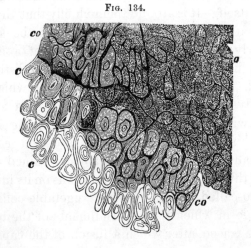

Fig. 134. Insular ossification in ricketty diaphysal cartilage. *c, c.* Ordinary growing (proliferating) cartilage, *c'*, increasing thickening of the capsules with formation of an indented cavity (osteoid cartilage-cells), *co'*, calcification of similar, still isolated cartilage-cells, *co*, commencing fusion of the capsules of calcified cartilage-cells, *o*, osseous substance. 300 diameters. (Cf. Archiv. f. path. Anat., Vol. XIV., Plate I.

* The following section, including the history of the formation of callus, has been transferred to this place from the next lecture, inasmuch as a better understanding of it is thus insured.

tance to the cellular theory in general. In this specimen (Fig. 134) the whole series of these processes is
seen at a glance. Where the completely ossified portion, in which the bone-corpuscles are developed with
perfect regularity, adjoins the cartilage, you see a zone
where the conversion of cartilage-corpuscles into perfect
osseous substance may be viewed within the limits of a
very short space. At the point of transition a number
of corpuscles are found lying close to one another like
hazel-nuts—distinguished from ordinary cartilage-corpuscles by their dark contours, hard appearance, and
unusually great brilliancy, and enclosing in a small,
indented cavity a little cell; these little cells are the
still isolated* bone-corpuscles with calcified capsules
which they have retained from that earlier period in
their existence when they were cartilage-cells. It is
especially important that you should see these bodies
thus isolated—in situ, in order that you may comprehend those other processes, in which in bone the terri-
tories† belonging to the bone-cells fall out (p. 462, Fig.
129). When an object of this kind has once been accurately examined, it is impossible that doubts can any
longer arise as to whether cartilage-cells can become
bone-corpuscles, and I cannot conceive how it is that
even the most recent (and those very careful) observers
still start the question, whether bone-corpuscles are not
in all cases structures obtained by a circuitous route, and
not directly produced from cartilage-corpuscles. It is

* Isolated, because their capsules have not yet become fused with the basis-substance.—*From a MS. Note by the Author.*

† In bone formed *directly* (i. e., without the intervention of medullary tissue) out
of cartilage, the territories of the bone-cells correspond to the cartilage-capsules.
But when bone is developed out of any other tissue, the limits of these territories
cannot be distinguished at all during growth, and it is only when gaps arise (through
disease) in the bone around the bone-cells that these limits are defined.—*From a
MS. Note by the Author.*

no doubt true, that in the case of the normal growth in length of bone most of the bone-corpuscles do not directly proceed from cartilage-corpuscles, but are immediately derived from marrow-cells and only mediately from cartilage-cells ; but it is just as true that cartilage-cells also can be transformed straightway into bone-corpuscles. It is now a long time since I called attention to one spot in particular, where the conversion of cartilage into osteoid tissue can be very distinctly viewed, namely at the points of transition from cartilage to perichondrium in the neighbourhood of the border of calcification of growing bones. Here the boundaries between the different forms of tissue are completely obliterated, and all sorts of transitions between round (cartilaginous) and jagged (osteoid) cells are seen.

The next preparations have reference to the *pathological new formation of bone*, or, if you will, to the *physiological formation of callus*. They are derived from a very recent fracture of the ribs, around which a thick mass of callus has been deposited. In reference to this process I will add a few words, as it is one that has been much discussed and is very important in a surgical point of view.

You have seen from what I have just been describing to you, that there are several ways in which the new formation of bone is effected, and that the old supposition that either the one or the other mode must be considered as the only prevailing one, is incorrect. The pre-existence of cartilage is by no means necessary for the formation of bone ; on the contrary, an osteoid substance is very frequently formed by a direct sclerosis in connective tissue, nay, ossification is thus really more easily effected than when it takes place in real cartilage. We see also by the history of the theories concerning callus, that the endeavour to show that it is always developed in the same way or out of the same substance (*e. g.* extravasated blood, periosteum, medullary tissue, exuded fluids, etc.) has proved the greatest obstacle to the true perception of the real state of things, and that all have really had right upon their side, inasmuch as new bone in fact builds itself up out of the most different materials. Unquestionably, when the case runs a very favourable course, that path is chosen in which the new formation can be most conveniently effected, and it is by far the most convenient way, when the periosteum produces a very large portion of the whole. This takes place in the following manner : the periosteum grows dense towards the edges of the fracture, and there gradually swells up, the swelling being of such a nature, that separate layers or strata can afterwards pretty clearly be distinguished in it. These continually become thicker and more numerous, in consequence of the constant proliferation of the innermost parts of the periosteum—and of the formation, by means of a multiplication of their cellular elements, of new layers, which accumulate between the bone and the relatively still normal parts of the periosteum. These layers may become cartilage, but it is not necessary, nor yet the rule. For we find that, in the greater number of favourable cases of fracture, where cartilage is produced, not the whole mass of the periosteal callus is produced from cartilage, but a greater or less portion of it is always formed out of connective tissue. The layers of cartilage generally lie next to the bone, whilst the farther we proceed outwards, the less does the formation out of cartilage, and the more a direct transformation of connective tissue, prevail.

The formation of bone is, however, by no means restricted to the limits of the periosteum—very commonly it extends beyond them in an outward direction,

and often penetrates, in the form of spicula, nodules,
and protuberances, to a very considerable depth into
the neighbouring soft parts. It is self-evident that in
these cases we have by no means to deal with any proliferation of the periosteum in any outward direction, but
that an ossifiable tissue arises out of the interstitial connective tissue of the neighbouring parts. Of this it is
very easy to convince oneself, because osseous spicula
are found shooting up in the interstitial tissue of the
neighbouring muscles. In the preparation from the
fractured ribs places are still to be found in the external

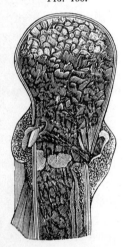

FIG. 135.

parts, where fat has been included
in the ossification. It cannot be said
therefore that the formation of callus
around fractured parts is altogether
a periosteal formation; in all cases
where it takes place with a certain
abundance, it transgresses the limits
of the periosteum, and invades the
connective tissue of the surrounding
soft parts.

There is a second kind of callus-
formation completely different to
this — that namely, which takes
place in the midst of the bone *from
the medullary tissue*.

At the moment when the bone in a case of fracture

Fig. 135. Transverse fracture of the humerus with formation of callus, about
fourteen days old. On the outside is seen the porous capsule of the callus produced from the periosteum and soft parts, the innermost layer on the right side
being still cartilaginous. On the left lies detached a fragment shivered off from
the cortex of the bone. The two fractured ends are connected by a (dark-red)
fibrinous layer of hæmorrhagic origin; the medulla on both sides is very dark
(owing to hyperæmia and extravasation), in the lower fragment several porous
islands of callus are seen which have been produced by the ossification of the
medulla.

is shivered, a number of little medullary spaces are naturally opened. In the neighbourhood of these, the still closed medullary spaces are seen nearly invariably, when matters follow a regular course, to become filled with callus, new lamellæ of bone attaching themselves to the internal surface of the osseus trabeculæ which bound the spaces, just as in the ordinary growth of bone in thickness, the originally pumicestone-like layers become compact by the deposition of concentric lamellæ. In this manner it happens, that after some time a larger or smaller new layer of bone is found, filling up the end of the medullary canal of each fragment, so as to occasion its occlusion. This is a kind of a new formation which has nothing in common with the former one, as far as their starting points are concerned, but has its origin in quite another tissue, and is altogether different in its palpable result, inasmuch as it produces, within the confines of its own bone, a condensation of that portion of the marrow which lies in the immediate vicinity of the fracture. Even in cases where the ends of the bones perfectly coincide, an internal formation of bone such as I have described takes place in the medullary canal of each fragment, producing its occlusion.

These two kinds are the usual and normal ones. Around the two fractured ends the swelling takes place, in the interior, the condensation. Gradually, in proportion as the extravasated blood is absorbed—the new masses of tissue which have been developed between the broken ends draw nearer to one another, and round about the fracture forms a bridge- or capsule-like communication by means of the ossification of the soft parts. There is therefore but little reason to ask whether the callus proceeds from free exuded or extravasated matter. No doubt an extravasation takes place in the first instance into the space between the fractured ends, but the extravasated blood is generally pretty completely reabsorbed, and it contributes comparatively but very little to the real formation of the subsequent uniting media.

We discussed, gentlemen, last time, the chief points in the history of new-formations. You remember that, according to our ideas, every kind of new-formation—inasmuch as it has its origin in pre-existing cellular elements and takes their place—must necessarily be connected with a change in the given part of the body. It is no longer possible to defend an hypothesis such as that which, based upon the supposed existence of plastic matters, was formerly maintained, namely, that a substance was deposited *between and upon* the existing elements of the body, which produced a new tissue out of itself and thus represented a clear accession to the body. If it is true that every new-formation proceeds from definite elements, and that usually divisions of the cells are the means by which the new-formation is produced, it becomes of course self-evident that *where a new-formation takes place, certain histological elements of the body must generally also cease to exist*. Even a cell, which simply divides and out of itself produces two new cells like itself, thereby ceases to exist, even though the whole result is only the apparent apposition of a cell. This holds good for all kinds of new-formations, both for benignant as well as for malignant ones, and it may therefore in a certain sense be said, that *every kind of new-formation is really destructive, and that it destroys something of what previously existed*. But we are, as it is well-known, accustomed to judge of destruction according to the more obvious effects produced, and when we speak of destructive formations, we do not so much mean those, in which the result of the new-formation is analogous to the old one, as some product or other deviating more or less from the original type of the part. This is the point of view to which I have already (p. 93) directed your attention when treating of the classification of pathological new-formations. By it is a reason, sensible and in correspondence with the facts, afforded for the separation of *all new-formations into homologous and heterologous ones.*

Heterologous we may call not only malignant, degenerative neoplasms, but we must also thus designate every tissue which deviates from the recognized type of the part, whilst we should call all that homologous, which, although new-formed, still reproduces the type of its parent soil. We find, for example, that the so extremely common form of uterine tumour, which has been designated fibrous or fibroid, has in every respect the same structure that the walls of the "hypertrophied" uterus have, inasmuch as it consists not only of fibrous connective tissue and vessels, but also of muscular fibre-cells. The tumour may, as it is well-known, become so large, as not only to embarrass the uterus in all its functions in an extreme degree, but also to exercise through pressure the most injurious influence upon the neighbouring parts. In spite of this, it must always be considered an homologous structure. On the other hand we cannot help employing the term heterologous formation, as soon as, by means of a process which at first seems to represent a simple multiplication of the parts, a result is obtained which is essentially different from the original condition of the spot. A catarrh for example in its simple form may be attended by a multiplication of the cellular elements on the surface of the mucous membrane, without the new cells' being essentially different from the pre-existing ones. Thus I brought along with me for you last time a vagina

with very marked leucorrhœa. You saw there no
doubt that the cells in leucorrhœa very closely resemble
those of epithelium of the part, although they no longer
entirely retain the typical form of pavement epithelium.
The less, however, they approach in their development
the typical forms of the epithelium of the part, the more
incapable do they become of performing their functions.
They are moveable upon a surface, to which they ought
properly to adhere, they flow down* and produce results which are incompatible with the integrity of the
parts.

In the narrower sense of the word heterologous new-
formations are no doubt alone destructive. The homologous ones may accidentally bec ome veryinjurious, but
still they do not possess what can properly be called a
destructive (in the unscientific and traditional sense of
the word), or malignant character. On the other hand
every kind of heterologous formation, whenever it has
not its seat in the entirely superficial parts, has a certain
degree of malignity clinging to it. And even superficial
affections, though entirely confined to the most external
layers of epithelium, may gradually exercise a very
prejudicial influence. Let us only reflect what happens
when a large surface of mucous membrane continually
secretes, and heterologous products are constantly engendered upon it which do not become persistent epithelium,
but continually keep flowing down from the surface of
the mucous membrane. In such a case, in addition to
the blennorrhœa (and its consequences, anæmia, neural-
gia, etc.), we find erosions.

It seems to me important that I should bring before
you a definite example of the mode in which destruction
in its more obvious forms is effected, in order that you

---

* Καταρρέω (catarrh).

may see how it leads to ulceration and to the formation of cavities in the interior of parts. It does indeed appear like a contradiction to say that a process, which produces new elements, destroys, but this contradiction nevertheless is merely a seeming one. If you imagine in a part, which had previously been firm, a new-formation to arise of which the individual constituents are loose and easily moveable one upon the other, the process will of course always be attended by a very important change in the usefulness of the part. The simple conversion of bone into medullary tissue (pp. 452, 453) may become the cause of great fragility in the bones, and *osteomalacia* [mollities ossium] essentially depends upon nothing else than the conversion of compact osseous substance into medullary tissue. An excessive formation of medullary spaces gradually advances from the interior of the bone towards the surface, deprives the bone of its firmness, gives rise to a tissue in itself quite normal, but of no service in maintaining the necessary firmness of the parts, and thus in some sort inevitably leads to a loss of cohesion. Marrow is an extraordinarily soft tissue, which in those conditions, where it is red and rich in cell, or atrophied and gelatinous, becomes nearly fluid. From marrow to perfectly fluid tissues is only a short step, and the boundaries separating marrow and pus cannot in many places be assigned with any degree of certainty. Pus is in our eyes a young tissue, in which, amidst the rapid development of cells, all solid intercellular substance is gradually dissolved. A single connective-tissue cell may in an extremely short space of time produce some dozens of pus-cells, for the development of pus follows an extremely hurried course. But the result is of no service to the body, *proliferation becomes luxuriation.* Suppuration is a pure process of luxuriation, by means of which

superfluous parts are produced, which do not acquire
that degree of consolidation, or permanent connection
with one another and with the neighbouring parts, which
is necessary for the existence of the body.

If now in the next place we investigate the *history of
suppuration*, we immediately discover that we must distinguish two different modes of pus-formation, according
namely as the pus proceeds from tissues of the first two
kinds mentioned in our classification (p. 55),
i. e., *from epithelium or from connective*
tissue. Whether there are also forms of
suppuration proceeding from a tissue of the
third class, from muscles, nerves, vessels,
etc., is at least doubtful, because of course
the elements of connective tissue which
enter into the composition of the larger
vessels, the muscles and the nerves, must
be eliminated from the really muscular, nervous and vascular (capillary) elements. With this reservation we can for the present only maintain the possibility of two modes of pus-formation.

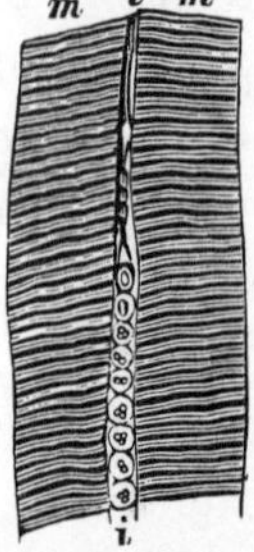

As long as the pus is formed out of epithelium, it is
naturally produced without any considerable loss of substance and without ulceration. But this is in every
instance the case, where pus is produced in connective
tissue. The real state of the matter therefore is exactly
the reverse of what it was previously imagined to be,
when a solvent property was ascribed to pus. *Pus is not
the dissolving, but the dissolved, i. e., the transformed, tissue.*
A part becomes soft, and liquefies whilst suppurating,
but it is not the pus which occasions this softening, on

FIG. 136.

Fig. 136. Interstitial purulent inflammation of muscle in a puerperal woman.
m, m. Primitive muscular fibres. *i, i.* Development of pus-corpuscles by means of
the proliferation of the corpuscles of the interstitial connective tissue. 280 diameters.

the contrary, it is the pus which is produced as the result of the proliferation of the tissue.

The development of pus we daily see upon different surfaces, both on the skin, and on mucous and serous membranes. We can observe its development most surely where stratified epithelium naturally exists. If you follow the development of pus upon the *skin*, when the process is unaccompanied by ulceration, you will constantly see that the suppuration proceeds from the rete Malpighii. It consists in a growth and development of new cells in this part of the cuticle. In proportion as these cells proliferate, a separation of the harder layers of the epidermis ensues, and they are lifted up in the form of a vesicle or pustule. The place where the suppuration chiefly occurs corresponds to the superficial layers of the rete, which are already in process of conversion into epithelium ; if the membrane of the vesicle be stripped off, these (layers) usually adhere to the epidermis and are stripped off with it. In the deeper layers we may watch how the cellular elements, which originally have only a single nuclei, divide, how the nuclei become more abundant, and single cells have their places taken by several, which in their turn again provide themselves with dividing nuclei. Here too people have generally helped themselves out of the difficulty by assuming that in the first instance an exudation was poured out, which produced the pus in itself, and this is the reason why, as you well know, most investigators into the development of pus especially selected fluids which were secreted from injured surfaces. It was very conceivable that, as long as no doubts were entertained with regard to the discontinuous formation of cells, the young cells should without more ado be looked upon as independent new-formations, and that the notion should be entertained that germs arose in the exuded fluids, and gradually becoming more numerous, supplied the pus. But the matter is on this wise, that, the longer the suppuration lasts, the more certainly is one series of cells after the other in the rete involved in the process of proliferation, and that, whilst the vesicle is rising up, the quantity of the cells which grow into its cavity is constantly becoming greater. When a variolous pustule forms, there is at first only a drop of clear fluid present, but nothing arises in it; it only loosens the neighbouring parts of the rete Malpighii.

Precisely the same is the case with *mucous membranes*. There is not a single mucous membrane which may not under certain circumstances furnish puriform elements. But here too a certain difference always presents itself. A mucous membrane is all the more in a condition to produce pus without ulceration, the more completely the epithelium it possesses is stratified. All mucous membranes with a single layer of cylindrical epithelium (intestines),* are much less adapted for the production of pus; that which is produced on them, even though it have quite the appearance of pus, frequently turns out upon close examination to be only epithelium. The intestinal mucous membrane, especially that of the small intestine, scarcely ever produces pus without ulceration. The mucous membrane of the uterus, and of the fallopian tubes, though it is frequently covered with a thick mass of quite a puriform appearance, almost always secretes †

---

* In the air passages (nose, larynx, trachea, bronchi) we commonly find several layers of cylindrical epithelium lying one above the other.—*From a MS. Note by the Author.*

† *Secrete* in this and similar places does not of course mean to separate from the *blood*, but from the *tissue itself*, whose elements (cells) are *separated* (detached) at the surface, and, when mixed with the serous effusion from the blood, **removed**. The detachment of the cells is effected sometimes by means of the fluid which transudes from the blood, sometimes by the continual growth of a succession of new cells beneath them, and sometimes in consequence of their own round form. In desquamation of the cuticle the second of these methods, in several forms of catarrh the

epithelial cells only, whilst on the other mucous membranes, as for example on that of the urethra, we see enormous quantities of pus secreted, as in gonorrhœa (Fig. 63) without even the slightest ulceration being present on the surface. This depends essentially upon the presence of several strata of cells, the upper forming a kind of protection to the deeper ones, of which the proliferation is thus for a time secured. The pus is at last either borne away by the production of new masses of pus beneath it, or there occurs simultaneously a transudation of fluid, which removes the pus-cells from the surface, just as in the secretion of semen the epithelial elements of the seminal tubules furnish the spermatozoa, and in addition a fluid transudes which sweeps them away. But the spermatozoa do not arise in the fluid—this is only the vehicle for their onward movement. In this manner we frequently see fluid exude on the surface of the body, without our being able to regard it as a *cyto*blastema. If a proliferation of epithelium simultaneously takes place upon the surface, the elements detached by the transuded fluid will also be found to consist of nothing but proliferating epithelium.

If now *pus-*, *mucus-* and *epithelial cells* be compared with one another, it appears that there certainly does exist a series of transitional forms, or intermediate stages, between pus-corpuscles and the ordinary epithelial structures. By the side of perfectly formed pus-corpuscles, provided with several nuclei, are very commonly found somewhat larger, round, granular cells with single nuclei, the so-called mucus-corpuscles (Fig. 11 *B*) ; a little further on we see perhaps still larger cells of a typical form and with single, large nuclei, and these we call epithelial cells. But the epithelial cells are flat, angular, or cylindrical,

third, on many serous membranes, the first, is the one pursued. Any two, or all three of them, however, may of course coincide.—*From a MS. Note by the Author.*

whilst mucus- and pus-corpuscles under all circumstances remain round. Even from this circumstance may be derived an explanation of the fact that, whilst the epithelial cells, which cover, and are in close apposition to, one another, acquire a certain firmness of cohesion, mucus- and pus-corpuscles which lie but loosely one against the other, and are of a spherical shape, retain a great degree of mobility and are easily displaced.

It has been said before now that mucus-corpuscles are nothing more than young epithelium ; another step and pus-corpuscles would be nothing more than young mucus-corpuscles. This is a somewhat erroneous notion. It cannot be maintained that a cell, which up to the point when it becomes a so-called mucus corpuscle has preserved its form as a spherical body, is still in a condition to assume the typical form of the epithelium, which ought to exist in the part ; and just as little can it be said that a pus-corpuscle, after it has developed itself in the regular manner, is capable of again entering upon a course of development calculated to produce a relatively permanent element of the body. The cells, in which the development of epithelial, mucus-, and pus-cells originates, are young forms, but they are not pus-corpuscles. In pus every new cell at a very early period sets about dividing its nucleus ; after a short time the division of the nucleus reaches a high pitch, without any further growth on the part of the cell. In mucus the cells are wont merely to grow, and in some instances to become very large, but they do not pass certain limits, and above all they do not assume any typical form. In epithelium, on the contrary, the elements begin even at a very early period, to assume their particular form, for " what is to become a hook, right early gets a crook." The very youngest elements however, which are found in pathological conditions, cannot be called epithelial cells, or at least they have as yet nothing typical about them, but are indifferent formative cells, which might also become mucus- or pus-corpuscles. Pus-, mucus- and epithelial cells are therefore pathologically equivalent parts which may indeed replace one another, but cannot perform each other's functions.

Even from this it follows that the distinction which it has been sought to establish between mucus- and pus-corpuscles, and for the discovery of which prizes were proposed in the last century, really could not be found out, and that the " tests " could never be otherwise than insufficient, inasmuch as the cells developed upon mucous membranes do not always possess a purely purulent, purely mucous, or purely epithelial character, but on the contrary in a great majority of cases a mixed condition exists. Nearly always, when a catarrhal process developes itself upon a large mucous surface, as, for example, in the urinary passages, quantities of puriform matter are produced, but its production is confined within certain limits, beyond which only mucus is secreted, and the secretion of mucus also at some point changes into a formation of epithelium. This mode of suppuration must of course always have for its result, that, in places where it reaches a certain height, the natural coverings of the surface do not attain their full development, or that, where they possess a certain degree of solubility, they are removed and destroyed. A pustule on the skin destroys the epidermis, and so far we may assign a degenerative character to these forms of suppuration also.

But degeneration in the usual sense of the word, only occurs when deeper parts are attacked. This more deeply seated pus-formation regularly takes place in the *connective tissue*. In it there first occurs an enlargement of the cells (connective-tissue corpuscles), the nuclei divide and for some time multiply excessively. The first stage is then very soon followed by divisions of the cells themselves. Round about the irritated parts, where before single cells lay, pairs or groups of cells are subsequently found, out of which a new-formation of an homologous kind (connective tissue) usually constructs itself. More in the interior on the contrary, where the cells were early abundantly filled with nuclei, heaps of little cells soon appear, which at first still preserve the direction and forms of the previous connective-tissue corpuscles. Somewhat later we find here roundish collections, or diffuse "infiltrations," in which the intermediate tissue is extremely

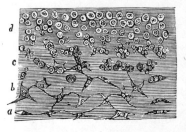

Fig. 137.

scanty and continually liquefies * more and more, in proliferation of the cells extends.

If this process takes place beneath a surface which does not participate in the morbid change, the layers of epithelium are sometimes seen, still perfectly coherent, to run over the irritated and somewhat swollen part. The outermost layer of the intercellular substance is also often long preserved, whilst all the deeper parts of the connective tissue are already filled with pus-corpuscles, are "infiltrated," or "absceded" † (abscedirt). At last the

---

Fig. 137. Purulent granulation from the subcutaneous tissue of a rabbit, round about a ligature. *a.* Connective-tissue corpuscles. *b.* Enlargement of the corpuscles with division of the nuclei. *c.* Division of the cells (granulation). *d,* Development of the pus-corpuscles. 300 diameters.

* This liquefaction (and the same is true of the liquefaction we have described as occurring in bone, p. 465) is a purely chemical process; the collagenous (gelatine-yielding) substance is first transformed into mucus, and then, becoming converted into an albuminous fluid, liquefies.—*From a MS. Note by the Author.*

† *I.e.*, converted into an abscess.—*Transl.*

surface gives way, or without giving way is directly transformed into a soft, diffluent mass. This mode of suppuration gradually yields the so-called *granulations* which always consist of a tissue, where, in a small quantity of soft intercellular substance, more or less numerous, and, at least in the strictly proliferating stage of the granulations, round, cellular elements are imbedded. The nearer we come to the surface, the more do the cells, which in the deeper parts were mostly uni-nucleated, present divisions in their nuclei, and on the extreme confines they can no longer be distinguished from pus-corpuscles. Then a detachment of the epithelium is wont to take place, and finally it may be that the basis-substance liquefies and the individual elements are set free. If the proliferation continues abundant, the mass keeps constantly breaking up, the cells pour themselves out upon the surface, and a destruction takes place, which makes deeper and deeper inroads into the tissue, and throws up more and more of its cells upon the surface. This is an *ulcer* properly so called.

According to the common notion, which supposed the pus to be derived from some exudation or other, this kind of ulceration was not at all easy of comprehension ; people always found themselves obliged to assume a special kind of transformation in the tissue in addition to the suppuration, and at last they went so far as to attribute a certain chemical solvent power to pus. But by surgical experiments the conviction has long since been acquired in the most manifold ways that pus has no solvent power. Bones have been placed in cavities full of pus and left there for weeks, and when they were afterwards weighed, they had if anything become heavier, through the absorption of fluid matters, but no softening had been produced excepting that occasioned by decomposition. How far the tissue is destroyed by real solution, chiefly depends upon whether the basis-substance which surrounds the young cells, becomes completely fluid. If it retains a certain degree of consistence, the process is confined to the production of granulations, and these may just as well proceed from a surface whose continuity is perfect, as from one where there is a breach of it. In surgery it is generally assumed that granulations form upon the walls of the breach occasioned by a loss of substance, but in every case they arise directly out of the tissue. They are found directly seated upon bone without any loss of substance in it having preceded them. They are found also in direct contact with the cutis under the intact epidermis, and with mucous membranes. Only in proportion as they become developed, do the mucous membranes lose their normal character.

Every development of the kind gives rise, as it proceeds, to separate masses (foci—Heerde) of new tissue, just in the same way indeed that growing cartilage produces, in the immediate vicinity of the margin of ossification, those large groups of cells (Fig. 124), each of which corresponds to a single pre-existing cartilage-cell. We have in fact to do with a process which finds its counterpart in the ordinary phenomena of growth. As a cartilage, when it does not calcify, as for example, in rickets, at last becomes so moveable that it can no longer perform its functions as a supporting structure, so we see everywhere that the firmness of a tissue gradually disappears through the development of granulations, and during suppuration. However different therefore these processes of destruction apparently are from the processes of growth, at a certain point nevertheless they entirely coincide. *There is a stage, when it is impossible to decide with certainty, whether we have in a part to deal with simple processes of growth, or with the development of a heteroplastic, destructive form.*

This mode of development, which I have just described to you, is not, however, in any way peculiar to pus alone, but characterizes every heteroplastic formation ; the first changes which we have shown to take place are found occurring in exactly the same manner in heteroplasms of every sort up to the most extreme and malignant forms. The first development of cancer, of cancroid and of sarcoma exhibits the same stages ; if

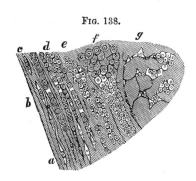

FIG. 138.

the course of their development be traced sufficiently far back, we at last always come across a stage, in which, in the younger and deeper layers, indifferent cells are met with, which do not until a later period, according to the particular nature of the irritation to which they are exposed, assume the one or the other type. We may therefore, taking new-formations in general, consider the history of the greater number, and especially of those which principally consist of cells, from an entirely similar point of view. The form of ulceration which is presented by cancer in its latest stages, bears so great a resemblance to its suppurative ulceration, that the two things have long since been compared, and quite in the olden time a parallel

Fig. 138. Development of cancer from connective-tissue in carcinoma of the breast. *a.* Connective-tissue corpuscles, *b*, division of the nuclei, *c*, division of the cells, *d*, accumulation of the cells in rows. *e*, enlargement of the young cells and formation of the groups of cells* (foci—Zellenheerde) which fill the alveoli of cancer, *f*, further enlargement of the cells and the groups. *g*. The same developmental process seen in transverse section. 300 diameters.

* When these groups of cells fall out, the alveoli (loculi) of cancer appear, the relation of the group to the alveolus being the same as that of the bone-cell to the lacuna.—*From a MS. Note by the Author.*

was drawn between the eroding form of suppuration, or chancre, and the "suppuration" or sanious ulceration* (Verjauchung) of cancer.

But there are essential differences between the individual species of new-formations in consequence of their elements' attaining to very different degrees of development, or to express myself otherwise, in consequence of the length of time their elements are calculated to last—*the average duration of the life of the individual elements*—being extremely different. We know, that if we examine a spot a month after suppuration has taken place in it, although the pus is apparently still present, we can no longer rely upon finding unaltered pus in the collection. Pus which has lain anywhere for weeks and months is, strictly speaking, no longer pus, but disintegrated matter, débris, dissolving particles of pus, which have become altered by fatty degeneration, putrefying processes, calcareous deposits and the like. On the contrary we find that a cancerous tumour may last for months, yet still contain the whole of its elements intact. We can therefore positively affirm, that a cancer-cell is capable of existing longer than a pus-corpuscle, just as we know that the thyroid body exists longer than the thymus gland, and that certain organs, for example individual parts of the sexual organs, early perish in the course of ordinary life, whilst others retain their existence throughout the whole of life. So it is also with pathological new-formations. At a time when certain forms have long since entered upon their course of retrogressive metamorphosis, others are just begin-

---

* Jauche (sanies) always conveys the idea of decomposition. We call Mist jauche the fluid obtained by the maceration of manure. Verjauchung is the process during which the substances are decomposed which subsequently furnish the Jauche. The French *putrilage* is nearly equivalent to Jauche in its pathological acceptation, only the latter is rather thinner and more liquid.—*From a MS. Note by the Author.*

ning to attain their full development. In the case of many new-formations, retrograde metamorphosis begins comparatively so early, nay constitutes to such a degree what is ordinarily met with, that the best investigators have looked upon its different stages as the really characteristic ones. In the case of tubercle, for example, we find that the majority of all modern observers who have made it their professed study, have taken its stage of retrograde metamorphosis for the real typical one, and that inferences have hence been drawn with regard to the nature of the whole process, which with equal right might have been drawn with regard to the different stages of the retrograde metamorphosis of pus and cancer.

We are as yet able in the case of very few elements to give in numbers with absolute certainty the average length of their life. There manifestly exist variations similar to those we meet with in normal organs. But among all pathological new-formations with fluid inter-cellular substance there is not a single one, which is able to preserve its existence for any length of time, not a single one, whose elements can become permanent constituents of the body, or exist as long as the individual. This may no doubt seem doubtful, because many forms of malignant tumours subsist for many years, and the individual retains them from the time of their development until his death, which may perhaps occur at a very advanced age. *But the tumour as a whole must be distinguished from its individual parts.* In a cancerous tumour which lasts for many years, the same elements do not last the whole time, but within its limits there occurs a frequently very numerous succession of fresh formations. The first development of a tumour takes place at a definite point, but its subsequent growth does not consist in the production of a

constant succession of new-formations from this point,
and in the occurrence there is an intus-susception (absorption) of material, by means of which the existing
parts enlarge and so the whole tumour grows. On the
contrary around the original focus* (Heerd), little new foci
are formed, which increasing in size, group themselves
around the first, and so gradually give rise to a continually
progressing enlargement of the existing tuber.† If the
tuber is seated on the surface, we find on section a semicir-
cular zone of the most recently formed matter, at its
periphery ; if it is in the middle of an organ, the newly
apposed foci form a spherical cortex around the older
centre. If we examine a tumour after it has existed
perhaps a year, it usually turns out that the elements first
formed no longer exist in the centre. There we find the
elements disintegrating, dissolved by fatty changes. If
the tumour is seated on a surface, it often presents in
the centre of its most prominent part a navel-shaped
depression, and the portions immediately under this
display a dense cicatrix which no longer bears the original character of the new-formation. These retrograde
forms I have described as occurring in cancer, especially
in the liver, lungs and intestines, where they are not
unfrequently met with, and can readily be demonstrated.

It is always possible to convince oneself, that, *what is
called a tumour, constitutes a conglomerate mass, often
extraordinarily large, made up of a number of little miliary foci* (lobules), of which every single one must be
referred to a single or a few parent elements. Inasmuch as the formations progress in this manner, no

---

* *Focus* here signifies the first rudiment of a tumour, produced by the proliferation of a limited group of cells. See note on Heerd, p. 381.—*From a MS. Note by
the Author.*

† Tuber = tuberous tumour. See note, p. 471.

matter whether they consist of pus, tubercle or cancer, new young zones are being constantly added on to the old ones, and we may, if we intend to trace the course of development, calculate with great certainty upon always finding the young parts at the extreme circumference, the old ones always in the centre. *But the zone produced at the latest period of the disease extends to a considerable distance beyond the zone of degeneration that can be discerned by the naked eye.* If we examine any proliferating tumour of a cellular character, we often find, three to five lines beyond its apparent limits, the tissues already in a state of disease, and exhibiting the first traces of a new zone. This is the chief source of local recurrence after extirpation, for it proceeds from the zone that cannot be detected by the naked eye, beginning to grow in consequence of the increased supply of nutritive material which results from the removal of the original tumour. No new deposit from the blood takes place there, but the new-formed germs, which already lie in the neighbouring tissue, run through their further development in the same manner that it would otherwise have taken place, or perhaps even still more quickly.

This fact I regard as extremely important, because it shows us that all these formations have essentially a *contagious character*. As long as it was imagined that the mass once formed increased only by the growth of its constituents, it would of course look as if all one had to do for the purpose of getting rid of it was merely to cut off from the tumour all further supply of material. But there is manifestly a contagious matter formed in the tumour itself, and when the cells, which are in its immediate neighbourhood and are connected by anastomoses with the diseased cells, likewise enter upon the heterologous proliferation, it is impossible, I think, to come to any other conclusion in the matter, than that the degeneration of the neighbouring parts arises in precisely the same manner as that of the nearest lymphatic glands which lie in the course of the stream of lymph which proceeds from the diseased part. The more anastomoses the parts possess, the more readily do they become diseased, and *vice versâ*. In cartilage malignant affections are so rare, that it is usually assumed to be altogether insusceptible of them. Thus in a joint the cartilaginous investment alone is sometimes found intact, whilst everything else has been destroyed. Thus too we see that fibrous parts which are rich in elastic elements, are very little disposed to become diseased by contagion. On the other hand, the softer a basis-substance is and the better the conveyance can take place, the more certainly we may expect, that, when occasion offers, new foci of disease will arise in the part. I have therefore come to the conclusion—the only one I think the facts warrant—that the infection is directly transferred by the means of the morbid juices from the original seat of the disease to the anastomosing elements in the neighbourhood, *without the intervention of vessels and nerves*. The nerves are indeed often the best conductors for the propagation of contagious newformations, only not as nerves, but as parts with soft interstitial tissue.

Here we have the importance of the anastomosing cellular elements of tissues, and the value of the cellular theory most clearly exhibited, and, when once we have become acquainted with this mode of conduction, we are afterwards able with a certain degree of probability to foresee in what direction, in parts possessing this means of conveyance, the disease will extend, and where finally the greater or less danger lies. It has hitherto been impossible to prove whether the infection of remote parts is effected by the conveyance of juices, in the same way that the infection of neighbouring parts is, and especially whether the blood takes up anything noxious from the diseased spot and conveys it to a distant place. I must confess that I am acquainted with no sufficiently convincing facts bearing upon the matter, and must still allow it to be possible that the diffusion by means of vessels may depend upon a dissemination of cells from the tumours themselves. There are, however, many facts, which speak but little in favour of the infection's taking place by means of really detached cells, for example, the circumstance that certain processes advance in a direction contrary to that of the current of lymph, so that after a cancer of the breast, disease of the liver takes place whilst the lung remains unaffected. Here it seems pretty probable that juices are taken up, which occasion a further propagation (p. 254).

Allow me still to add a few words upon a subject which can here be dispatched off hand, namely, the so-called *parasitism* of new-formations.

It is self-evident, that the view taken of parasitism by the old writers who held it to be applicable to a large proportion of new-formations, is completely borne out by facts, and that in reality every new-formation which contributes to the body no serviceable structures, must be regarded as a parasitical element in the body. Only bear in mind that the idea conveyed by parasitism does not differ from that conveyed by the autonomy of every part of the body excepting in degree, and that every single epithelial and muscular fibre-cell leads a sort of parasitical existence in relation to the rest of the body, just as much as every individual cell in a tree has in relation to the others a special existence, appertaining to itself alone, and deprives the remaining cells of certain matters. Parasitism in a narrower sense of the word, develops itself out of this idea of the independence of individual parts. As long as the requirements of the remaining parts demand the existence of a part, as long as this part is in any way useful to the other parts, so long will it not be termed a parasite ; but it becomes so from the moment that it becomes foreign or injurious to the body. The epithet, parasitical, must therefore not be restricted to a single class of tumours, but applies to all heteroplastic forms, which do not in the course of their further metamorphoses give rise to homologous products, but furnish neoplasms which in a greater or less degree are alien to the composition of the body. Every one of their elements will withdraw matters from the body which might be used for other purposes, and as it has at the very outset destroyed normal parts and even its first development presupposes the destruction of its parent structures it both plays a destructive part at the commencement of its career, and a depredatory one throughout its course.

LECTURE XX.

APRIL 27, 1858.

FORM AND NATURE OF PATHOLOGICAL NEW-FORMATIONS.

IF, gentlemen, we prosecute the train of thought which we have pursued in the last lectures, it seems to me that the question which you will perhaps next ask me, is, at what point the differentiation of new-formations really begins. You will remember that, according to our views the great majority of new-formations have their origin in connective tissue or parts equivalent to connective tissue, and that the first rudiments of all new-formations are nearly of the same nature, and that in particular the division of the nuclei, their multiplication, and the final

division of the cells show themselves in nearly all new-
formations, in the benignant as well as in the malignant,
in the hyperplastic as well as in the heteroplastic ones,
in the self-same manner. Unquestionably, however, this
similarity of nature is transitory ; it is not long before
some one characteristic feature displays itself in each individual structure, whereby we are enabled distinctly to
recognize its nature.

With regard to this question of the criteria of new-
formations, no agreement in opinion has indeed even at
the present moment been come to, and here too therefore it is incumbent upon me now to show how I have
arrived at my views, which in many respects so widely
differ from those generally held, and for what reasons I
have deemed myself obliged to quit the beaten track.

The names which have been bestowed upon individual
new-formations, have, as you know, often been based
pretty much upon accidental peculiarities, and not so very
unfrequently selected in quite an arbitrary manner. The
attempts to establish a regular nomenclature, which were
formerly made, were really only based upon the consistence of tumours, reasons for classification having been
derived from the circumstance that the substance of new-
formations was found to be sometimes hard, at others
soft, fluid, pultaceous, gelatinous, etc., and thus meliceris,
atheromata, steatomata, scirrhi, etc., were separated from
one another.   It is self-evident that the ideas which are
now attached to several of these things must be done
away with, if it be wished to understand the original
meaning of these designations. When the presence of
an atheromatous process is now-a-days spoken of, something is meant thereby of which the old observers were
far from having any idea.   When the tumour anatomists
of the present day labour hard to revive the name steatoma and would have it designate a firm fatty tumour,

you must remember that the manufacture of stearine was not known at the time when the term steatoma first came into use, and that the old observers never entertained the notion, which the tumour teachers of the present day cannot get out of their heads—that a steatoma* was a stearine- or indeed a fatty, tumour at all.

The improved nomenclature which was introduced at the commencement of this century, was based more upon comparisons which were instituted between the new-formations and individual parts or tissues of the body. The term "medullary fungus" (Markschwamm) originally arose out of the idea that medullary cancers originated in the nervès and resembled nervous matter in their composition. These comparisons have, however, until recently been always very arbitrary, because they were founded upon more or less rough resemblances in external appearance, without a due appreciation of the more delicate peculiarities of structure, and particularly of the really histological composition.

Recently attempts have been made, and here and there even with great affectation, to make use of normal structures as aids in terminology. Many attach a certain degree of importance to this, and consider it more scientific to say epithelioma, where others say cancroid or epithelial cancer. Thus in France great stress has, it is well known, been laid upon calling sarcomata fibro-plastic tumours, because Schwann and his followers looked upon caudate corpuscles as directly producing the fibres of connective tissue—which, in my opinion (p. 70), is an error. But in spite of these errors we must consider the histological point of view as the true one, only it is not, I think, advisable, in accordance with this principle, at once to proceed to create new names for everything, and

---

* The ancients called any firm tumour (e. g., an enchondroma) a steatoma.— *From a MS. Note by the Author.*

by means of these new names to render things which
have long been known strange to the minds of people in
general. Even new-formations which very evidently follow the type of some definite normal tissue, still for the
most part possess peculiarities, whereby they may be
more or less distinguished from this tissue, so that in the
majority of cases, at least, it is by no means necessary to
see the whole of the new-formation in order to know
that this is not the normal, regular development of the
tissue, but that on the contrary there is something in it,
although it does not lose the type, which deviates from
the ordinary course of homologous development. Besides there still remain even at the present time a certain
number of new-formations, the external appearance or
clinical character of which has, in part from the want of
known physiological types, been retained as the basis for
their names.

We still continue to speak of tubercle, and the name
which Fuchs has invented as a substitute, the only new
one, as far as I know, which it has been attempted to
introduce in its stead, Phyma, is so very indefinite, so
readily applicable to every "growth," that it has met
with no great favour. Several other names have been
recently used to a continually increasing extent, which
are also nothing more than stop-gags, as for example that
of Colloid. This name was invented at the commencement of the present century by Laennec to designate a
form of tumour which he described as analogous in consistence to half-set glue ; in its well-developed form it
constitutes a half-trembling gelly, colourless or of slightly
yellowish hue, which on the whole conveys the impression of a nearly complete absence of all structure. Whilst
people formerly declared themselves perfectly content,
when tumours of this kind were designated jelly-like, or
gelatinous, to many of the more recent observers it has

appeared a proof of superior penetration to say, instead of gelatinous tumour or gelatinous mass, colloid tumour or colloid mass. But you must not think that those, who have these denominations the most constantly in their mouths, intend to express anything else by them, than what most others call simply a jelly-like tumour, or only jelly. It is just the same with it, as, in the time of Homer, with the herb Μῶλυ, which was so called in the language of the gods, but by another name by men.* It is, however, very advisable, that these really unmeaning and only high-sounding expressions should not be unnecessarily diffused, and that the habit should be acquired of conveying a precise meaning by every expression, and that therefore from the moment one really aspires to make histological divisions, one should no longer employ, when speaking of every jelly-like tumour, the term colloid which has no histological value whatever, but merely designates an external appearance which tissues of the most different nature may under certain circumstances present. Laennec himself inaugurated the somewhat pernicious practice, by speaking of a colloid transformation of fibrinous exudations of the pleura.

The chief difficulty, which here presents itself, consists in this, that people do not know how to discover any difference between *the mere form and the true nature*. The form ought only to be admitted as a decisive criterion for the diagnosis of new-formations, when it is conjoined with a real difference in the tissue, and does not result from accidental peculiarities of situation or position. If, for example, you wish to make use of the name colloid, you can do so in two ways. You can either employ it to designate nothing more than a kind of appearance, and then you will certainly be able to find

---

* Odyss. X. 305. Note of the Stenograph.

different tumours which you can distinguish from other
tumours of the same genus by means of the addition
"colloid." You may therefore say : colloid cancer, colloid sarcoma, colloid fibroma [fibrous (connective-tissue)
tumour]. Here colloid means nothing more than jelly-
like. Or you must have a distinct notion of the nature,
of the chemical or physical peculiarities of the colloid
substance, or of the morphological nature of the colloid
tissue, and then it will be impossible for you to class
together two, chemically and morphologically, entirely
different products, such as the colloid of the thyroid body
and colloid cancer.

In just the same manner we see that a great number
of tumours, when they are seated on the surface, give
rise to excretions, which, according to the nature of the
surface, appear in the form of villi, papillæ or warts. All
these tumours may be comprised under one name and
called papillomata, but the tumours which have this form
often differ toto cœlo from one another. Whilst in the
one case we have a true hyperplastic development, we
find in another, at the base of these villi where they rest
upon the skin or mucous membrane, some specific form
of tumour. In many cases even the villi themselves are
filled with a substance analogous to that of the tumour.
This is a very important difference. If, for example, you
examine a *broad condyloma*, the mucous tubercle or
plaque muqueuse of Ricord, you will find, under the
epidermis which still remains smooth, the papillæ enlarging and ultimately growing out into branched figures so
as to represent regular trees. Cancer, however, may give
rise to excrescences of the same shape as these condylomata. This we see comparatively less frequently occur
on the skin than on the different mucous surfaces. In
these cases it may happen that real cancer is seated in
the villi. Nor is this in itself indeed at all surprising.

The papillæ consists of connective tissue like the skin, or the mucous membrane, upon which they are seated; within the papillæ therefore a cancerous mass may develop itself out of the connective tissue, as out of the connective tissue of the skin or mucous membrane. Moreover, it cannot be denied that this peculiarity of superficial formation very frequently explains certain peculiarities in the course of the disease, whereby a papillary tumour is strikingly distinguished from the same kind of tumour when not papillary. Any one may have a cancer of the bladder—if it be merely seated in the parietes—for a very long time, without any other changes being necessarily displayed in the nature of the secretion, which must be evacuated with the urine, than those exhibited in a simple catarrh. As soon, on the contrary, as a formation of villi takes place upon the surface, nothing is more common than for hematuria to arise as a complication, from the simple reason, that every villus upon the walls of the urinary bladder is not clothed with a firm layer of epidermis, but lies almost bare under a loose epithelial covering. Into the interior of the villi ascend large vascular loops which reach quite up to the surface, and therefore very considerable mechanical irritation supplies a condition for the production of hyperæmia and the rupture of the villi. A spasmodic contraction of the bladder drives the blood up into the apices of the villi, in consequence of the shortening of the surface on which they are seated, and when to this is added the mechanical friction of the surfaces, nothing is more likely to ensue than a sometimes more, sometimes less considerable effusion of blood. But in order that such hæmorrhage should take place it is altogether unnecessary that the papillary tumour should be cancerous. I have seen cases in which, for years, uncontrollable bleedings recurred from time to time, through which at last the

patients died anæmic, and yet no trace of any cancerous
infiltration of the base of the growth or of the villi existed, but the tumour was quite a simple papillary one, a
benignant formation, which on the surface of the skin
could easily have been removed by the knife or ligature,
but which, owing to its concealed position, was in these
cases attended with a series of phenomena, which during
life it seemed impossible to refer to anything else than a
really malignant new formation.

Just the same is the case with the much-discussed
cauliflower-tumours, as they are seen on the surface of the
genital organs, both in man and woman. In men, these
papillary tumours, which proceed from the prepuce and
surround the corona glandis, are for the most part covered
by a very thick layer of epidermis, so that, when they
ulcerate, they yield but a very trifling amount of secretion. In women, on the contrary, the tumour being
seated on the neck of the uterus—a very vascular part,
provided with a thin stratum of epithelium, and naturally beset with a thick layer of numerous and large
papillæ—for the most part very early occasions abundant transudations and occasionally hæmorrhagical exudations of a fluid, like water in which raw meat has been
soaked, or really red and bloody. In these cases there
frequently exists doubts as to the nature of the disease.
I myself was present when a very renowned surgeon
came to Dieffenbach's operating room, just as that ope-
rator had amputated a penis on account of a " carcinoma "
—and when the stranger afterwards declared it to have
been a simple condyloma. On the other hand I have
examined cases, in which growths of this sort had been
doctored about for years as if they had been syphilitic
condylomata, because the external appearance is so extremely analogous, and it is so extremely difficult to discover a criterion by which it can be accurately determined

whether the formation only involves the surface, or whether it is complicated with disease of the subjacent tissue. There are certainly at the present time very many anatomists and surgeons who entertain the notion that cells may grow on the surface exactly similar to those which are usually only found in the interior of diseased organs—that, for example, a villous tumour must be termed cancerous, if it is covered over with cancer-cells as with an epithelium, without any development of cancerous matter having shown itself in the interior of the villi. In fact, villi, which are very delicate and scarcely contain enough connective-tissue to envelop the vessels that run up in them, are sometimes met with, enclosed in a thick layer of cells which, from the irregularity of their form, the size of their nuclei, and their own large dimensions, present rather the character of cancer than that of epithelium. But I must confess that I have not as yet been able to convince myself that cancer-cells are able to arise upon the free surfaces of membranes, and that they can be produced simply from epithelium; on the contrary, I believe from all that I have seen, that a very strict line of demarcation must be drawn between the cases, where masses of cells, however abundant and curiously shaped they may be, are found seated upon a basis-tissue in itself unaltered, and those, where the cells have been formed in the parenchyma of the parts themselves.

The pathological importance of a papillary tumour is, at least as far as I know, determined by the condition of its basis-substance, or by that of the parenchyma of the villi themselves; and a formation can only be pronounced to be cancroid or carcinoma when, in addition to the growth of the surface, the peculiar degenerations which characterize these two kinds of tumours, take place also in the deeper layers or in the villi themselves. I think, therefore, that all these external differences of form can only serve to distinguish different species of the same genus of tumours, but by no means different tumours, from one another.   There are connective-tissue [fibrous] tumours of the surface, which manifest themselves in the form of simple tubera (Knoten*), others which show themselves in the form of warts and papillary tumours. In just the same manner, there are cancerous formations

Fig. 139.

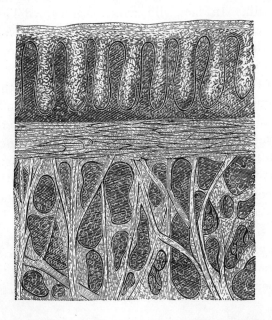

Fig. 139. Vertical section through a commencing cauliflower growth (cancroid) of the neck of the uterus. On the still unchanged surface the tolerably large papillæ of the os uteri are seen invested by a homogeneous, stratified layer of epithelium. The disease begins first on the other side of the mucous membrane in the real parenchyma of the cervix, where large, roundish or irregular, scattered groups of cells (contained in alveoli) are disseminated throughout the tissue. 150 diameters.

* The term Knoten (Eng. knot, Lat. tuber) having reference rather to the form than to the size of the tumour, is used in this work as a designation for all sorts of tuberiform tumors, even the largest.—Trans.

and cancroid formations which may assume this form, and others again, which do not do so.

With reference to the relation of form and nature, there is a question of really cardinal importance, concerning which, in the interest of mankind, a certain degree of unanimity ought soon to be arrived at, namely, what is properly to be understood by the term *tubercle*. The same difficulties which I have just described to you, are again encountered in the case of tubercle in a still higher degree. The old writers introduced the name tubercle merely to express an external form. Everything was called a tubercle which manifested itself in the shape of a small knot. It is, as you are no doubt aware, by no means so very long since this term was employed in the most loose manner. Carcinomatous and scirrhous tubercles were talked about, scrofulous and syphilitic tubercles were distinguished from one another, and these terms are still preserved in France. Cancer too, you know, in old times was not by any means exclusively employed to designate a real tumour, but noma (cancer aquaticus) was considered to have as much right to the appellation as a chancre (cancer syphiliticus).

Now in the course of the present century endeavours have been made gradually to exchange these somewhat superficial views for more accurate conceptions, and here also it is to Laennec especially that credit is due for having sought for precise denominations. Still he himself in his turn has been the cause of this matter's having fallen into a state of nearly irremediable confusion. For, as you no doubt recollect, he asserted that tubercle presented itself in the lungs under two different aspects, the so-called *tubercular infiltration*, and *tubercular granulation*. Now, inasmuch as infiltration signifies something completely at variance with the old notion of tubercle, since it does not at all imply the presence of small knots

(Knötchen), but expresses an equable pervasion of the whole parenchyma, a track was hereby opened, in following which the old idea of tubercle has more and more been departed from. As soon as the infiltration of tubercle had once been created and the form of the neoplasm had thereby been abandoned, the infiltration was generally, as being more extensive and therefore more instructive, taken as the basis of subsequent descriptions, and attempts were made to find out in what respects it really agreed with the other, previously known forms of tubercle. It was in this way, that the cheesy stage of tubercle came to be gradually adopted as the common generic characteristic of all tuberculous products, not merely as the principal aid in diagnosis, but as the starting-point for the interpretation of the process in general. It was in this way, in particular, that the idea came to be entertained, that tubercles could arise simply by any exudation's losing its water constituents, growing thick, turbid, opaque, cheesy, and remaining in this condition.

The term, tubercle-corpuscles (corpuscules tuberculeux), which is, you know, still in very frequent use, has reference to just this cheesy stage, and the accurate description which Lebert has given of them amounts to this —that they are formations which correspond with none of the known organic forms, and are neither cells, nor nuclei, nor anything else of an analogous nature, but appear in the form of little, roundish, solid corpuscles, which frequently have particles of fat scattered through them (Fig. 64). But if the development of these corpuscles be investigated, it is easy to convince oneself that, wherever they occur, they arise out of previous organic morphological elements, and that they are not by any means the first bungling products, unfortunate essays of organization, but that they were once well-grown elements, which by an unhappy chance were early checked in their

development and early succumbed to a process of shrivelling. You may with certainty assume that, where
you meet with a largish corpuscle of this description, a
cell had previously existed, and where you find a small
one, there once had been a nucleus, enclosed perhaps
within a cell.

Upon examining the point which has been the leading
one in the doctrine of tuberculosis recently advanced,
namely tubercular infiltration of the lungs, we readily
arrive at the result which Reinhardt has set down as the
final one, namely, that tuberculosis is nothing more than
one of the forms presented by inflammatory products
when undergoing transformation, and especially that all
tuberculous matter is really inspissated pus. In fact,
what has been termed tubercular infiltration, can with
few exceptions be traced to an originally inflammatory,
purulent or catarrhal mass which has gradually, in consequence of incomplete reabsorption, fallen into the shrivelled and shrunken state in which it afterwards remains.
But Reinhardt was deceived when he thought he was examining tubercle. He was led astray by the false direction which had been given to the whole doctrine of tuberculosis from the time of Laennec until his own, especially through the fault of the Vienna school. If he had
confined himself in his investigations to the form of old
assigned to tubercle, and knot (granule), if he had examined the constitution of the knot in its different stages
and had afterwards compared the different organs in
which knotted (granular) tubercle occurs, he would unquestionably have arrived at a different result.

It may, at least according to what I consider to be the
correct view of the matter, certainly be said, that the
greatest part of whatever in the course of tuberculosis
does not appear in the form of granules, is an inspissated
inflammatory product, and has at any rate no direct rela-

tion to tubercle. But by the side of these inflammatory
products, or also independently of them, we find a peculiar structure [the knot, granule] which, if they are to
be regarded as real tubercle, would no longer be included
in the ordinary classification ; and it is certainly an extremely characteristic circumstance that in France, where
the terminology of Lebert has become the prevailing one,
and the *corpuscules tuberculeux* are wont to be regarded
as the necessary accompaniments of tuberculosis—bodies,
concerning the tuberculous nature of which there can be
no doubt, have quite recently been set down as something altogether peculiar and which had hitherto remained undescribed. For one of the best, nay perhaps
the best, micrographer France possesses, Robin, has, in
his examinations of cases of tubercular meningitis, deemed
it impossible to regard the little granules in the arachnoid* [pia mater] which every body looks upon as tubercles, as being really tubercles, because the dogma
now prevails in France that tubercle consists of solid
non-cellular corpuscles, and in the tubercles of the cerebral membrane cells in a state of perfect preservation are
met with. To such curious aberrations does this track
lead that one ends by being unable to find a name for
real tubercle, because so many accidental objects have
been confounded with it, that what was sought for, or
even what had been found and was already grasped, has,

* The so-called visceral (cerebral) layer of the arachnoid is only the superficial
layer of the pia mater which is spread evenly over, and does not dip in between,
the convolutions, and being (as the name, arachnoid, implies), of a reticulated texture contains spaces (subarachnoid spaces). The so-called parietal layer of the
arachnoid is only the inner superficial layer of the dura mater with the epithelium
lining it. The Author employs the term arachnoid in general only for the purpose
of making himself more intelligible to others, but as this superficial layer of the
dura mater does not possess a reticulated structure and is everywhere insepara bly
connected with the rest of the membrane, and as epithelial coverings are not wont
to be designated by special names, he of course always uses the term of the pia
mater. Such expressions, therefore, as the "sac" or "cavity of the arachnoid"
are incorrect.—*Based upon MS. Notes by the Author.*

in consequence of the attention of observers being diverted by these objects, been allowed to slip out of one's hand again. I am of opinion that a tubercle is a granule, or a knot, and that this knot constitutes a new-formation, and indeed one, which from the time of its earliest development is necessarily of a cellular nature, and generally, just like all other new-formations, has its origin in connective tissue, and which, when it has reached a certain degree of development, constitutes a minute knot within this tissue, that, when it is at the sur-face, projects in the form of a little protuberance, and consists throughout its whole mass of small uni- or multi-nuclear cells. What especially characterizes this forma-tion is the circumstance, that it is extremely rich in nu-clei, so that when it is examined as it lies imbedded in

Fig. 140.

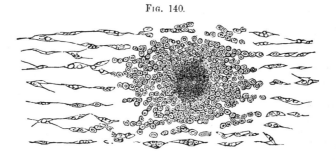

the tissue which invests it, at the first glance there seems to be scarcely anything else than nuclei. But upon iso-lating the constituents of the mass, either very small cells provided with one nucleus are obtained—and these are often so small that the membrane closely invests the nu-cleus—or larger cells with a manifold division of the nu-

Fig. 140. Development of tubercle from connective tissue in the pleura. The whole succession of transitions is seen from the simple connective-tissue corpuscles, the division of the nuclei and cells up to the production of the tubercle-granule, the cells of which in the middle are disintegrating into fatty granular débris. 300 diameters.

clei, so that from twelve to twenty-four or thirty are contained in one cell, in which case, however, the nuclei are always small and have a homogeneous and somewhat shining appearance.

This structure, which in its development is comparatively most nearly related to pus, inasmuch as it has the smallest nuclei and relatively the smallest cells, is distinguished from all the more highly organized forms of cancer, cancroid and sarcoma, by the circumstance, that these contain large, voluminous, nay often gigantic corpuscles with highly developed nuclei and nucleoli. Tubercle, on the contrary, is always a pitiful production, a new-formation from its very outset miserable. From its very commencement it is, like other new-formations, not unfrequently pervaded by vessels, but when it enlarges, its many little cells throng so closely together, that the vessels gradually become completely impervious and only the larger ones, which merely traverse the tubercle, remain intact. Generally fatty degeneration sets in very early in the centre of the knot (granule), where the oldest cells lie (Fig. 140), but usually does not become complete. Then every trace of fluid disappears, the corpuscles begin to shrivel, the centre becomes yellow and opaque, and a yellowish spot is seen in the middle of the grey translucent granule. This is the commencement of the *cheesy metamorphosis* which subsequently characterizes the tubercle. This change advances from cell to cell farther and farther outwards, and it not unfrequently happens that the whole granule is gradually involved in it.

Now, the reason why I think that the name of tubercle must be specially retained for this formation as being extremely characteristic of it, is this—that the tubercle-granule never attains any considerable size, and that a tuber never arises out of it. Those which are wont to be termed large tubercles, and attain the size of a walnut, or

a Borsdorf apple,* as for example in the brain—those
are not simple tubercles. You will generally find the
tubercles in the brain described as being solitary, but
they are not simple bodies ; every such mass (tuber)
which is as large as an apple, or even not larger than a
walnut, contains many thousands of tubercles ; it is quite
a nest of them which enlarges, not by the growth of the
original focus (granule), but rather by the continual formation and adjunction of new foci (granules) at its circumference. If we examine one of these perfectly yellowish white, dry, cheesy tubera, we find immediately
surrounding it a soft, vascular layer which marks it off
from the adjoining cerebral substance—a closely investing areola of connective tissue and vessels. In this layer
lie the small, young granules, now in greater, now in
less, number. They establish themselves externally [to
the previously existing ones] and the large tuber grows
by the continual apposition of new granules (tubercles),
of which every one singly becomes cheesy ; the whole
mass, therefore, cannot in its entirety be regarded as a
simple tubercle. The tubercles themselves remain really
minute, or as we are wont to say, *miliary*. Even when
on the pleura, by the side of quite small granules, large
yellow plates, looking as if they were deposited upon the
surface, are met with, these too are not simple tubercles,
but masses composed of a large aggregate of originally
separate granules.

Here, you see, form and nature are in reality inseparably connected. The form is produced by the growth of
the tubercle from single cells of connective tissue, by the
degenerative proliferation of single groups of connective-
tissue corpuscles. Thus, without more ado, it appears

---

* Borsdolf apples are very constant in their size, and measure from an inch and a
half to an inch and three quarters (1½″—1¾″) in diameter.—*From a MS. Note by
the Author.*

at once in the shape of a granule. As soon as it has
once attained a certain size, as soon as the generation of
new corpuscles which develop themselves out of the old
histological elements by a continual succession of divisions, at last lie so close to one another as to cause a
mutual arrest of development, gradually to induce the
disappearance of the vessels of the tubercle, and thereby
to cut off their own supplies, then they begin to break up,
they die away and nothing remains behind but débris—
shrunken, disintegrated, cheesy material.

The cheesy transformation is the regular termination
of tubercle, but, on the one hand, it is not the necessary
one, inasmuch as there are rare cases, in which tubercles,
in consequence of their undergoing a complete fatty metamorphosis, become capable of reabsorption ; and, on
the other hand, the same cheesy metamorphosis befalls
other kinds of cellular new-formations ; for pus may become cheesy, and likewise cancer and sarcoma. This
metamorphosis, therefore, being common to more than
one formation, cannot well be set down as a criterion for
the diagnosis of any particular structure, such as tubercle ; on the contrary, there are certain stages in its retrograde metamorphosis, where one cannot help confess-
ing that it is not always possible to come to a decision.
If a lung be laid before you with cheesy masses scattered
through it, and you are asked if that be tubercle or no,
you will frequently be unable to say with certainty what
the individual masses originally were. There are periods
in the course of development, when that which is inflammatory and that which is tuberculous can with precision
be distinguished from one another ; but, at last, there
comes a time, when both products become confounded,
and when, if one does not know how the whole arose, no
opinion can any longer be formed as to what its nature
is. In the midst of cancerous masses also cheesy spots

occur which look exactly like tubercles. I have demonstrated that it is by the gradual transformation of the elements of cancer that this cheesy matter is produced. But if we did not positively know from the history of their development that cancer-cells disintegrate step by step, and that no tubercles form in the middle of cancer, we should in many cases be altogether unable to arrive at any decision from merely examining the specimen.

If those difficulties be surmounted which lie in the external appearance of the formation, and lead the observer astray not only when he considers its grosser features, but also when he investigates its more intimate composition, there remains nothing else to assist us in coming to a right conclusion than the investigation of the type of development displayed by the individual new-formations during the stages of their actual development, not during those of their retrograde metamorphosis. The nature of tubercle cannot be studied after the period when it becomes cheesy, for from that time its history is identical with the history of pus which is becoming cheesy; an earlier period must be chosen when it is really engaged in proliferation. So in the case of other formations, that period must be studied which is comprised between their origin and their culminating point, and we must see with what normal physiological types they agree. Then it is, I think, certainly possible for us to arrive at a just conclusion with the aid of the simple principles of histological classification, which I have already propounded to you (p. 91). *Heterologous tissues also have physiological types.*

A colloid growth, if we really take it to mean what Laennec did—a gelatinous organized new-formation—must necessarily correspond to some type to be met with in the body when in its normal condition. Thus there are a series of tumours, that have been included in the colloid class, which have altogether the structure of the umbilical cord, and which, like this part, essentially contain mucus in their intercellular substance. Now since I had named the tissue of the umbilical cord and analogous parts, mucous tissue, it is a very simple step for me to call these tumours *Mucous tumours* (Schleimgeschwülste), Myxomata. When we demonstrate the occurrence of tumours exhibiting the histological type of the umbilical cord in the midst of the adult body, the striking character of the phenomenon is in no wise lessened, but we have found for them a type among the normal tissues of the body. Another form of colloid, or as Johannes Müller has called it, *Collonema*, turns out to be merely œdematous connective tissue. We find nothing more than a very soft tissue, soaked in an albuminous fluid. Such a tumour cannot be separated from connective-tissue [fibrous] tumours generally, whether they be denominated gelatinous, œdematous, or sclerematous* connective-tissue tumours, and I think there is no occasion to estrange it from the mind by bestowing upon it the name of collonema. So, again, we find certain forms of cancer, in which the stroma, instead of being composed simply of connective tissue, consists of the same mucous tissue which we meet with in a simple mucous tumour. These we may simply name *Mucous Cancer* (Gelatinous or Colloid Cancer). We then know exactly what we have before us. We know it is a cancer, but that its stroma differs in its containing mucus and in its gelatinous nature from the ordinary stroma of cancers.

To revert once more to the consideration of tubercle— it would certainly be something completely abnormal if it were composed of *corpuscles tuberculeux ;* but if you compare the cells which are, as at least I must assume to

---

* Sclerema=œdema durum.

be the case, the real constituents of the granule, with normal tissues of the body, you will remark the most complete correspondence between them and the corpuscles of the *lymphatic glands*, and this is a correspondence which is neither accidental nor unimportant, for was it not known even of old, that lymphatic glands have an especial tendency to undergo the cheesy degeneration? Even the old writers have stated that a lymphatic constitution disposes to processes of this kind.

With regard to pus, I need only remind you that we have been occupied during several lectures in discussing the question of the possibility of diagnosing between pyæmia and leucocytosis, and that we have recognized in the colourless corpuscles of the blood bodies so perfectly analogous to pus-corpuscles, that some have thought they saw pus when they had colourless blood-corpuscles before them, whilst Addison and Zimmermann, on the contrary, imagined they had found colourless blood-corpuscles when they really were looking upon pus. Both have a like type of formation. It may therefore be said that pus has a *hæmatoid* form, nay, the old doctrine may be revived afresh, namely, that pus is the blood of pathology. But if one would seek a distinction, if one would be able to say in individual cases what is pus and what blood-corpuscles, there is no other criterion than to determine whether the cell arose at a spot where a colourless blood-corpuscle might be expected to arise, or at one where it ought not be produced.

So, moreover, we find amongst pathological new-formation a large category, the natural type of which is epithelium—*Epitheliomata*, if you will. But the term epithelioma, which has recently been introduced by Hannover, is completely inadmissible in the case of the particular kind of tumour which it was intended to designate, because the epithelioma is by no means the only tumour whose elements bear the character of epithelial cells.

Epithelioma cannot be distinguished from other tumours
by its elements' having the character of epithelium whilst
those of the others have it not. The tumour that
[Johannes] Müller called Cholesteatoma, Cruveilhier,
tumeur perlée—which I have translated *Perlgeschwulst*
[pearly tumour]—this tumour has exactly the same epi-

FIG. 141.

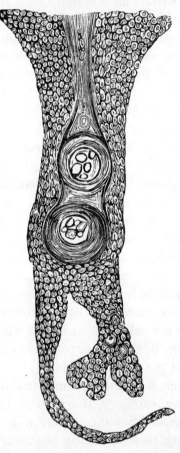

Fig. 141. Solid mass of cancroid from a tumour of the underlip. Closely packed
layers of cells at the circumference, presenting all the characters of the rete Malpighii : in one of the processes, globules glistening like fat ; in the middle of the body
of the growth, a horny, epidermoidal, hair-like structure, with onion-like globules
(pearls, globes épidermiques). 300 diameters.

thelial structure as that which Hannover has called epithelioma, nay, ordinary epithelioma very commonly engenders in itself little pearly globules in an often astonishingly great number. Yet both exhibit very essential points of difference. Never as yet have any pearly tumours been seen which, after existing in one place, recurred in remote places, and behaved like malignant tumours ; never did anything else occur than a slight extension—and that at an extremely slow rate—to the immediate neighborhood of the tumour. In the case of epitheliomata on the other hand, or as they are otherwise called, epithelial cancer or cancroid, we see a very marked malignity, for not only are they liable to recur at their original site, but they also reproduce themselves in distant parts. In many cases nearly all the organs of the body are metastatically filled with masses of cancroid.

Again, if you attempt to distinguish cancroid growths from real cancer by the epithelial structure of their elements, you will herein too give yourselves trouble in vain. Cancer proper has also elements of an epithelial character, and you need only turn to those parts of the body, where the epithelial cells are irregularly developed, as for example in the urinary passages (Fig. 15), and you will meet with the same curious bodies, provided

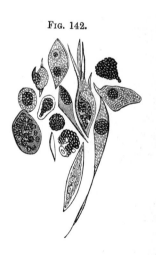

Fig. 142.

with large nuclei and nucleoli, which are described as the specific, polymorphous cells of cancer. Cancer, cancroid or epithelioma, pearly tumours or cholesteatoma, nay

Fig. 142. Various, polymorphous cancer-cells, some of them in a state of fatty degeneration, two with multiplication of nuclei. 300 diameters.

perhaps the dermoid growths which produce hairs, teeth, and sebaceous glands, and so frequently occur in the ovary —all these are formations in which there is a pathological production of epithelial cells, but they constitute a graduated series of different kinds, which extend from those which are entirely local, and, in the usual meaning of the word, perfectly benignant, to the extremest malignity. The mere form of the cells which compose a structure, is of no decisive value. Cancer is not malignant because it contains heterologous cells, nor cancroid benignant because its cells are homologous—they are both malignant, and their malignity only differs in degree.

The forms which yield dry, juiceless masses, are relatively benignant. Those which produce succulent tissues have always more or less a malignant character (p. 251). The pearly tumour, for example, yields perfectly dry epithelial masses, almost without a trace of moisture, and it only infects locally. Cancroid remains for a very long

Fig. 143.

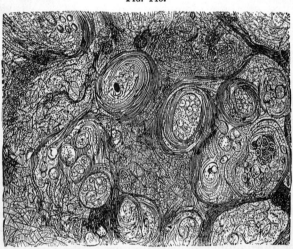

Fig. 143. Section through a cancroid of the orbit. Large epidermic globules (pearls), laminated after the manner of an onion, in a closely packed mass of cells, which have partly the character of epidermis, partly that of rete Malpighii. 150 diameters.

time local, so that the nearest lymphatic glands often do not become affected until after the lapse of years, and then again the process is for a long time confined to the disease of the lymphatic glands, so that a general outbreak of the disease in all parts of the body does not take place until late, and only in rare instances. In cancer proper the local progress is often very rapid and the disease early becomes general ; a cure, even for a short, time is so rare, that in France the complete incurability of cancer properly so called has been asserted and maintained with success.

Among the formations also which are analogous to the ordinary connective tissues, and are therefore apparently perfectly homologous and benignant, the succulent ones prove to be much more capable of communicating infection than the dry ones. A myxoma which has always a good deal of juice about it, is at all times a suspicious tumour, and, in proportion to the quantity of juice it contains, is its liability to recur. Cartilaginous tumours (Enchondromata) which were formerly described as unquestionably benignant, sometimes occur in soft and rather gelatinous forms, which may occasion just such internal metastases as cancer properly so-called. Even connective-tissue * [fibrous] tumours become, under certain circumstances, richer in cells and enlarge, whilst their interstitial connective tissue becomes

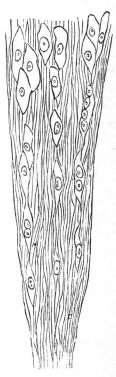

Fig. 144.

Fig. 144. Diagrammatic representation of the development of sarcoma, as it may very well be seen in sarcoma of the breast. 350 diameters.

* Fibrous tissue is *dense* connective tissue. It is not a special tissue, but only a

more succulent, nay in many cases disappears so completely, that at last scarcely anything but cellular elements remain. This is the kind of tumour which, according to my opinion, ought to be designated by the old name of *Sarcoma*. These sarcomata are frequently, indeed benignant, still they do not unfrequently recur, like epithelial cancer, at their original site, whilst under certain circumstances they appear secondary in the lymphatic glands, and in many cases occur throughout the whole body metastatically to such an extent, that scarcely any organ is spared by them.

In the case of all these formations, every one of which corresponds more or less completely to a normal tissue, investigations ought not to be conducted with a view to determine whether they have a physiological type, or whether they bear a specific stamp impressed upon them ; our final decision depends upon the answer to the question, *whether they arise at a spot to which they belong, or not, and whether they produce a fluid, which, when brought into contact with the neighbouring parts, may there exercise an unfavourable, contagious or irritative influence.*

It is with these formations as with vegetable ones. The nerves and vessels have not the slightest *direct* influence. They are only of importance so far as they determine the greater or less abundance of supply ; they are altogether unable to impel to the development of tumours, to produce them or to modify them in a direct manner. A pathological tumour in man forms in exactly the same way that a swelling on a tree does, whether on the bark, or on the surface of the trunk or a leaf, where any pathological irritation has occurred. The gall-nut which arises

---

form of connective tissue. Periosteum, perichondrium, tendons &c. all of them consist of connective tissue, in which, however, the cells have in part become converted into elastic fibres and network. In Germany indeed connective (cellular) tissue has ever since the time of Treviranus (1835) been divided into *formed* and *formless*, the former including tendons, fasciæ, ligaments, &c.—*From a MS. Note by the Author.*

in consequence of the puncture of an insect, the tuberous swellings which mark the spots on a tree where a bough has been cut off, and the wall-like elevation which forms around the border of the wounded surface produced by cutting down a tree, and which ultimately covers in the surface—all of them depend upon a proliferation of cells just as abundant and often just as rapid as that which we perceive in a tumour of a proliferating part of the human body. The pathological irritation acts in both cases precisely in the same manner ; the processes in plants conform entirely to the same type, and just as little as the tree produces on its bark or leaves cells of a kind, which it could not bring forth at other times, just as little does the animal body do this.

But if you consider the history of a vegetable tumour, you will see there also that it is above all the diseased spots which become unusually rich in specific constituents, and absorb and store up the peculiar substances which the tree produces, in more than average quantity. The vegetable cells which form on an oak-leaf round the puncture made by an insect contains much more tannic acid than any other part of the tree. The tumour-cells which form with such exuberance in a pine at the spot where an insect has buried itself in the young trunk, are stuffed completely full of resin. The peculiar formative energy which is developed at these spots, occasions also an unusually abundant accumulation of juices. There is no need of any nerves or vessels to instigate the cells to an increased absorption of matter. It is by their own action—by means of the attraction which they exercise upon the neighboring fluids—that they draw in the most serviceable materials. The great importance, which a knowledge of botany possesses for the pathologist also, lies in this—that it enables him to discover in all these processes the existence of an inward correspondence in the whole series of vital phenomena, and to show how the lowest formations may serve to explain the history of the most perfect and complex parts.

I have in the course of these lectures, gentlemen, developed to you as completely as it was possible for me here to do, the principles by means of which alone it is, according to my experience, possible to come to any correct decision in the case of pathological processes. I heartily thank you for the lively interest which you have testified to me up to the last moment. I perfectly know how to appreciate the fact that men like you, whose time is taken up by such manifold labours, still retain a taste for discussions of this kind, and I only wish that many a useful view of recent date may have been rendered more intelligible to you by these lectures, and that the facts I have laid before you may furnish you with recollections which may prove of service in your practice.

INDEX.

———•••———

by when irritated, 336, &c ; anastomosing, of tissues, importance of, in
conveyance of infection, 504-505.

Cellular Pathology, contrasted with Humoral and Solidistic, 40-42, 162, 504
et passim. See Humoralism and Solidism.

Cellular Tissue. See Connective Tissue.

Cellulose, reaction of, with iodine and
sulphuric acid, 31, similar to that of
cholestearine with same reagents, 400,
414 ; analogy of, to amyloid substance,
414.

Cerebellum, bacillar layer of, 301, 307-
308.

Cerebrum, bacillar layer of, 301, 307-
308 ; ganglion-cells of, 295, 298-299 ;
see Brain.

Chancre, 500, 517.

Cheesy metamorphosis, of pus, 213-215 ;
of tubercle, 522 524 ; of cancer, 524 ;
of sarcoma, 524.

Chlorosis, 260-261 ; distinction between,
and leukæmia, 261 ; imperfect development of different organs in, 261 ;
congenital, or coming on in early
youth, 261.

Cholepyrrhine, allied to Hæmatoidine,
177.

Cholera, leucocytosis in, 228 ; retention
of fat in intestinal villi in, 369.

Cholestearine, in atheromatous deposits,
382, 399-400 ; its reaction with iodine
and sulphuric acid, 400, similar to
that of cellulose with the same reagents, 400, 414.

Cholesteatoma, 528.

Chyle, absorption of, 367, 368 ; retention
of, 369.

Ciliary movement, persistence of, after
death, 331 ; provoked by soda and
potash, 331.

Classification, of normal tissues, the author's, 55, Bichat's, 56 ; of pathological new-formations, 91-92, 508-510.

Cloudy Swelling, 335 ; in cornea, 344 ;
in kidney and muscle, 392 ; &c.

Club-foot, fatty degeneration of muscles
in different kinds of, 384.

Cochlea, terminations of auditory nerve
in, 285 ; bodies found in, allied to
corpora amylacea, 319-320.

Colloid, definition of the term, 510-512 ;
different forms of, 525-526.

Collonema, 526.

Colostrum, 376-377 ; compared with sebaceous matter, 376, with milk, 377.

Condylomata, acuminate (non-syphilitic)
and broad, flat (plaques muqueuses—
syphilitic), 282, 512.

Connective substance, 98.

Connective Tissue, 69-70 ; fibres of, 69-
70, 138 ; Reichert's theory of formation of, 70-72, Henle's, 71-62,
Schwann's, 71-72, the author's, 71-72 ;
nutrition of, 131 ; interstitial, in muscles, 131 ; loose, in dartos, 136-137 ;
structure of, 137-139 ; resemblance of
intercellular substance of, to fibrine,
169 ; action of vegetable, and diluted
mineral acids upon, 169 ; of intestinal
villi, 366-367 ; and its equivalents,
common stock of germs of body, 441 ;
general source of pathological new-
formations, 441 ; transformation of,
into osteoid tissue and bone, 467-469,
472-475 ; formation of callus out of,
483-484 ; development of pus out of,
495 ; development of cancer out of,
499, of tubercle out of, 522, of sarcoma
out of, 531.

Connective-Tissue Corpuscles, 35, 72-73,
138 ; at base of papillæ in corium, 61,
277 ; anastomosing systems of, a supplement to blood- and lymphatic vessels, 79, in bone, 111-112, in teeth,
115, in semilunar cartilages, 116-117,
in tendons, 121-124, in cornea, 125,
342-344, in umbilical cord, 130, in dartos, 136, 137, in melanotic tumour from
parotid gland, 346, in periosteum,
468, 473 ; proliferation of (in suppuration) in interstices of muscle, 489,
in subcutaneous tissue, 495-496, in
development of cancer, 499, in development of tubercle, 521, in development of sarcoma, 531.

Connective Tissues, 69-76 ; connective
tissue proper, 69-72 ; cartilage, 74-75 ;
mucous tissue, 75 ; reticular arrangement of cells in (connective tissue,
bone, mucous tissue, &c.), 76 ; its object, 76 ; kind of neutral ground, 99 ;
strictly speaking, scarcely any real
function, 327 ; source of nearly all
new-formations, 441.

Connective-Tissue Tumours. See Fibrous
Tumours.

Consciousness, 323-324.

Contagious Juices, infection by means
of, 254, 504-505.

Continuity of Tissues, law of (Reichert's),
97-99.

Continuous Development, law of, 54-55 ;
in opposition to blastema and exudation doctrine, 439.

Contractility, of muscle, 81, 84-85 ; of
arteries, 147.

Contraction, of muscle, 81-82 ; of arteries and its effects, 147-151. See p. 85.

Cord, umbilical. See Umbilical cord.

Corium, 60, 62 ; papillary portion of,

the production of every vital action, 325 ; results of, either functional, nutritive, or formative, 326-327 ; functional, 330 ; nutritive, 334-345 ; formative, 345-350 ; inflammatory, a compound phenomenon, 354 ; the starting-point in every form of inflammation, 430-431 ; definition of, 431.

Ischæmia, result of action of arteries, 151.

Jacubowitsch, on the presence of a ganglion-cell in the bulbous swelling in which the nerve of a Pacinian body terminates, 276 ; on the three kinds of ganglion-cells met with in the spinal cord, 297, 298, 315.

Jauche (sanies) definition of, 500.

Jelly of Wharton, 126 ; its close relationship to vitreous body, 129.

Jones, Mr. Wharton, on rhythmical movements of veins of bat's wing, 148 ; on irregular contraction of small vessels in frog's web, 149.

Juice-conveying Canals or Tubes, in papillæ of skin, 62, 277 ; a supplement to blood- and lymphatic vessels, 76 ; in bone, 115 ; in teeth, 115 ; in semilunar cartilages, 116 ; in cornea, 116 ; in tendon, 120-124 ; in umbilical cord (mucous tissue), 130-131 ; in dartos, 136-137 ; in connective tissues, 131 ; in connective tissue-proper, 138 ; see 346, 504.

Juices, conveyance of infection by means of morbid, 257, 504-505. Cf. 254, 530-531.

Kekule, his analysis of amyloid spleens, 415.

Keratitis (parenchymatous), 340-341, 343-344.

Kidney, epithelium of vessels of, 145 ; action of, due to its epithelium, 158 ; minute metastatic deposits in, from endocarditis, 244 ; swelling of, and changes in, from infectant matters in blood, 246 ; deposition of silver in Malpighian bodies and medullary substance of, 247 ; deposition of urate of soda in, in gout, 248 ; changes in, in Bright's disease, 335-336 ; appearance of convoluted tubules in fatty degeneration of, 389 ; inflammatory (secondary) fatty degeneration of epithelium of (392), leading to atrophy, 393 ; amyloid degeneration of Malpighian bodies of, with their afferent arteries, 423 ; circulation in, 424.

Kirkes, Dr., 406.

Kluge, on independent vascular system of new-formations, 89.

Kölliker, 67, 68 ; on contractile substances of muscle, 85 ; on muscular fibres of umbilical vessels, 127 ; on Hæmato-crystalline, 179 ; on lymphatic glands, 207 ; on many-nucleated cells in marrow of bones, 347 ; on striated border of cylindrical epithelium of intestinal villi, 366-367 ; on physiological fatty liver in sucking animals, 370.

Kunde, on production of cataract in frogs by introduction of salt into intestinal canal or subcutaneous tissue, 154 ; on Hæmato-crystalline, 179.

Lactic acid, in leukæmic blood, 205 ; in spleen, 205.

Lacunæ, no real existence in living bone, in which entirely filled up by bone-cells, 458-460 ; see Bone.

Laennec, on colloid, 510-511, 525 ; on tubercle, 517, 519.

Lardaceous (Bacony) Degeneration. See Amyloid Degeneration.

Lebert, his fibro-plastic corpuscles, 70-71 ; on the corpuscles tuberculeux, 518-519.

Lecanu, on presence of fibrine in red blood-corpuscles, 174.

Lecithine. See Myeline.

Lehmann, on Syntonin, 84 ; on Hæmato-crystalline, 179.

Lens, Crystalline, origin of, 65 ; fibres of, epidermoidal cells, 66 ; reproduction of, after extraction for cataract, 66 ; see Cataract.

Lereboullet, on the fatty livers of geese, 370.

Leucine, in leukæmic blood, 205 ; in contents of intestines, 205 ; in spleen, 205.

Leucocytosis, definition of, 201 ; confounded with pyæmia, 223 ; physiological, in digestion, 224 ; in pregnancy, 224-225 ; pathological, in scrofulosis, 226, typhoid-fever, cancer, malignant erysipelas, 226 ; see 526-527.

Leucorrhœa, heterologous nature of secretion in, 488-489.

Leukæmia, 201-205 ; accompanied either by hyperinosis or hypinosis, 201 ; blood in, how distinguished from chylous blood, 202 ; fatal tendency of, 203 ; hæmorrhagic diathesis in, 203 ; epistaxis, apoplexy, melæna in, 203 ; splenic and lymphatic forms, 204 ; difference of morphological elements in blood in these two forms, 204 ; is a permanent, progressive leucocytosis, 205 ; substances found in blood in, 205 ; confounded with pyæmia, 223 ;

distinction between, and chlorosis, 261.

Leydig, on structure of muscle, 80, 83.

Life, characteristics of, 324 ; duration of in different elements, 500-501.

Lipomata, 363.

Liquefaction, of bone, 464, 496 ; of intercellular substance of connective tissue, 496.

Liver, hypertrophy and hyperplasy of, 94 ; arrangement of capillary vessels in acini of, and their relation to hepatic cells, 102-103 ; the three constituents of capillary network in acini, 103 ; secretion of, due to hepatic cells, 159 ; its connection with the hæmorrhagic diathesis, 164 ; enlargement of, and changes in, from infectant matters in blood, 246 ; secondary cancer more frequent in, than in lungs, 253, 505 ; increased secretion provoked in, by injection of irritating substances into blood, 331 ; fatty physiological and pathological, 370-374 ; intermediate interchange of matter in, by means of biliary ducts, 371-372 ; three zones of change (fat, amyloid matter, pigment), in acini of, 371-372 ; persistence of cells, in fatty, 373-374 ; curability of fatty condition of, 374 ; amyloid degeneration of, 417-418.

Lobstein, 93.

Loculi, of cancer, how produced, 499.

Locus Niger, 295.

Long Bones (i. e., osseous tissue of), growth in length of, from cartilage, in thickness, from periosteum, 451-452.

Ludwig, on molecules of nerves when at rest, 328 ; on salivary glands, 329.

Lungs, metastases (metastatic deposits) in, as a rule due to peripheral thrombosis, 240, deposition of bone-earth in, in mollities ossium, 249 ; secondary cancer less frequent in, than in liver, 253-505 ; myeline in, 270 ; fatty and pigmentary degeneration of epithelium of air-cells of, 387 ; gangrene of, from gangrenous metamorphosis of thrombus in transverse sinus after caries of internal ear, 387 ; laminated bodies in, 412.

Luxuriation, 489.

Luys, on excretion of starch through skin, 420.

Lymph, conveys corpuscular elements to blood, 191 ; fibrine of, how it differs from fibrine of blood, 192, not perfect fibrine, 192.

Lymph-corpuscles, 209.

Lymphatic Glands, how distinguished from ordinary secreting glands, 78 ; supply blood with its corpuscular elements, 191, 204 ; affection of, in erysipelas and diffuse phlegmonous inflammation, 200, in typhoid fever, 200 ; leucocytosis due to affection of, 201 ; swelling of, in leukæmia, 203-204 ; structure of, 206-210 ; no passage for pus-corpuscles through, 218 ; deposits in, from tattooing, 218-220 ; deposition of cancerous matter in, 221, of syphilitic virus in, 221 ; irritation of, in what consists, 222 ; physiological irritation of, in digestion, 224, in pregnancy, 224-225 ; affection of, in scrofulosis, 226 ; category of, extended, 227 ; diseases of, from action of infectant fluids, 245 ; amyloid degeneration of (minute arteries and gland-cells) 425-427 ; scrofulous changes in, 439 ; complete correspondence between corpuscles of, and constitutents of tubercle, 526.

Lymphatic Vessels, connection of, with phlogistic crasis or hyperinosis, 196 ; introduction of pus into, 217.

Lymphoid Organs, 226-228 ; diseases of, from action of infectant fluids, 245.

Magnetic needle, action of nerves upon, 325.

Malignity, not to be confounded with heterology, 92, 529.

Malpighi, on fibrine, 167.

Malpighian Bodies, (spleen) equivalen to follicles of lymphatic glands, 227 ; amyloid degeneration of, 411, 415.

—— (kidney) deposition of silver in, 247 ; amyloid degeneration of, and of their afferent arteries, 421-424.

Marrow, multi-nuclear cells in, 346-347 ; a connective tissue, 452 ; formed from osseous tissue, 452 ; ultimate product of development of bone, 452 ; formed from cartilage either directly, 457-459, or indirectly (through osseous tissue) 457 ; fatty, formation of, 458, normal in long bones, 458 ; in bodies of vertebræ nearly always only small cells of, without fat, 458 ; inflammatory, 458 ; very close correspondence between, and granulations, 464 ; formation of osteoid tissue and bone from, 465-466 ; young (granulations) starting-point of all heteroplastic development, 470 ; formation of bone out of, in fractures, 483-484 ; undue formation of, in osteomalacia, 489-490 ; very close relation of, to pus, 490.

Marrow-cells, throw out processes (become jagged) during ossification, 461,

blood-corpuscles from, 235; detachment of fragments from softening, 238, 406; prolonged, and their import, 239; autochthonous, 239; condition of, important in determining character of metastatic deposits arising from, 241, cf. 387.

Thrombosis, 232-238; may arise from phlebitis, arteritis, endocarditis, 236; of transverse sinus, from caries of internal ear, 387.

Thymus Gland, essentially a lymphatic gland, 227; endogenous cell-formation in, 444-445.

Tigri, on melanæmia, 257.

Tissues, classification of normal, 55-56, of pathological, 91-92, 509-510.

Tongue, follicles of root of, equivalent to follicles of lymphatic glands, 227; terminations of nerves in mucous membrane of, 285.

Tonsils, really lymphatic glands, 227.

Traer, Mr. James, on contraction of alæ vespertilionum, 147.

Traube, on section of pneumogastric nerve, 332.

Trigeminus (fifth pair of nerves) effects of section of, explained, 351-352.

Tuber, definition of, 502.

Tubercle, neglected as being a crude product, 90; cheesy products regarded as, in great measure really derived from pus, 215, cf. 520; phyma, as a new name for, 510; as a designation for an external form, 517; infiltration and granulation of, 517; corpuscles of, 518; real, only exist in a knotted or granular form, 519-520; its origin from connective tissue, 520-521; nuclei and cells of, how they resemble those of pus and differ from those of cancer, 522; fatty degeneration (cheesy metamorphosis) of, 522; solitary, of brain, 522-523; obliteration of vessels of, 523-524; lymphoid nature of, 527.

Tubercle, mucous, 512.

Tubercle-corpuscles, 518.

Tubercular Infiltration of lungs, due to presence within alveoli of shrivelled-up pus-cells, 215, 518; inflammatory origin and non-tuberculous nature of, 519.

Tubercular Meningitis, 520.

Tuberculization, of Pus, 215.

Tumeur perlée, 528.

Tumours: see the specific names; tuberous and infiltrated, 471; compound nature of tuberous, and mode of their enlargement, 501-502; local recurrence of, after extirpation, its cause, 503; vegetable, 533.

Typhoid-fever, hypinosis in, 200; in-

crease of colourless corpuscles in, 200; swelling of mesenteric glands and spleen in, 201, cf. 226; melanic corpuscles in blood in, 260; deposition of pigment in ganglia of sympathetic in, 295. See 439.

Typhoid fevers, diminution of respiratory power of red blood-corpuscles in, 262.

Typhous matter, not an exudation, 440.

Tyrosine, on liver, 205; in contents of intestines, 205; in spleen, 205.

Ulcer, atheromatous, 382; description of, 404.

Ulceration, 497; sanious, 500.

Umbilical Cord, 125-130; really non-vascular, 125; capillaries of, 126; persistent portion of, its limits, how determined, 127; deciduous portion of, 127; mucous tissue of, 128-130; nutrition of, 128-130; structure of, 128-129.

—— Vessels, their relation to umbilical cord, 126; great thickness of muscular coat of, 127.

Urate of Soda, in gout, 248; deposition of, in kidney, 248.

Urea, diminution of secretion of, in amyloid degeneration of kidney, 423-424.

Uric acid, in leukæmic blood, 205; in spleen, 205.

Uterus, creatine in muscular fibres of, 84; ciliated epithelium of mucous membrane of, replaced by squamous, epithelium in pregnancy, 100; new formation of muscular fibres, in fibrous tumours of, 487; cauliflower tumours of neck of, 514-516.

Utricle, primordial, 31; 45-46.

Vagina, substitution, in prolapsed, of epidermis for epithelium, 100.

Vagus (pneumogastric nerve) effects of section of, explained, 351-352.

Valentin, on lining membrane of cerebral ventricles, 311; on ciliary movement, 331.

Varicose veins, how produced, 153.

Vasa Serosa, substitute for, 75, 114.

Vascular canals of bone. See Haversian or Medullary canals.

—— System, everywhere closed by membranes, 144.

—— territories. See Vessel-territories.

—— theory (of inflammation) 428.

Vascularity, import of, 87-88.

Vegetable Tumours, 532-533.

Veins, longitudinal muscular layers in, 86; muscular tissue in superficial cutaneous, 142; small, formation and

A CATALOGUE OF SELECTED DOVER BOOKS
IN ALL FIELDS OF INTEREST

A CATALOGUE OF SELECTED DOVER BOOKS
IN ALL FIELDS OF INTEREST

AMERICA'S OLD MASTERS, James T. Flexner. Four men emerged unexpectedly from provincial 18th century America to leadership in European art: Benjamin West, J. S. Copley, C. R. Peale, Gilbert Stuart. Brilliant coverage of lives and contributions. Revised, 1967 edition. 69 plates. 365pp. of text.

21806-6 Paperbound $2.75

FIRST FLOWERS OF OUR WILDERNESS: AMERICAN PAINTING, THE COLONIAL PERIOD, James T. Flexner. Painters, and regional painting traditions from earliest Colonial times up to the emergence of Copley, West and Peale Sr., Foster, Gustavus Hesselius, Feke, John Smibert and many anonymous painters in the primitive manner. Engaging presentation, with 162 illustrations. xxii + 368pp.

22180-6 Paperbound $3.50

THE LIGHT OF DISTANT SKIES: AMERICAN PAINTING, 1760-1835, James T. Flexner. The great generation of early American painters goes to Europe to learn and to teach: West, Copley, Gilbert Stuart and others. Allston, Trumbull, Morse; also contemporary American painters—primitives, derivatives, academics—who remained in America. 102 illustrations. xiii + 306pp. 22179-2 Paperbound $3.00

A HISTORY OF THE RISE AND PROGRESS OF THE ARTS OF DESIGN IN THE UNITED STATES, William Dunlap. Much the richest mine of information on early American painters, sculptors, architects, engravers, miniaturists, etc. The only source of information for scores of artists, the major primary source for many others. Unabridged reprint of rare original 1834 edition, with new introduction by James T. Flexner, and 394 new illustrations. Edited by Rita Weiss. 6⅝ x 9⅝.

21695-0, 21696-9, 21697-7 Three volumes, Paperbound $13.50

EPOCHS OF CHINESE AND JAPANESE ART, Ernest F. Fenollosa. From primitive Chinese art to the 20th century, thorough history, explanation of every important art period and form, including Japanese woodcuts; main stress on China and Japan, but Tibet, Korea also included. Still unexcelled for its detailed, rich coverage of cultural background, aesthetic elements, diffusion studies, particularly of the historical period. 2nd, 1913 edition. 242 illustrations. lii + 439pp. of text.

20364-6, 20365-4 Two volumes, Paperbound $5.00

THE GENTLE ART OF MAKING ENEMIES, James A. M. Whistler. Greatest wit of his day deflates Oscar Wilde, Ruskin, Swinburne; strikes back at inane critics, exhibitions, art journalism; aesthetics of impressionist revolution in most striking form. Highly readable classic by great painter. Reproduction of edition designed by Whistler. Introduction by Alfred Werner. xxxvi + 334pp.

21875-9 Paperbound $2.25

INCIDENTS OF TRAVEL IN YUCATAN, John L. Stephens. Classic (1843) exploration of jungles of Yucatan, looking for evidences of Maya civilization. Stephens found many ruins; comments on travel adventures, Mexican and Indian culture. 127 striking illustrations by F. Catherwood. Total of 669 pp.

20926-1, 20927-X Two volumes, Paperbound $5.00

INCIDENTS OF TRAVEL IN CENTRAL AMERICA, CHIAPAS, AND YUCATAN, John L. Stephens. An exciting travel journal and an important classic of archeology. Narrative relates his almost single-handed discovery of the Mayan culture, and exploration of the ruined cities of Copan, Palenque, Utatlan and others; the monuments they dug from the earth, the temples buried in the jungle, the customs of poverty-stricken Indians living a stone's throw from the ruined palaces. 115 drawings by F. Catherwood. Portrait of Stephens. xii + 812pp.

22404-X, 22405-8 Two volumes, Paperbound $6.00

A NEW VOYAGE ROUND THE WORLD, William Dampier. Late 17-century naturalist joined the pirates of the Spanish Main to gather information; remarkably vivid account of buccaneers, pirates; detailed, accurate account of botany, zoology, ethnography of lands visited. Probably the most important early English voyage, enormous implications for British exploration, trade, colonial policy. Also most interesting reading. Argonaut edition, introduction by Sir Albert Gray. New introduction by Percy Adams. 6 plates, 7 illustrations. xlvii + 376pp. $6\frac{1}{2}$ x $9\frac{1}{4}$.

21900-3 Paperbound $3.00

INTERNATIONAL AIRLINE PHRASE BOOK IN SIX LANGUAGES, Joseph W. Bátor. Important phrases and sentences in English paralleled with French, German, Portuguese, Italian, Spanish equivalents, covering all possible airport-travel situations; created for airline personnel as well as tourist by Language Chief, Pan American Airlines. xiv + 204pp.

22017-6 Paperbound $2.00

STAGE COACH AND TAVERN DAYS, Alice Morse Earle. Detailed, lively account of the early days of taverns; their uses and importance in the social, political and military life; furnishings and decorations; locations; food and drink; tavern signs, etc. Second half covers every aspect of early travel; the roads, coaches, drivers, etc. Nostalgic, charming, packed with fascinating material. 157 illustrations, mostly photographs. xiv + 449pp.

22518-6 Paperbound $4.00

NORSE DISCOVERIES AND EXPLORATIONS IN NORTH AMERICA, Hjalmar R. Holand. The perplexing Kensington Stone, found in Minnesota at the end of the 19th century. Is it a record of a Scandinavian expedition to North America in the 14th century? Or is it one of the most successful hoaxes in history? A scientific detective investigation. Formerly *Westward from Vinland*. 31 photographs, 17 figures. x + 354pp.

22014-1 Paperbound $2.75

A BOOK OF OLD MAPS, compiled and edited by Emerson D. Fite and Archibald Freeman. 74 old maps offer an unusual survey of the discovery, settlement and growth of America down to the close of the Revolutionary war: maps showing Norse settlements in Greenland, the explorations of Columbus, Verrazano, Cabot, Champlain, Joliet, Drake, Hudson, etc., campaigns of Revolutionary war battles, and much more. Each map is accompanied by a brief historical essay. xvi + 299pp. 11 x $13\frac{3}{4}$.

22084-2 Paperbound $6.00

ADVENTURES OF AN AFRICAN SLAVER, Theodore Canot. Edited by Brantz Mayer. A detailed portrayal of slavery and the slave trade, 1820-1840. Canot, an established trader along the African coast, describes the slave economy of the African kingdoms, the treatment of captured negroes, the extensive journeys in the interior to gather slaves, slave revolts and their suppression, harems, bribes, and much more. Full and unabridged republication of 1854 edition. Introduction by Malcom Cowley. 16 illustrations. xvii + 448pp. 22456-2 Paperbound $3.50

MY BONDAGE AND MY FREEDOM, Frederick Douglass. Born and brought up in slavery, Douglass witnessed its horrors and experienced its cruelties, but went on to become one of the most outspoken forces in the American anti-slavery movement. Considered the best of his autobiographies, this book graphically describes the inhuman treatment of slaves, its effects on slave owners and slave families, and how Douglass's determination led him to a new life. Unaltered reprint of 1st (1855) edition. xxxii + 464pp. 22457-0 Paperbound $2.50

THE INDIANS' BOOK, recorded and edited by Natalie Curtis. Lore, music, narratives, dozens of drawings by Indians themselves from an authoritative and important survey of native culture among Plains, Southwestern, Lake and Pueblo Indians. Standard work in popular ethnomusicology. 149 songs in full notation. 23 drawings, 23 photos. xxxi + 584pp. 6⅝ x 9⅜. 21939-9 Paperbound $4.00

DICTIONARY OF AMERICAN PORTRAITS, edited by Hayward and Blanche Cirker. 4024 portraits of 4000 most important Americans, colonial days to 1905 (with a few important categories, like Presidents, to present). Pioneers, explorers, colonial figures, U. S. officials, politicians, writers, military and naval men, scientists, inventors, manufacturers, jurists, actors, historians, educators, notorious figures, Indian chiefs, etc. All authentic contemporary likenesses. The only work of its kind in existence; supplements all biographical sources for libraries. Indispensable to anyone working with American history. 8,000-item classified index, finding lists, other aids. xiv + 756pp. 9¼ x 12¾. 21823-6 Clothbound $30.00

TRITTON'S GUIDE TO BETTER WINE AND BEER MAKING FOR BEGINNERS, S. M. Tritton. All you need to know to make family-sized quantities of over 100 types of grape, fruit, herb and vegetable wines; as well as beers, mead, cider, etc. Complete recipes, advice as to equipment, procedures such as fermenting, bottling, and storing wines. Recipes given in British, U. S., and metric measures. Accompanying booklet lists sources in U. S. A. where ingredients may be bought, and additional information. 11 illustrations. 157pp. 5⅝ x 8⅛.
(USO) 22090-7 Clothbound $3.50

GARDENING WITH HERBS FOR FLAVOR AND FRAGRANCE, Helen M. Fox. How to grow herbs in your own garden, how to use them in your cooking (over 55 recipes included), legends and myths associated with each species, uses in medicine, perfumes, etc.—these are elements of one of the few books written especially for American herb fanciers. Guides you step-by-step from soil preparation to harvesting and storage for each type of herb. 12 drawings by Louise Mansfield. xiv + 334pp. 22540-2 Paperbound $2.50

JIM WHITEWOLF: THE LIFE OF A KIOWA APACHE INDIAN, Charles S. Brant, editor. Spans transition between native life and acculturation period, 1880 on. Kiowa culture, personal life pattern, religion and the supernatural, the Ghost Dance, breakdown in the White Man's world, similar material. 1 map. xii + 144pp.
22015-X Paperbound $1.75

THE NATIVE TRIBES OF CENTRAL AUSTRALIA, Baldwin Spencer and F. J. Gillen. Basic book in anthropology, devoted to full coverage of the Arunta and Warramunga tribes; the source for knowledge about kinship systems, material and social culture, religion, etc. Still unsurpassed. 121 photographs, 89 drawings. xviii + 669pp.
21775-2 Paperbound $5.00

MALAY MAGIC, Walter W. Skeat. Classic (1900); still the definitive work on the folklore and popular religion of the Malay peninsula. Describes marriage rites, birth spirits and ceremonies, medicine, dances, games, war and weapons, etc. Extensive quotes from original sources, many magic charms translated into English. 35 illustrations. Preface by Charles Otto Blagden. xxiv + 685pp.
21760-4 Paperbound $3.50

HEAVENS ON EARTH: UTOPIAN COMMUNITIES IN AMERICA, 1680-1880, Mark Holloway. The finest nontechnical account of American utopias, from the early Woman in the Wilderness, Ephrata, Rappites to the enormous mid 19th-century efflorescence; Shakers, New Harmony, Equity Stores, Fourier's Phalanxes, Oneida, Amana, Fruitlands, etc. "Entertaining and very instructive." *Times Literary Supplement*. 15 illustrations. 246pp.
21593-8 Paperbound $2.00

LONDON LABOUR AND THE LONDON POOR, Henry Mayhew. Earliest (c. 1850) sociological study in English, describing myriad subcultures of London poor. Particularly remarkable for the thousands of pages of direct testimony taken from the lips of London prostitutes, thieves, beggars, street sellers, chimney-sweepers, street-musicians, "mudlarks," "pure-finders," rag-gatherers, "running-patterers," dock laborers, cab-men, and hundreds of others, quoted directly in this massive work. An extraordinarily vital picture of London emerges. 110 illustrations. Total of lxxvi + 1951pp. 6⅝ x 10.
21934-8, 21935-6, 21936-4, 21937-2 Four volumes, Paperbound $14.00

HISTORY OF THE LATER ROMAN EMPIRE, J. B. Bury. Eloquent, detailed reconstruction of Western and Byzantine Roman Empire by a major historian, from the death of Theodosius I (395 A.D.) to the death of Justinian (565). Extensive quotations from contemporary sources; full coverage of important Roman and foreign figures of the time. xxxiv + 965pp. 21829-5 Record, book, album. Monaural. $2.75

AN INTELLECTUAL AND CULTURAL HISTORY OF THE WESTERN WORLD, Harry Elmer Barnes. Monumental study, tracing the development of the accomplishments that make up human culture. Every aspect of man's achievement surveyed from its origins in the Paleolithic to the present day (1964); social structures, ideas, economic systems, art, literature, technology, mathematics, the sciences, medicine, religion, jurisprudence, etc. Evaluations of the contributions of scores of great men. 1964 edition, revised and edited by scholars in the many fields represented. Total of xxix + 1381pp. 21275-0, 21276-9, 21277-7 Three volumes, Paperbound $7.75

THE PHILOSOPHY OF THE UPANISHADS, Paul Deussen. Clear, detailed statement of upanishadic system of thought, generally considered among best available. History of these works, full exposition of system emergent from them, parallel concepts in the West. Translated by A. S. Geden. xiv + 429pp.

21616-0 Paperbound $3.00

LANGUAGE, TRUTH AND LOGIC, Alfred J. Ayer. Famous, remarkably clear introduction to the Vienna and Cambridge schools of Logical Positivism; function of philosophy, elimination of metaphysical thought, nature of analysis, similar topics. "Wish I had written it myself," Bertrand Russell. 2nd, 1946 edition. 160pp.

20010-8 Paperbound $1.35

THE GUIDE FOR THE PERPLEXED, Moses Maimonides. Great classic of medieval Judaism, major attempt to reconcile revealed religion (Pentateuch, commentaries) and Aristotelian philosophy. Enormously important in all Western thought. Unabridged Friedländer translation. 50-page introduction. lix + 414pp.

(USO) 20351-4 Paperbound $2.50

OCCULT AND SUPERNATURAL PHENOMENA, D. H. Rawcliffe. Full, serious study of the most persistent delusions of mankind: crystal gazing, mediumistic trance, stigmata, lycanthropy, fire walking, dowsing, telepathy, ghosts, ESP, etc., and their relation to common forms of abnormal psychology. Formerly *Illusions and Delusions of the Supernatural and the Occult*. iii + 551pp. 20503-7 Paperbound $3.50

THE EGYPTIAN BOOK OF THE DEAD: THE PAPYRUS OF ANI, E. A. Wallis Budge. Full hieroglyphic text, interlinear transliteration of sounds, word for word translation, then smooth, connected translation; Theban recension. Basic work in Ancient Egyptian civilization; now even more significant than ever for historical importance, dilation of consciousness, etc. clvi + 377pp. 6½ x 9¼.

21866-X Paperbound $3.75

PSYCHOLOGY OF MUSIC, Carl E. Seashore. Basic, thorough survey of everything known about psychology of music up to 1940's; essential reading for psychologists, musicologists. Physical acoustics; auditory apparatus; relationship of physical sound to perceived sound; role of the mind in sorting, altering, suppressing, creating sound sensations; musical learning, testing for ability, absolute pitch, other topics. Records of Caruso, Menuhin analyzed. 88 figures. xix + 408pp.

21851-1 Paperbound $2.75

THE I CHING (THE BOOK OF CHANGES), translated by James Legge. Complete translated text plus appendices by Confucius, of perhaps the most penetrating divination book ever compiled. Indispensable to all study of early Oriental civilizations. 3 plates. xxiii + 448pp. 21062-6 Paperbound $2.75

THE UPANISHADS, translated by Max Müller. Twelve classical upanishads: Chandogya, Kena, Aitareya, Kaushitaki, Isa, Katha, Mundaka, Taittiriyaka, Brhadaranyaka, Svetasvatara, Prasna, Maitriyana. 160-page introduction, analysis by Prof. Müller. Total of 826pp. 20398-0, 20399-9 Two volumes, Paperbound $5.00

PLANETS, STARS AND GALAXIES: DESCRIPTIVE ASTRONOMY FOR BEGINNERS, A. E. Fanning. Comprehensive introductory survey of astronomy: the sun, solar system, stars, galaxies, universe, cosmology; up-to-date, including quasars, radio stars, etc. Preface by Prof. Donald Menzel. 24pp. of photographs. 189pp. $5\frac{1}{4}$ x $8\frac{1}{4}$.
21680-2 Paperbound $1.50

TEACH YOURSELF CALCULUS, P. Abbott. With a good background in algebra and trig, you can teach yourself calculus with this book. Simple, straightforward introduction to functions of all kinds, integration, differentiation, series, etc. "Students who are beginning to study calculus method will derive great help from this book." Faraday House Journal. 308pp. 20683-1 Clothbound $2.00

TEACH YOURSELF TRIGONOMETRY, P. Abbott. Geometrical foundations, indices and logarithms, ratios, angles, circular measure, etc. are presented in this sound, easy-to-use text. Excellent for the beginner or as a brush up, this text carries the student through the solution of triangles. 204pp. 20682-3 Clothbound $2.00

TEACH YOURSELF ANATOMY, David LeVay. Accurate, inclusive, profusely illustrated account of structure, skeleton, abdomen, muscles, nervous system, glands, brain, reproductive organs, evolution. "Quite the best and most readable account,' *Medical Officer.* 12 color plates. 164 figures. 311pp. $4\frac{3}{4}$ x 7.
21651-9 Clothbound $2.50

TEACH YOURSELF PHYSIOLOGY, David LeVay. Anatomical, biochemical bases; digestive, nervous, endocrine systems; metabolism; respiration; muscle; excretion; temperature control; reproduction. "Good elementary exposition," *The Lancet.* 6 color plates. 44 illustrations. 208pp. $4\frac{1}{4}$ x 7. 21658-6 Clothbound $2.50

THE FRIENDLY STARS, Martha Evans Martin. Classic has taught naked-eye observation of stars, planets to hundreds of thousands, still not surpassed for charm, lucidity, adequacy. Completely updated by Professor Donald H. Menzel, Harvard Observatory. 25 illustrations. 16 x 30 chart. x + 147pp. 21099-5 Paperbound $1.25

MUSIC OF THE SPHERES: THE MATERIAL UNIVERSE FROM ATOM TO QUASAR, SIMPLY EXPLAINED, Guy Murchie. Extremely broad, brilliantly written popular account begins with the solar system and reaches to dividing line between matter and nonmatter; latest understandings presented with exceptional clarity. Volume One: Planets, stars, galaxies, cosmology, geology, celestial mechanics, latest astronomical discoveries; Volume Two: Matter, atoms, waves, radiation, relativity, chemical action, heat, nuclear energy, quantum theory, music, light, color, probability, antimatter, antigravity, and similar topics. 319 figures. 1967 (second) edition. Total of xx + 644pp. 21809-0, 21810-4 Two volumes, Paperbound $4.00

OLD-TIME SCHOOLS AND SCHOOL BOOKS, Clifton Johnson. Illustrations and rhymes from early primers, abundant quotations from early textbooks, many anecdotes of school life enliven this study of elementary schools from Puritans to middle 19th century. Introduction by Carl Withers. 234 illustrations. xxxiii + 381pp.
21031-6 Paperbound $2.50

THE PRINCIPLES OF PSYCHOLOGY, William James. The famous long course, complete and unabridged. Stream of thought, time perception, memory, experimental methods—these are only some of the concerns of a work that was years ahead of its time and still valid, interesting, useful. 94 figures. Total of xviii + 1391pp.
20381-6, 20382-4 Two volumes, Paperbound $6.00

THE STRANGE STORY OF THE QUANTUM, Banesh Hoffmann. Non-mathematical but thorough explanation of work of Planck, Einstein, Bohr, Pauli, de Broglie, Schrödinger, Heisenberg, Dirac, Feynman, etc. No technical background needed. "Of books attempting such an account, this is the best," Henry Margenau, Yale. 40-page "Postscript 1959." xii + 285pp.
20518-5 Paperbound $2.00

THE RISE OF THE NEW PHYSICS, A. d'Abro. Most thorough explanation in print of central core of mathematical physics, both classical and modern; from Newton to Dirac and Heisenberg. Both history and exposition; philosophy of science, causality, explanations of higher mathematics, analytical mechanics, electromagnetism, thermodynamics, phase rule, special and general relativity, matrices. No higher mathematics needed to follow exposition, though treatment is elementary to intermediate in level. Recommended to serious student who wishes verbal understanding. 97 illustrations. xvii + 982pp.
20003-5, 20004-3 Two volumes, Paperbound $5.50

GREAT IDEAS OF OPERATIONS RESEARCH, Jagjit Singh. Easily followed non-technical explanation of mathematical tools, aims, results: statistics, linear programming, game theory, queueing theory, Monte Carlo simulation, etc. Uses only elementary mathematics. Many case studies, several analyzed in detail. Clarity, breadth make this excellent for specialist in another field who wishes background. 41 figures. x + 228pp.
21886-4 Paperbound $2.25

GREAT IDEAS OF MODERN MATHEMATICS: THEIR NATURE AND USE, Jagjit Singh. Internationally famous expositor, winner of Unesco's Kalinga Award for science popularization explains verbally such topics as differential equations, matrices, groups, sets, transformations, mathematical logic and other important modern mathematics, as well as use in physics, astrophysics, and similar fields. Superb exposition for layman, scientist in other areas. viii + 312pp.
20587-8 Paperbound $2.25

GREAT IDEAS IN INFORMATION THEORY, LANGUAGE AND CYBERNETICS, Jagjit Singh. The analog and digital computers, how they work, how they are like and unlike the human brain, the men who developed them, their future applications, computer terminology. An essential book for today, even for readers with little math. Some mathematical demonstrations included for more advanced readers. 118 figures. Tables. ix + 338pp.
21694-2 Paperbound $2.25

CHANCE, LUCK AND STATISTICS, Horace C. Levinson. Non-mathematical presentation of fundamentals of probability theory and science of statistics and their applications. Games of chance, betting odds, misuse of statistics, normal and skew distributions, birth rates, stock speculation, insurance. Enlarged edition. Formerly "The Science of Chance." xiii + 357pp.
21007-3 Paperbound $2.00

AMERICAN FOOD AND GAME FISHES, David S. Jordan and Barton W. Evermann. Definitive source of information, detailed and accurate enough to enable the sportsman and nature lover to identify conclusively some 1,000 species and sub-species of North American fish, sought for food or sport. Coverage of range, physiology, habits, life history, food value. Best methods of capture, interest to the angler, advice on bait, fly-fishing, etc. 338 drawings and photographs. 1 + 574pp. 6⅝ x 9⅜.

22383-1 Paperbound $4.50

THE FROG BOOK, Mary C. Dickerson. Complete with extensive finding keys, over 300 photographs, and an introduction to the general biology of frogs and toads, this is the classic non-technical study of Northeastern and Central species. 58 species; 290 photographs and 16 color plates. xvii + 253pp.

21973-9 Paperbound $4.00

THE MOTH BOOK: A GUIDE TO THE MOTHS OF NORTH AMERICA, William J. Holland. Classical study, eagerly sought after and used for the past 60 years. Clear identification manual to more than 2,000 different moths, largest manual in existence. General information about moths, capturing, mounting, classifying, etc., followed by species by species descriptions. 263 illustrations plus 48 color plates show almost every species, full size. 1968 edition, preface, nomenclature changes by A. E. Brower. xxiv + 479pp. of text. 6½ x 9¼.

21948-8 Paperbound $5.00

THE SEA-BEACH AT EBB-TIDE, Augusta Foote Arnold. Interested amateur can identify hundreds of marine plants and animals on coasts of North America; marine algae; seaweeds; squids; hermit crabs; horse shoe crabs; shrimps; corals; sea anemones; etc. Species descriptions cover: structure; food; reproductive cycle; size; shape; color; habitat; etc. Over 600 drawings. 85 plates. xii + 490pp.

21949-6 Paperbound $3.50

COMMON BIRD SONGS, Donald J. Borror. 33⅓ 12-inch record presents songs of 60 important birds of the eastern United States. A thorough, serious record which provides several examples for each bird, showing different types of song, individual variations, etc. Incstimable identification aid for birdwatcher. 32-page booklet gives text about birds and songs, with illustration for each bird.

21829-5 Record, book, album. Monaural. $2.75

FADS AND FALLACIES IN THE NAME OF SCIENCE, Martin Gardner. Fair, witty appraisal of cranks and quacks of science: Atlantis, Lemuria, hollow earth, flat earth, Velikovsky, orgone energy, Dianetics, flying saucers, Bridey Murphy, food fads, medical fads, perpetual motion, etc. Formerly "In the Name of Science." x + 363pp.

20394-8 Paperbound $2.00

HOAXES, Curtis D. MacDougall. Exhaustive, unbelievably rich account of great hoaxes: Locke's moon hoax, Shakespearean forgeries, sea serpents, Loch Ness monster, Cardiff giant, John Wilkes Booth's mummy, Disumbrationist school of art, dozens more; also journalism, psychology of hoaxing. 54 illustrations. xi + 338pp.

20465-0 Paperbound $2.75

How to Know the Wild Flowers, Mrs. William Starr Dana. This is the classical book of American wildflowers (of the Eastern and Central United States), used by hundreds of thousands. Covers over 500 species, arranged in extremely easy to use color and season groups. Full descriptions, much plant lore. This Dover edition is the fullest ever compiled, with tables of nomenclature changes. 174 full-page plates by M. Satterlee. xii + 418pp.   20332-8 Paperbound $2.50

Our Plant Friends and Foes, William Atherton DuPuy. History, economic importance, essential botanical information and peculiarities of 25 common forms of plant life are provided in this book in an entertaining and charming style. Covers food plants (potatoes, apples, beans, wheat, almonds, bananas, etc.), flowers (lily, tulip, etc.), trees (pine, oak, elm, etc.), weeds, poisonous mushrooms and vines, gourds, citrus fruits, cotton, the cactus family, and much more. 108 illustrations. xiv + 290pp.   22272-1 Paperbound $2.00

How to Know the Ferns, Frances T. Parsons. Classic survey of Eastern and Central ferns, arranged according to clear, simple identification key. Excellent introduction to greatly neglected nature area. 57 illustrations and 42 plates. xvi + 215pp.   20740-4 Paperbound $1.75

Manual of the Trees of North America, Charles S. Sargent. America's foremost dendrologist provides the definitive coverage of North American trees and tree-like shrubs. 717 species fully described and illustrated: exact distribution, down to township; full botanical description; economic importance; description of subspecies and races; habitat, growth data; similar material. Necessary to every serious student of tree-life. Nomenclature revised to present. Over 100 locating keys. 783 illustrations. lii + 934pp. 20277-1, 20278-X Two volumes, Paperbound $6.00

Our Northern Shrubs, Harriet L. Keeler. Fine non-technical reference work identifying more than 225 important shrubs of Eastern and Central United States and Canada. Full text covering botanical description, habitat, plant lore, is paralleled with 205 full-page photographs of flowering or fruiting plants. Nomenclature revised by Edward G. Voss. One of few works concerned with shrubs. 205 plates, 35 drawings. xxviii + 521pp.   21989-5 Paperbound $3.75

The Mushroom Handbook, Louis C. C. Krieger. Still the best popular handbook: full descriptions of 259 species, cross references to another 200. Extremely thorough text enables you to identify, know all about any mushroom you are likely to meet in eastern and central U. S. A.: habitat, luminescence, poisonous qualities, use, folklore, etc. 32 color plates show over 50 mushrooms, also 126 other illustrations. Finding keys. vii + 560pp.   21861-9 Paperbound $3.95

Handbook of Birds of Eastern North America, Frank M. Chapman. Still much the best single-volume guide to the birds of Eastern and Central United States. Very full coverage of 675 species, with descriptions, life habits, distribution, similar data. All descriptions keyed to two-page color chart. With this single volume the average birdwatcher needs no other books. 1931 revised edition. 195 illustrations. xxxvi + 581pp.   21489-3 Paperbound $3.25

"ESSENTIAL GRAMMAR" SERIES

All you really need to know about modern, colloquial grammar. Many educational shortcuts help you learn faster, understand better. Detailed cognate lists teach you to recognize similarities between English and foreign words and roots—make learning vocabulary easy and interesting. Excellent for independent study or as a supplement to record courses.

ESSENTIAL FRENCH GRAMMAR, Seymour Resnick. 2500-item cognate list. 159pp.
(EBE) 20419-7 Paperbound $1.25

ESSENTIAL GERMAN GRAMMAR, Guy Stern and Everett F. Bleiler. Unusual shortcuts on noun declension, word order, compound verbs. 124pp.
(EBE) 20422-7 Paperbound $1.25

ESSENTIAL ITALIAN GRAMMAR, Olga Ragusa. 111pp.
(EBE) 20779-X Paperbound $1.25

ESSENTIAL JAPANESE GRAMMAR, Everett F. Bleiler. In Romaji transcription; no characters needed. Japanese grammar is regular and simple. 156pp.
21027-8 Paperbound $1.25

ESSENTIAL PORTUGUESE GRAMMAR, Alexander da R. Prista. vi + 114pp.
21650-0 Paperbound $1.25

ESSENTIAL SPANISH GRAMMAR, Seymour Resnick. 2500 word cognate list. 115pp.
(EBE) 20780-3 Paperbound $1.25

ESSENTIAL ENGLISH GRAMMAR, Philip Gucker. Combines best features of modern, functional and traditional approaches. For refresher, class use, home study. x + 177pp.
21649-7 Paperbound $1.25

A PHRASE AND SENTENCE DICTIONARY OF SPOKEN SPANISH. Prepared for U. S. War Department by U. S. linguists. As above, unit is idiom, phrase or sentence rather than word. English-Spanish and Spanish-English sections contain modern equivalents of over 18,000 sentences. Introduction and appendix as above. iv + 513pp.
20495-2 Paperbound $2.00

A PHRASE AND SENTENCE DICTIONARY OF SPOKEN RUSSIAN. Dictionary prepared for U. S. War Department by U. S. linguists. Basic unit is not the word, but the idiom, phrase or sentence. English-Russian and Russian-English sections contain modern equivalents for over 30,000 phrases. Grammatical introduction covers phonetics, writing, syntax. Appendix of word lists for food, numbers, geographical names, etc. vi + 573 pp. 6⅛ x 9¼.
20496-0 Paperbound $3.00

CONVERSATIONAL CHINESE FOR BEGINNERS, Morris Swadesh. Phonetic system, beginner's course in Pai Hua Mandarin Chinese covering most important, most useful speech patterns. Emphasis on modern colloquial usage. Formerly *Chinese in Your Pocket.* xvi + 158pp.
21123-1 Paperbound $1.50

Two Little Savages; Being the Adventures of Two Boys Who Lived as Indians and What They Learned, Ernest Thompson Seton. Great classic of nature and boyhood provides a vast range of woodlore in most palatable form, a genuinely entertaining story. Two farm boys build a teepee in woods and live in it for a month, working out Indian solutions to living problems, star lore, birds and animals, plants, etc. 293 illustrations. vii + 286pp.

20985-7 Paperbound $1.95

Peter Piper's Practical Principles of Plain & Perfect Pronunciation. Alliterative jingles and tongue-twisters of surprising charm, that made their first appearance in America about 1830. Republished in full with the spirited woodcut illustrations from this earliest American edition. 32pp. 4½ x 6⅜.

22560-7 Paperbound $1.00

Science Experiments and Amusements for Children, Charles Vivian. 73 easy experiments, requiring only materials found at home or easily available, such as candles, coins, steel wool, etc.; illustrate basic phenomena like vacuum, simple chemical reaction, etc. All safe. Modern, well-planned. Formerly *Science Games for Children*. 102 photos, numerous drawings. 96pp. 6⅛ x 9¼.

21856-2 Paperbound $1.25

An Introduction to Chess Moves and Tactics Simply Explained, Leonard Barden. Informal intermediate introduction, quite strong in explaining reasons for moves. Covers basic material, tactics, important openings, traps, positional play in middle game, end game. Attempts to isolate patterns and recurrent configurations. Formerly *Chess*. 58 figures. 102pp. (USO) 21210-6 Paperbound $1.25

Lasker's Manual of Chess, Dr. Emanuel Lasker. Lasker was not only one of the five great World Champions, he was also one of the ablest expositors, theorists, and analysts. In many ways, his Manual, permeated with his philosophy of battle, filled with keen insights, is one of the greatest works ever written on chess. Filled with analyzed games by the great players. A single-volume library that will profit almost any chess player, beginner or master. 308 diagrams. xli x 349pp.

20640-8 Paperbound $2.50

The Master Book of Mathematical Recreations, Fred Schuh. In opinion of many the finest work ever prepared on mathematical puzzles, stunts, recreations; exhaustively thorough explanations of mathematics involved, analysis of effects, citation of puzzles and games. Mathematics involved is elementary. Translated by F. Göbel. 194 figures. xxiv + 430pp. 22134-2 Paperbound $3.00

Mathematics, Magic and Mystery, Martin Gardner. Puzzle editor for Scientific American explains mathematics behind various mystifying tricks: card tricks, stage "mind reading," coin and match tricks, counting out games, geometric dissections, etc. Probability sets, theory of numbers clearly explained. Also provides more than 400 tricks, guaranteed to work, that you can do. 135 illustrations. xii + 176pp.

20338-2 Paperbound $1.50

EAST O' THE SUN AND WEST O' THE MOON, George W. Dasent. Considered the best of all translations of these Norwegian folk tales, this collection has been enjoyed by generations of children (and folklorists too). Includes True and Untrue, Why the Sea is Salt, East O' the Sun and West O' the Moon, Why the Bear is Stumpy-Tailed, Boots and the Troll, The Cock and the Hen, Rich Peter the Pedlar, and 52 more. The only edition with all 59 tales. 77 illustrations by Erik Werenskiold and Theodor Kittelsen. xv + 418pp.   22521-6 Paperbound $3.00

GOOPS AND HOW TO BE THEM, Gelett Burgess. Classic of tongue-in-cheek humor, masquerading as etiquette book. 87 verses, twice as many cartoons, show mischievous Goops as they demonstrate to children virtues of table manners, neatness, courtesy, etc. Favorite for generations. viii + 88pp. 6½ x 9¼.
22233-0 Paperbound $1.25

ALICE'S ADVENTURES UNDER GROUND, Lewis Carroll. The first version, quite different from the final *Alice in Wonderland,* printed out by Carroll himself with his own illustrations. Complete facsimile of the "million dollar" manuscript Carroll gave to Alice Liddell in 1864. Introduction by Martin Gardner. viii + 96pp. Title and dedication pages in color.   21482-6 Paperbound $1.00

THE BROWNIES, THEIR BOOK, Palmer Cox. Small as mice, cunning as foxes, exuberant and full of mischief, the Brownies go to the zoo, toy shop, seashore, circus, etc., in 24 verse adventures and 266 illustrations. Long a favorite, since their first appearance in St. Nicholas Magazine. xi + 144pp. 6⅝ x 9¼.
21265-3 Paperbound $1.50

SONGS OF CHILDHOOD, Walter De La Mare. Published (under the pseudonym Walter Ramal) when De La Mare was only 29, this charming collection has long been a favorite children's book. A facsimile of the first edition in paper, the 47 poems capture the simplicity of the nursery rhyme and the ballad, including such lyrics as I Met Eve, Tartary, The Silver Penny. vii + 106pp. 21972-0 Paperbound $1.25

THE COMPLETE NONSENSE OF EDWARD LEAR, Edward Lear. The finest 19th-century humorist-cartoonist in full: all nonsense limericks, zany alphabets, Owl and Pussycat, songs, nonsense botany, and more than 500 illustrations by Lear himself. Edited by Holbrook Jackson. xxix + 287pp.   (USO) 20167-8 Paperbound $1.75

BILLY WHISKERS: THE AUTOBIOGRAPHY OF A GOAT, Frances Trego Montgomery. A favorite of children since the early 20th century, here are the escapades of that rambunctious, irresistible and mischievous goat—Billy Whiskers. Much in the spirit of *Peck's Bad Boy,* this is a book that children never tire of reading or hearing. All the original familiar illustrations by W. H. Fry are included: 6 color plates, 18 black and white drawings. 159pp.   22345-0 Paperbound $2.00

MOTHER GOOSE MELODIES. Faithful republication of the fabulously rare Munroe and Francis "copyright 1833" Boston edition—the most important Mother Goose collection, usually referred to as the "original." Familiar rhymes plus many rare ones, with wonderful old woodcut illustrations. Edited by E. F. Bleiler. 128pp. 4½ x 6⅜.   22577-1 Paperbound $1.25

THE RED FAIRY BOOK, Andrew Lang. Lang's color fairy books have long been children's favorites. This volume includes Rapunzel, Jack and the Bean-stalk and 35 other stories, familiar and unfamiliar. 4 plates, 93 illustrations x + 367pp.
21673-X Paperbound $1.95

THE BLUE FAIRY BOOK, Andrew Lang. Lang's tales come from all countries and all times. Here are 37 tales from Grimm, the Arabian Nights, Greek Mythology, and other fascinating sources. 8 plates, 130 illustrations. xi + 390pp.
21437-0 Paperbound $1.95

HOUSEHOLD STORIES BY THE BROTHERS GRIMM. Classic English-language edition of the well-known tales — Rumpelstiltskin, Snow White, Hansel and Gretel, The Twelve Brothers, Faithful John, Rapunzel, Tom Thumb (52 stories in all). Translated into simple, straightforward English by Lucy Crane. Ornamented with headpieces, vignettes, elaborate decorative initials and a dozen full-page illustrations by Walter Crane. x + 269pp.
21080-4 Paperbound $1.75

THE MERRY ADVENTURES OF ROBIN HOOD, Howard Pyle. The finest modern versions of the traditional ballads and tales about the great English outlaw. Howard Pyle's complete prose version, with every word, every illustration of the first edition. Do not confuse this facsimile of the original (1883) with modern editions that change text or illustrations. 23 plates plus many page decorations. xxii + 296pp.
22043-5 Paperbound $2.00

THE STORY OF KING ARTHUR AND HIS KNIGHTS, Howard Pyle. The finest children's version of the life of King Arthur; brilliantly retold by Pyle, with 48 of his most imaginative illustrations. xviii + 313pp. 6⅛ x 9¼.
21445-1 Paperbound $2.00

THE WONDERFUL WIZARD OF OZ, L. Frank Baum. America's finest children's book in facsimile of first edition with all Denslow illustrations in full color. The edition a child should have. Introduction by Martin Gardner. 23 color plates, scores of drawings. iv + 267pp.
20691-2 Paperbound $1.95

THE MARVELOUS LAND OF OZ, L. Frank Baum. The second Oz book, every bit as imaginative as the Wizard. The hero is a boy named Tip, but the Scarecrow and the Tin Woodman are back, as is the Oz magic. 16 color plates, 120 drawings by John R. Neill. 287pp.
20692-0 Paperbound $1.75

THE MAGICAL MONARCH OF MO, L. Frank Baum. Remarkable adventures in a land even stranger than Oz. The best of Baum's books not in the Oz series. 15 color plates and dozens of drawings by Frank Verbeck. xviii + 237pp.
21892-9 Paperbound $2.00

THE BAD CHILD'S BOOK OF BEASTS, MORE BEASTS FOR WORSE CHILDREN, A MORAL ALPHABET, Hilaire Belloc. Three complete humor classics in one volume. Be kind to the frog, and do not call him names . . . and 28 other whimsical animals. Familiar favorites and some not so well known. Illustrated by Basil Blackwell. 156pp.
(USO) 20749-8 Paperbound $1.25

INCIDENTS OF TRAVEL IN YUCATAN, John L. Stephens. Classic (1843) exploration of jungles of Yucatan, looking for evidences of Maya civilization. Stephens found many ruins; comments on travel adventures, Mexican and Indian culture. 127 striking illustrations by F. Catherwood. Total of 669 pp.
20926-1, 20927-X Two volumes, Paperbound $5.00

INCIDENTS OF TRAVEL IN CENTRAL AMERICA, CHIAPAS, AND YUCATAN, John L. Stephens. An exciting travel journal and an important classic of archeology. Narrative relates his almost single-handed discovery of the Mayan culture, and exploration of the ruined cities of Copan, Palenque, Utatlan and others; the monuments they dug from the earth, the temples buried in the jungle, the customs of poverty-stricken Indians living a stone's throw from the ruined palaces. 115 drawings by F. Catherwood. Portrait of Stephens. xii + 812pp.
22404-X, 22405-8 Two volumes, Paperbound $6.00

A NEW VOYAGE ROUND THE WORLD, William Dampier. Late 17-century naturalist joined the pirates of the Spanish Main to gather information; remarkably vivid account of buccaneers, pirates; detailed, accurate account of botany, zoology, ethnography of lands visited. Probably the most important early English voyage, enormous implications for British exploration, trade, colonial policy. Also most interesting reading. Argonaut edition, introduction by Sir Albert Gray. New introduction by Percy Adams. 6 plates, 7 illustrations. xlvii + 376pp. 6½ x 9¼.
21900-3 Paperbound $3.00

INTERNATIONAL AIRLINE PHRASE BOOK IN SIX LANGUAGES, Joseph W. Bátor. Important phrases and sentences in English paralleled with French, German, Portuguese, Italian, Spanish equivalents, covering all possible airport-travel situations; created for airline personnel as well as tourist by Language Chief, Pan American Airlines. xiv + 204pp.
22017-6 Paperbound $2.00

STAGE COACH AND TAVERN DAYS, Alice Morse Earle. Detailed, lively account of the early days of taverns; their uses and importance in the social, political and military life; furnishings and decorations; locations; food and drink; tavern signs, etc. Second half covers every aspect of early travel; the roads, coaches, drivers, etc. Nostalgic, charming, packed with fascinating material. 157 illustrations, mostly photographs. xiv + 449pp.
22518-6 Paperbound $4.00

NORSE DISCOVERIES AND EXPLORATIONS IN NORTH AMERICA, Hjalmar R. Holand. The perplexing Kensington Stone, found in Minnesota at the end of the 19th century. Is it a record of a Scandinavian expedition to North America in the 14th century? Or is it one of the most successful hoaxes in history. A scientific detective investigation. Formerly *Westward from Vinland*. 31 photographs, 17 figures. x + 354pp.
22014-1 Paperbound $2.75

A BOOK OF OLD MAPS, compiled and edited by Emerson D. Fite and Archibald Freeman. 74 old maps offer an unusual survey of the discovery, settlement and growth of America down to the close of the Revolutionary war: maps showing Norse settlements in Greenland, the explorations of Columbus, Verrazano, Cabot, Champlain, Joliet, Drake, Hudson, etc., campaigns of Revolutionary war battles, and much more. Each map is accompanied by a brief historical essay. xvi + 299pp. 11 x 13¾.
22084-2 Paperbound $6.00

POEMS OF ANNE BRADSTREET, edited with an introduction by Robert Hutchinson. A new selection of poems by America's first poet and perhaps the first significant woman poet in the English language. 48 poems display her development in works of considerable variety—love poems, domestic poems, religious meditations, formal elegies, "quaternions," etc. Notes, bibliography. viii + 222pp.

22160-1 Paperbound $2.00

THREE GOTHIC NOVELS: THE CASTLE OF OTRANTO BY HORACE WALPOLE; VATHEK BY WILLIAM BECKFORD; THE VAMPYRE BY JOHN POLIDORI, WITH FRAGMENT OF A NOVEL BY LORD BYRON, edited by E. F. Bleiler. The first Gothic novel, by Walpole; the finest Oriental tale in English, by Beckford; powerful Romantic supernatural story in versions by Polidori and Byron. All extremely important in history of literature; all still exciting, packed with supernatural thrills, ghosts, haunted castles, magic, etc. xl + 291pp.

21232-7 Paperbound $2.00

THE BEST TALES OF HOFFMANN, E. T. A. Hoffmann. 10 of Hoffmann's most important stories, in modern re-editings of standard translations: Nutcracker and the King of Mice, Signor Formica, Automata, The Sandman, Rath Krespel, The Golden Flowerpot, Master Martin the Cooper, The Mines of Falun, The King's Betrothed, A New Year's Eve Adventure. 7 illustrations by Hoffmann. Edited by E. F. Bleiler. xxxix + 419pp. 21793-0 Paperbound $2.25

GHOST AND HORROR STORIES OF AMBROSE BIERCE, Ambrose Bierce. 23 strikingly modern stories of the horrors latent in the human mind: The Eyes of the Panther, The Damned Thing, An Occurrence at Owl Creek Bridge, An Inhabitant of Carcosa, etc., plus the dream-essay, Visions of the Night. Edited by E. F. Bleiler. xxii + 199pp. 20767-6 Paperbound $1.50

BEST GHOST STORIES OF J. S. LeFANU, J. Sheridan LeFanu. Finest stories by Victorian master often considered greatest supernatural writer of all. Carmilla, Green Tea, The Haunted Baronet, The Familiar, and 12 others. Most never before available in the U. S. A. Edited by E. F. Bleiler. 8 illustrations from Victorian publications. xvii + 467pp. 20415-4 Paperbound $2.50

THE TIME STREAM, THE GREATEST ADVENTURE, AND THE PURPLE SAPPHIRE—THREE SCIENCE FICTION NOVELS, John Taine (Eric Temple Bell). Great American mathematician was also foremost science fiction novelist of the 1920's. *The Time Stream,* one of all-time classics, uses concepts of circular time; *The Greatest Adventure,* incredibly ancient biological experiments from Antarctica threaten to escape; The *Purple Sapphire,* superscience, lost races in Central Tibet, survivors of the Great Race. 4 illustrations by Frank R. Paul. v + 532pp.

21180-0 Paperbound $2.50

SEVEN SCIENCE FICTION NOVELS, H. G. Wells. The standard collection of the great novels. Complete, unabridged. *First Men in the Moon, Island of Dr. Moreau, War of the Worlds, Food of the Gods, Invisible Man, Time Machine, In the Days of the Comet.* Not only science fiction fans, but every educated person owes it to himself to read these novels. 1015pp. 20264-X Clothbound $5.00

AGAINST THE GRAIN (A REBOURS), Joris K. Huysmans. Filled with weird images, evidences of a bizarre imagination, exotic experiments with hallucinatory drugs, rich tastes and smells and the diversions of its sybarite hero Duc Jean des Esseintes, this classic novel pushed 19th-century literary decadence to its limits. Full unabridged edition. Do not confuse this with abridged editions generally sold. Introduction by Havelock Ellis. xlix + 206pp. 22190-3 Paperbound $2.00

VARIORUM SHAKESPEARE: HAMLET. Edited by Horace H. Furness; a landmark of American scholarship. Exhaustive footnotes and appendices treat all doubtful words and phrases, as well as suggested critical emendations throughout the play's history. First volume contains editor's own text, collated with all Quartos and Folios. Second volume contains full first Quarto, translations of Shakespeare's sources (Belleforest, and Saxo Grammaticus), Der Bestrafte Brudermord, and many essays on critical and historical points of interest by major authorities of past and present. Includes details of staging and costuming over the years. By far the best edition available for serious students of Shakespeare. Total of xx + 905pp. 21004-9, 21005-7, 2 volumes, Paperbound $5.25

A LIFE OF WILLIAM SHAKESPEARE, Sir Sidney Lee. This is the standard life of Shakespeare, summarizing everything known about Shakespeare and his plays. Incredibly rich in material, broad in coverage, clear and judicious, it has served thousands as the best introduction to Shakespeare. 1931 edition. 9 plates. xxix + 792pp. (USO) 21967-4 Paperbound $3.75

MASTERS OF THE DRAMA, John Gassner. Most comprehensive history of the drama in print, covering every tradition from Greeks to modern Europe and America, including India, Far East, etc. Covers more than 800 dramatists, 2000 plays, with biographical material, plot summaries, theatre history, criticism, etc. "Best of its kind in English," New Republic. 77 illustrations. xxii + 890pp. 20100-7 Clothbound $7.50

THE EVOLUTION OF THE ENGLISH LANGUAGE, George McKnight. The growth of English, from the 14th century to the present. Unusual, non-technical account presents basic information in very interesting form: sound shifts, change in grammar and syntax, vocabulary growth, similar topics. Abundantly illustrated with quotations. Formerly Modern English in the Making. xii + 590pp. 21932-1 Paperbound $3.50

AN ETYMOLOGICAL DICTIONARY OF MODERN ENGLISH, Ernest Weekley. Fullest, richest work of its sort, by foremost British lexicographer. Detailed word histories, including many colloquial and archaic words; extensive quotations. Do not confuse this with the Concise Etymological Dictionary, which is much abridged. Total of xxvii + 830pp. 6½ x 9¼. 21873-2, 21874-0 Two volumes, Paperbound $5.50

FLATLAND: A ROMANCE OF MANY DIMENSIONS, E. A. Abbott. Classic of science-fiction explores ramifications of life in a two-dimensional world, and what happens when a three-dimensional being intrudes. Amusing reading, but also useful as introduction to thought about hyperspace. Introduction by Banesh Hoffmann. 16 illustrations. xx + 103pp. 20001-9 Paperbound $1.00

JOHANN SEBASTIAN BACH, Philipp Spitta. One of the great classics of musicology, this definitive analysis of Bach's music (and life) has never been surpassed. Lucid, nontechnical analyses of hundreds of pieces (30 pages devoted to St. Matthew Passion, 26 to B Minor Mass). Also includes major analysis of 18th-century music. 450 musical examples. 40-page musical supplement. Total of xx + 1799pp.
(EUK) 22278-0, 22279-9 Two volumes, Clothbound $15.00

MOZART AND HIS PIANO CONCERTOS, Cuthbert Girdlestone. The only full-length study of an important area of Mozart's creativity. Provides detailed analyses of all 23 concertos, traces inspirational sources. 417 musical examples. Second edition. 509pp.
(USO) 21271-8 Paperbound $2.50

THE PERFECT WAGNERITE: A COMMENTARY ON THE NIBLUNG'S RING, George Bernard Shaw. Brilliant and still relevant criticism in remarkable essays on Wagner's Ring cycle, Shaw's ideas on political and social ideology behind the plots, role of Leitmotifs, vocal requisites, etc. Prefaces. xxi + 136pp.
21707-8 Paperbound $1.50

DON GIOVANNI, W. A. Mozart. Complete libretto, modern English translation; biographies of composer and librettist; accounts of early performances and critical reaction. Lavishly illustrated. All the material you need to understand and appreciate this great work. Dover Opera Guide and Libretto Series; translated and introduced by Ellen Bleiler. 92 illustrations. 209pp.
21134-7 Paperbound $1.50

HIGH FIDELITY SYSTEMS: A LAYMAN'S GUIDE, Roy F. Allison. All the basic information you need for setting up your own audio system: high fidelity and stereo record players, tape records, F.M. Connections, adjusting tone arm, cartridge, checking needle alignment, positioning speakers, phasing speakers, adjusting hums, trouble-shooting, maintenance, and similar topics. Enlarged 1965 edition. More than 50 charts, diagrams, photos. iv + 91pp.
21514-8 Paperbound $1.25

REPRODUCTION OF SOUND, Edgar Villchur. Thorough coverage for laymen of high fidelity systems, reproducing systems in general, needles, amplifiers, preamps, loudspeakers, feedback, explaining physical background. "A rare talent for making technicalities vividly comprehensible," R. Darrell, *High Fidelity*. 69 figures. iv + 92pp.
21515-6 Paperbound $1.00

HEAR ME TALKIN' TO YA: THE STORY OF JAZZ AS TOLD BY THE MEN WHO MADE IT, Nat Shapiro and Nat Hentoff. Louis Armstrong, Fats Waller, Jo Jones, Clarence Williams, Billy Holiday, Duke Ellington, Jelly Roll Morton and dozens of other jazz greats tell how it was in Chicago's South Side, New Orleans, depression Harlem and the modern West Coast as jazz was born and grew. xvi + 429pp.
21726-4 Paperbound $2.00

FABLES OF AESOP, translated by Sir Roger L'Estrange. A reproduction of the very rare 1931 Paris edition; a selection of the most interesting fables, together with 50 imaginative drawings by Alexander Calder. v + 128pp. 6½x9¼.
21780-9 Paperbound $1.25

THE ARCHITECTURE OF COUNTRY HOUSES, Andrew J. Downing. Together with Vaux's *Villas and Cottages* this is the basic book for Hudson River Gothic architecture of the middle Victorian period. Full, sound discussions of general aspects of housing, architecture, style, decoration, furnishing, together with scores of detailed house plans, illustrations of specific buildings, accompanied by full text. Perhaps the most influential single American architectural book. 1850 edition. Introduction by J. Stewart Johnson. 321 figures, 34 architectural designs. xvi + 560pp.
22003-6 Paperbound $3.50

LOST EXAMPLES OF COLONIAL ARCHITECTURE, John Mead Howells. Full-page photographs of buildings that have disappeared or been so altered as to be denatured, including many designed by major early American architects. 245 plates. xvii + 248pp. 7⅞ x 10¾.
21143-6 Paperbound $3.00

DOMESTIC ARCHITECTURE OF THE AMERICAN COLONIES AND OF THE EARLY REPUBLIC, Fiske Kimball. Foremost architect and restorer of Williamsburg and Monticello covers nearly 200 homes between 1620-1825. Architectural details, construction, style features, special fixtures, floor plans, etc. Generally considered finest work in its area. 219 illustrations of houses, doorways, windows, capital mantels. xx + 314pp. 7⅞ x 10¾.
21743-4 Paperbound $3.50

EARLY AMERICAN ROOMS: 1650-1858, edited by Russell Hawes Kettell. Tour of 12 rooms, each representative of a different era in American history and each furnished, decorated, designed and occupied in the style of the era. 72 plans and elevations, 8-page color section, etc., show fabrics, wall papers, arrangements, etc. Full descriptive text. xvii + 200pp. of text. 8⅜ x 11¼.
21633-0 Paperbound $4.00

THE FITZWILLIAM VIRGINAL BOOK, edited by J. Fuller Maitland and W. B. Squire. Full modern printing of famous early 17th-century ms. volume of 300 works by Morley, Byrd, Bull, Gibbons, etc. For piano or other modern keyboard instrument; easy to read format. xxxvi + 938pp. 8⅜ x 11.
21068-5, 21069-3 Two volumes, Paperbound $8.00

HARPSICHORD MUSIC, Johann Sebastian Bach. Bach Gesellschaft edition. A rich selection of Bach's masterpieces for the harpsichord: the six English Suites, six French Suites, the six Partitas (Clavierübung part I), the Goldberg Variations (Clavierübung part IV), the fifteen Two-Part Inventions and the fifteen Three-Part Sinfonias. Clearly reproduced on large sheets with ample margins; eminently playable. vi + 312pp. 8⅛ x 11.
22360-4 Paperbound $5.00

THE MUSIC OF BACH: AN INTRODUCTION, Charles Sanford Terry. A fine, nontechnical introduction to Bach's music, both instrumental and vocal. Covers organ music, chamber music, passion music, other types. Analyzes themes, developments, innovations. x + 114pp.
21075-8 Paperbound $1.25

BEETHOVEN AND HIS NINE SYMPHONIES, Sir George Grove. Noted British musicologist provides best history, analysis, commentary on symphonies. Very thorough, rigorously accurate; necessary to both advanced student and amateur music lover. 436 musical passages. vii + 407 pp.
20334-4 Paperbound $2.25

A HISTORY OF COSTUME, Carl Köhler. Definitive history, based on surviving pieces of clothing primarily, and paintings, statues, etc. secondarily. Highly readable text, supplemented by 594 illustrations of costumes of the ancient Mediterranean peoples, Greece and Rome, the Teutonic prehistoric period; costumes of the Middle Ages, Renaissance, Baroque, 18th and 19th centuries. Clear, measured patterns are provided for many clothing articles. Approach is practical throughout. Enlarged by Emma von Sichart. 464pp. 21030-8 Paperbound $3.00

ORIENTAL RUGS, ANTIQUE AND MODERN, Walter A. Hawley. A complete and authoritative treatise on the Oriental rug—where they are made, by whom and how, designs and symbols, characteristics in detail of the six major groups, how to distinguish them and how to buy them. Detailed technical data is provided on periods, weaves, warps, wefts, textures, sides, ends and knots, although no technical background is required for an understanding. 11 color plates, 80 halftones, 4 maps. vi + 320pp. 6⅛ x 9⅛. 22366-3 Paperbound $5.00

TEN BOOKS ON ARCHITECTURE, Vitruvius. By any standards the most important book on architecture ever written. Early Roman discussion of aesthetics of building, construction methods, orders, sites, and every other aspect of architecture has inspired, instructed architecture for about 2,000 years. Stands behind Palladio, Michelangelo, Bramante, Wren, countless others. Definitive Morris H. Morgan translation. 68 illustrations. xii + 331pp. 20645-9 Paperbound $2.50

THE FOUR BOOKS OF ARCHITECTURE, Andrea Palladio. Translated into every major Western European language in the two centuries following its publication in 1570, this has been one of the most influential books in the history of architecture. Complete reprint of the 1738 Isaac Ware edition. New introduction by Adolf Placzek, Columbia Univ. 216 plates. xxii + 110pp. of text. 9½ x 12¾. 21308-0 Clothbound $10.00

STICKS AND STONES: A STUDY OF AMERICAN ARCHITECTURE AND CIVILIZATION, Lewis Mumford.One of the great classics of American cultural history. American architecture from the medieval-inspired earliest forms to the early 20th century; evolution of structure and style, and reciprocal influences on environment. 21 photographic illustrations. 238pp. 20202-X Paperbound $2.00

THE AMERICAN BUILDER'S COMPANION, Asher Benjamin. The most widely used early 19th century architectural style and source book, for colonial up into Greek Revival periods. Extensive development of geometry of carpentering, construction of sashes, frames, doors, stairs; plans and elevations of domestic and other buildings. Hundreds of thousands of houses were built according to this book, now invaluable to historians, architects, restorers, etc. 1827 edition. 59 plates. 114pp. 7⅞ x 10¾. 22236-5 Paperbound $3.00

DUTCH HOUSES IN THE HUDSON VALLEY BEFORE 1776, Helen Wilkinson Reynolds. The standard survey of the Dutch colonial house and outbuildings, with constructional features, decoration, and local history associated with individual homesteads. Introduction by Franklin D. Roosevelt. Map. 150 illustrations. 469pp. 6⅝ x 9¼. 21469-9 Paperbound $3.50

MATHEMATICAL PUZZLES FOR BEGINNERS AND ENTHUSIASTS, Geoffrey Mott-Smith. 189 puzzles from easy to difficult—involving arithmetic, logic, algebra, properties of digits, probability, etc.—for enjoyment and mental stimulus. Explanation of mathematical principles behind the puzzles. 135 illustrations. viii + 248pp.

20198-8 Paperbound $1.25

PAPER FOLDING FOR BEGINNERS, William D. Murray and Francis J. Rigney. Easiest book on the market, clearest instructions on making interesting, beautiful origami. Sail boats, cups, roosters, frogs that move legs, bonbon boxes, standing birds, etc. 40 projects; more than 275 diagrams and photographs. 94pp.

20713-7 Paperbound $1.00

TRICKS AND GAMES ON THE POOL TABLE, Fred Herrmann. 79 tricks and games— some solitaires, some for two or more players, some competitive games—to entertain you between formal games. Mystifying shots and throws, unusual caroms, tricks involving such props as cork, coins, a hat, etc. Formerly *Fun on the Pool Table*. 77 figures. 95pp.

21814-7 Paperbound $1.00

HAND SHADOWS TO BE THROWN UPON THE WALL: A SERIES OF NOVEL AND AMUSING FIGURES FORMED BY THE HAND, Henry Bursill. Delightful picturebook from great-grandfather's day shows how to make 18 different hand shadows: a bird that flies, duck that quacks, dog that wags his tail, camel, goose, deer, boy, turtle, etc. Only book of its sort. vi + 33pp. 6½ x 9¼. 21779-5 Paperbound $1.00

WHITTLING AND WOODCARVING, E. J. Tangerman. 18th printing of best book on market. "If you can cut a potato you can carve" toys and puzzles, chains, chessmen, caricatures, masks, frames, woodcut blocks, surface patterns, much more. Information on tools, woods, techniques. Also goes into serious wood sculpture from Middle Ages to present, East and West. 464 photos, figures. x + 293pp.

20965-2 Paperbound $2.00

HISTORY OF PHILOSOPHY, Julián Marias. Possibly the clearest, most easily followed, best planned, most useful one-volume history of philosophy on the market; neither skimpy nor overfull. Full details on system of every major philosopher and dozens of less important thinkers from pre-Socratics up to Existentialism and later. Strong on many European figures usually omitted. Has gone through dozens of editions in Europe. 1966 edition, translated by Stanley Appelbaum and Clarence Strowbridge. xviii + 505pp.

21739-6 Paperbound $2.75

YOGA: A SCIENTIFIC EVALUATION, Kovoor T. Behanan. Scientific but non-technical study of physiological results of yoga exercises; done under auspices of Yale U. Relations to Indian thought, to psychoanalysis, etc. 16 photos. xxiii + 270pp.

20505-3 Paperbound $2.50

Prices subject to change without notice.

Available at your book dealer or write for free catalogue to Dept. GI, Dover Publications, Inc., 180 Varick St., N. Y., N. Y. 10014. Dover publishes more than 150 books each year on science, elementary and advanced mathematics, biology, music, art, literary history, social sciences and other areas.